Computational Psychiatry

Computational Psychiatry

A Primer

edited by Peggy Seriès

The MIT Press
Cambridge, Massachusetts
London, England

This book was set in ITC Stone Serif Std and ITC Stone Sans Std by New Best-set Typesetters Ltd. Printed and bound in the United States of America.

Library of Congress Cataloging-in-Publication Data

Names: Seriès, Peggy, editor.
Title: Computational psychiatry : a primer / edited by Peggy Seriès.
Description: Cambridge, Massachusetts : The MIT Press, [2020] | Includes bibliographical
   references and index.
Identifiers: LCCN 2019059142 | ISBN 9780262044592 (hardcover)
Subjects: LCSH: Psychiatry—Data processing. | Psychiatry—Mathematical models. |
   Computational biology.
Classification: LCC RC455.2.D38 S47 2020 | DDC 616.8900285—dc23
LC record available at https://lccn.loc.gov/2019059142

10 9 8 7 6 5 4 3 2 1

Contents

Preface

I used to work in visual computational neuroscience and gradually moved toward computational psychiatry. This move was partly motivated by my own struggles, but ultimately by witnessing the suffering in some of our students, and even the suicide of two of them.

I felt we did not understand them, and what really mattered for all of us. In terms of our research in computational neuroscience, I felt that we were not putting the efforts where they mattered most, and that our research could be immensely more useful in the long term if we did. I became interested in understanding how mental illness is described and how to bridge advances in neurobiology, computational cognitive science, and psychiatric disorders. I was attracted as well by the idea that mental health and illness lie on a continuum that concerns all of us, to various degrees, since we are all potentially at risk for suffering that can become overwhelming.

I wanted to provide an accessible book for students starting in this new emerging field and coming from a wide variety of backgrounds. I am well aware, though, that there are no solid truths in this field yet. The field of computational psychiatry is being met with great enthusiasm and hopes for clinical usefulness, but it is still in its infancy. This book is very imperfect in that it only addresses a subset of questions, and often leads to more questions than answers. Still, I think it shows that computational psychiatry can provide important new insights and help bridge neuroscience and clinical applications.

I am immensely grateful to the brilliant contributors of this book, all international leaders in the field, who trusted me in this process, despite this being my first book and many of them being more established than I am.

I have been deeply inspired by my postdoctoral stay at the Gatsby Computational Neuroscience Unit and the research led by Peter Dayan with Nathaniel Daw, Yael Niv, and Quentin Huys at that time. I'm also very grateful to Eero Simoncelli for teaching me about scientific humility and our role in making our research accessible. More recently, I am very grateful for discussions with my collaborators, particularly Stephen Lawrie and Douglas Steele, Renaud Jardri, Sophie Deneve, Jonathan Roiser, Phil Corlett, Paul Fletcher, Andrew McIntosh, Andy Clark, and many others.

I would like to thank my very talented students, who chose a project in this field at a time when it was new to all of us: Vincent Valton, James Raymond, Aleks Stolicyn, Aistis Stankevicius, Frank Karvelis, Samuel Rupprechter, and Andrea D'Olimpio.

Many thanks to all the people who have supported me from close or far; my mother for the inspiration toward academia and psychiatry; my sister Emma; all my colleagues and friends, particularly Aaron Seitz, Matthias Hennig, Isabelle Duverne, Laetitia Pichevin and Robert Hamilton.

I am finally extremely grateful to the Simons Institute for the Theory of Computing and to the 2018 "Brain and Computation" program. Staying for a few months at UC Berkeley offered a wonderful environment to work on this book and discuss its very first drafts.

I am hoping the book can be useful as a textbook in this new field and inspire a generation of students who can make a difference.

1 Introduction: Toward a Computational Approach to Psychiatry

Janine M. Simmons, Bruce Cuthbert, Joshua A. Gordon, and Michele Ferrante
U.S. National Institute of Mental Health

1.1 A Brief History of Psychiatry: Clinical Challenges and Treatment Development

1.1.1 Clinical Burden

Mental health disorders affect up to one in five adults in the United States and contribute substantially to worldwide morbidity and mortality. The lives of individuals with mental disorders are cut short by 10 years on average (Walker, McGee, and Druss 2015). Mental illness accounts for 7–13% of all-cause disability-adjusted life years. Because of the young age at which they strike, as well as their chronicity and resistance to treatment, mental disorders account for an even greater proportion of all-cause years lived with disability (21–32%; Whiteford et al. 2015; Vigo, Thornicroft, and Atun 2016). To take just one example, major depressive disorder has become the second leading cause of noncommunicable disease disability worldwide (Mrazek et al. 2014). To lessen these burdens, we need new ways to understand and treat mental illnesses. Achieving this goal represents a substantial challenge. Therefore, it is imperative to utilize all tools at our disposal to make progress in psychiatric research.

1.1.2 Diagnostic Complexity

Although the behaviors associated with mental illness have been described for millennia (i.e., a description of depression and dementia can be found in the Ebers Papyrus, written in Egypt circa 1550 BC), psychiatry as a medical specialty emerged less than 150 years ago (Wilson 1993; Fischer 2012). As in all medical fields, clinicians and clinical researchers in psychiatry have attempted to establish discrete diagnostic categories to guide treatment and inform prognosis. However, the multifaceted nature of mental disorders has made this task extremely complex. At the turn of the twentieth century, Emil Kraepelin's (1856–1926) work captured the extent of this challenge in ways that are still echoing today. Importantly, he noted the difficulty of creating a complete nosology in the face of diverse, nonspecific clinical presentations, and in the absence of a clear understanding of natural causes (Kendler and Jablensky 2011). Kraepelin's approach emphasized detailed, longitudinal clinical assessments with a focus on *syndromes* of commonly co-occurring symptoms. Through this process, he made one of the first diagnostic classifications in psychiatry. Specifically, he differentiated manic-depressive illness (bipolar disorder, in today's terminology) from "dementia praecox" (Fischer 2012). Subsequently, Bleuler (1857–1939) recharacterized and renamed dementia praecox as schizophrenia (Maatz, Hoff, and Angst 2015). Although the diagnostic criteria and subtypes of these disorders have evolved over time, Kraepelin and Bleuler's fundamental clinical characterizations of different types of psychosis remain in use today.

In 1970, Robins and Guze sought to update the work of Kraepelin and Bleuler by establishing a method for achieving a more rigorous classification and improved diagnostic validity in psychiatry (Robins and Guze 1970). They recommended that psychiatric diagnoses be based upon five components. The first three of these reemphasized the features of a thorough clinical assessment: 1) symptoms, demographics, and precipitating factors; 2) longitudinal course; and 3) family history; while two additional elements would aid in the creation of homogeneous diagnostic subgroups: 4) laboratory studies and psychological tests; and 5) exclusion criteria. This work proved hugely influential, even though the fourth component was not actually available. As the authors note themselves: "Unfortunately, consistent and reliable laboratory findings have not yet been demonstrated in the more common psychiatric disorders" (Robins and Guze 1970). In the twenty-first century, psychiatry still lacks objective and robust laboratory testing.

Following on these early efforts, the publication of the third edition of the *Diagnostic and Statistical Manual of Mental Disorders* (*DSM-III*) in 1980 marked the modern age of psychiatric nosology (American Psychiatric Association 1980; Spitzer, Williams, and Skodol 1980; Wilson 1993; Hyman 2010; Fischer 2012). Facing the challenges of a field without objective diagnostic testing, Spitzer and the American Psychiatric Association (APA) recognized that diagnostic validity might be out of reach. Given the extent of the knowledge gap, they sought to address the critical needs by 1) defining boundaries of mental disorders; 2) stimulating progress in research and treatment development; and 3) increasing diagnostic reliability across research and treatment settings. The *DSM-III* intentionally and explicitly adopted a *theoretical*, descriptive approach that continues to serve as the bedrock of psychiatric diagnosis today (including *DSM-V*; American Psychiatric Association 2013). In the DSM, each disorder is characterized by a list of possible symptoms, and a minimum number of these symptoms are required to provide a diagnosis. For example, to meet criteria for major depressive disorder, at least five of nine possible symptoms must be present concurrently. The *DSM* has become the de facto guide of both clinical psychiatry and psychiatric research. Newer versions of the *DSM* have largely achieved APA's goals of providing clinicians with a common clinical language, improving diagnostic reliability, and allowing rough classification of patients for treatment (Hyman 2010).

The *DSM* has established a common framework within which clinical psychiatrists can operate. However, the current diagnostic system poses challenges for multiple reasons. The *DSM* groups patients into diagnostic categories based on subsets of symptoms selected from a longer checklist. Patient groups become heterogeneous because individuals grouped into one category can have different (and sometimes nonoverlapping) constellations of symptoms (table 1.1). Moreover, because many symptoms are shared by more than one syndrome, comorbidity becomes the rule rather than the exception. As a result, patients frequently receive multiple diagnoses. It remains unclear whether this apparent comorbidity arises from underlying biology or simply reflects a classification system that is ill-suited to capture the full complexity of human behavior and the brain (Lilienfeld, Waldman, and Israel 1994; Maj 2005; Kaplan et al. 2001; Sanislow et al. 2010). In addition, progress in genomics and neurobiology has revealed that different *DSM* diagnostic categories often share risk genes and, so far, cannot be differentiated by neuroimaging (Farah and Gillihan 2012; Cross-Disorder Group of the Psychiatric Genomics Consortium 2013; Mayberg 2014; Simmons and Quinn 2014). Ideally, our diagnostic nosology should be informed by a deeper understanding of pathophysiology. In the United States, the National Institute of Mental Health (NIMH) has sought to address these problems through the Research Domain Criteria (RDoC) initiative launched in 2010 (see section 1.4).

1.1.3 Treatment Development

In other areas of medicine, clinical advances have followed the availability of objective diagnostic tests, increased understanding of pathophysiological mechanisms, and the development of appropriate animal and computational models to rigorously test potential treatments. A prime example of this process can be seen in the improved treatments for cardiac arrhythmias resulting from identification and modeling of relevant cardiac ion channels (Bartos, Grandi, and Ripplinger 2015; Gomez, Cardona, and Trenor 2015). In psychiatry, treatment development has not yet followed such a path. Modern treatment options remain closely linked to psychotherapeutic and pharmacological approaches developed or discovered over 50 years ago.

Table 1.1

DSM-V depression symptom patterns in the Sequenced Treatment Alternatives to Relieve Depression (STAR*D) study

	Sad	Ene	Con	Ins	Int	App	Bla	Wei	Agi	Ret	Sui	Hyp	Ref (%)	Profile description
A													1.78	No symptoms
B	x	x	x	x	x	x	x	x	x	x			1.24	All but Sui and Hyp
C	x	x	x	x	x	x		x					1.19	Mixed profile
D	x	x	x	x	x	x	x	x					1.19	Mixed profile
E	x	x	x	x	x								1.13	Mixed profile
F	x	x	x	x	x			x					1.13	Mixed profile
G				x									1.08	Only Ins
H	x	x	x	x	x	x	x	x	x				1.00	All but Ret, Sui, and Hyp
I	x	x	x	x									0.92	Mixed profile
J	x	x	x	x	x	x		x	x	x			0.89	All but Hyp, Bla, and Sui

Reproduced from Fried and Nesse (2015).

Table 1.1 illustrates the 10 most frequent symptom profiles of 1,030 unique symptom profiles found in 3,703 patients diagnosed with major depressive disorder. Cells containing "x" indicate symptom presence. Abbreviations: Sad, sadness; Ene, energy loss; Con, concentration problems; Ins, insomnia; Int, interest loss; App, appetite problems; Bla, self-blame; Wei, weight problems; Agi, psychomotor agitation; Ret, psychomotor retardation; Sui, suicidal ideation; Hyp, hypersomnia; Freq, frequency of profiles.

Although there are a multitude of psychotherapy subtypes, three fundamental psychological models predominate. First, Sigmund Freud's (1856–1939) psychoanalytic theory emphasized the importance of the unconscious mind (see topographical model in figure 1.1). Freud and his followers proposed that intrapsychic conflict led to mental illness. Therefore, psychodynamic psychotherapy seeks to bring unconscious material to conscious awareness, uncover unexpressed emotions, and resolve past experiences (Freud 1966; Blagys and Hilsenroth 2002; Rawson 2005).

Second, behavior therapy grew from the early twentieth-century psychological tradition of behaviorism (Watson 1913; Skinner 1938). In contrast to the psychodynamic focus on internal states, behaviorism prioritizes observable actions and proposes that all behavior is fundamentally a learned response to environmental stimuli. Which

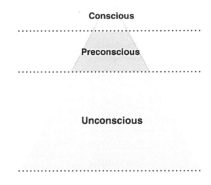

Figure 1.1
The three levels of consciousness. The conscious mind includes all thoughts, feelings, and actions of which we are aware. The preconscious mind includes all mental activities that are not presently active, but stored and accessible when required. The unconscious mind includes mental activity of which we are unaware. According to Freud, some of the feelings, thoughts, urges, and emotions that are actively buried in the unconscious mind influence some of our unexplained behavior.

behaviors are expressed depends on prior experience with environmental contingencies, and mental illnesses consist of maladaptive learned responses (Mowrer 1947; Foa and Kozak 1986; Foa 2011). Behavior therapy seeks to eliminate psychiatric symptoms by disconnecting maladaptive behaviors from their environmental triggers or by forming new, more adaptive responses. For example, behavior therapists commonly use exposure therapy to treat anxiety disorders such as phobias, obsessive-compulsive disorder, and post-traumatic stress disorder (PTSD; Foa and Kozak 1986; Foa 2011).

Third, in the 1950s and 1960s, Albert Ellis and Aaron Beck proposed new models for psychotherapy that integrated information processing and cognitive psychology (Ellis 1957; Beck 1991). In these models, automatic thoughts and core beliefs underlie emotions and behaviors (figure 1.2). Depressive mood and anxiety disorders result from irrational beliefs, distorted perceptions, and automatic negative thoughts. Therefore, the goal of this type of therapy is to identify and correct these cognitive distortions. Cognitive and behavioral therapy techniques are often combined as CBT (Blagys and Hilsenroth 2002).

Whatever the method, psychotherapy has been shown to significantly reduce psychiatric symptoms and improve mental well-being over the long term, with multiple meta-analyses demonstrating large effect sizes.[1] For psychodynamic psychotherapy, median effect sizes range from 0.69 to 1.8, depending on the targeted symptoms and length of treatment (Shedler 2010). A meta-analytic review of prolonged exposure

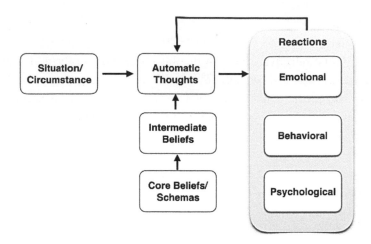

Figure 1.2
Beck's cognitive model. The cognitive model developed by A. Beck explains individuals' emotional, physiological, and behavioral responses to circumstances and situations as mediated by their automatic thoughts (see, e.g., Beck 1991). Automatic thoughts are influenced by underlying beliefs developed over time and through experience. Individuals' perceptions are often distorted and dysfunctional when they are distressed, leading to automatic negative thoughts. Through cognitive therapy, individuals can learn to identify, evaluate, and correct their automatic negative thinking. When they do so, distress usually decreases and psychological function increases.

therapy for PTSD demonstrated mean effect sizes of 1.08 for PTSD-specific symptoms and 0.77 for general symptoms of distress (Powers et al. 2010). Because CBT has been standardized, its benefits for depression and anxiety have been rigorously studied. Effect sizes are moderate to large, ranging from 0.58 to 1.0 (Shedler 2010). It should be noted, however, that very few psychotherapy outcome studies adequately assess the quality and fidelity of psychotherapy, even in research settings (Perepletchikova, Treat, and Kazdin 2007; Cox, Martinez, and Southam-Gerow 2019). In 2015, the Institute of Medicine found that psychosocial interventions proven effective in research settings have not been routinely integrated into clinical practice.

Whereas psychotherapeutic techniques have deep roots in historical theories of mental and/or behavioral processes, most breakthrough developments in psychiatric medications have occurred purely by chance (Preskorn 2010a). Serendipitous discoveries between the 1920s and 1960s led to early pharmacological treatments for mental disorders, including chlorpromazine and other typical antipsychotics, lithium for bipolar disorder, and tricyclic antidepressants. During the second half of the twentieth century, rational pharmaceutical development followed the accumulation of knowledge related to neurotransmitters. The greatest production of compounds targeting specific neurotransmitter systems occurred between the 1960s and 1990s (Preskorn 2010b). Fluoxetine, the first selective serotonin-reuptake inhibitor, received FDA approval for treatment of depression in 1987. Risperidone, an early "atypical" or second-generation antipsychotic, came on the market in 1993. Most recently, after a gap of more than 25 years, drugs that act at glutamate receptors have shown potential for acute treatment of depression and suicidality (Zanos et al. 2016; Lener et al. 2017).

Despite these advances, fundamental pharmacological treatment developments in psychiatry have stagnated (Hyman 2012; Insel 2015). First-line medication fails in approximately half of all patients, and the median effect size of treatment with any psychopharmacological agent is only 0.4. Moreover, for the last 25 to 30 years, almost all new psychiatric medications have been "me too" drugs—closely related to the original chemical compound and acting through the same mechanism of action (Fibiger 2012; Harrison et al. 2016). Although newer medications can provide important reductions in associated side effects and greater tolerability, they are not more effective. For example, modern antipsychotics are no more effective than first-generation drugs, according to recent meta-analyses (Geddes et al. 2000; Crossley et al. 2010). Antidepressant efficacy remains difficult to differentiate from placebo effects (Khin et al. 2011), and lithium remains the most effective option for bipolar disorder, despite its limited tolerability and unclear mechanisms of action (Harrison et al. 2016). After more than 100 years of psychological theories, psychopharmacological research, and clinical experience, the challenges of understanding and treating mental illness remain firmly in place. As a medical field, psychiatry faces two interrelated sticking points. The first is diagnostic complexity. Although *DSM* provides a foundation for clinical care in the face of limited treatment options, heterogeneous categories, individual differences, and comorbidity have stymied development of a principled pathophysiological understanding of psychiatric disorders. The second is stagnation in treatment development. Although both psychotherapeutic and pharmacological treatments have shown efficacy, morbidity and mortality for people with serious mental illness remain unacceptably high (Insel 2012; Walker, McGee, and Druss 2015; Whiteford et al. 2015; Vigo, Thornicroft, and Atun 2016). Solving these extremely difficult problems requires a set of novel conceptual approaches, including the integration of neuroscience findings and computational modeling.

1.1.4 Toward the Future of Psychiatric Research

In 2010, NIMH proposed a new conceptual model to guide clinical psychiatric research (Insel et al. 2010; Morris and Cuthbert 2012; Simmons and Quinn 2014). The RDoC

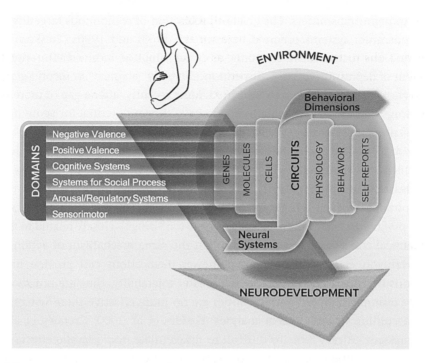

Figure 1.3
The RDoC matrix. RDoC is a research framework proposed by NIMH for new approaches to investigating mental disorders. It integrates many levels of information (from genomics and circuits to behavior and self-reports) in order to explore basic dimensions of functioning that span the full range of human behavior from normal to abnormal. RDoC is not meant to serve as a diagnostic guide, nor is it intended to replace current diagnostic systems. The goal is to understand the nature of mental health and illness in terms of varying degrees of dysfunction in general psychological/biological systems.

take a fundamentally different approach than *DSM* and address a different set of proximate questions. The RDoC framework seeks to further our understanding of psychopathology through pathophysiology by building upon ongoing advances in the behavioral and neurobiological sciences. The RDoC model proposes that human behavior can be parsed into fundamental domains of function (currently negative valence, positive valence, cognitive systems, social processes, arousal and regulatory processes, and sensorimotor systems; figure 1.3). These domains can be further subdivided into core psychological-level constructs (e.g., working memory; see MacCorquodale and Meehl 1948). RDoC hypothesizes that construct-level behaviors can be linked to the function of specific neural circuits and other biological processes, but also emphasizes the importance of developmental trajectories and environmental influences upon behavior. Constructs are conceptualized as dimensional, including the full continuum from illness to health, without specific clinical break points. The RDoC matrix provides a framework for investigations across multiple units of biological and behavioral analysis.

RDoC was created as an attempt to move beyond the stagnation in psychiatric diagnosis and treatment development. The intent was to provide a framework based upon mechanisms of dysregulation in normative functioning, thus better aligning psychopathology research with rapidly evolving knowledge about neural systems and behavior. The specific elements of the framework are expected to change as new knowledge accumulates. The overriding question is whether this framework can help characterize psychiatric dysfunction more robustly; the long-term goal is to identify underlying mechanisms and specific functions that might serve as targets for treatment.

As a heuristic, RDoC can readily serve as a basis for the emerging field of computational psychiatry. RDoC provides a conceptual framework within which specific theories can be applied and quantitative models tested. Rather than considering psychiatric diagnoses as clusters of symptoms, RDoC functional domains and constructs can be conceptualized as resulting from sets of underlying computations taking place across interacting neural circuits. In theory, these neural processes can, in turn, be described by algorithmic representations that describe information processing in the system (Marr 1982; Hofstadter 2007, 2008; Churchland and Sejnowski 1994; Damasio 2010; Redish 2013). Questions regarding the underlying neural circuits that perform those computations can then be asked. Stated differently, RDoC constructs can be considered latent constructs linking neurophysiological processes to behavioral observations (Huys, Moutsoussis, and Williams 2011; Maia and Frank 2011; Wang and Krystal 2014; Redish and Gordon 2016). Environmental factors and neurodevelopmental status can also be formally included in these algorithms. Ongoing RDoC experiments have begun to produce results that computational modelers can use as the basis for formalizing models that will better inform clinical practice. As such, applying computational approaches to RDoC-like frameworks may even transcend psychiatry and be used for advancing all kinds of translational neuroscience research (Sanislow et al. 2019): for example, computational neurology, computational vision, and computational neuroscience of drug addiction. The goals of computational psychiatry and how computational models might best be applied to questions in behavioral neuroscience and psychiatry will be discussed in the following section.

1.2 Computational Approaches in Neuroscience and Psychiatry

1.2.1 Computational Neuroscience

Computational neuroscience formalizes the biological structures and mechanisms of the nervous system in terms of information processing. Computational neuroscience is a highly interdisciplinary field at the intersections of fields such as neuroscience, cognitive science, psychology, engineering, computer science, mathematics, and biophysics. The last 25 years have seen significant growth in this field. From 1991 to 2016, the field grew more than 200 times, from two peer-reviewed scientific articles published per year to more than 400 publications per year. During the mid-1980s, two key factors led to this booming growth (Abbott 2008). The first factor was linked to the implementation and wide adoption of the back-propagation algorithm in artificial neural networks (Rumelhart, Hinton, and Williams 1986; see section 2.1). Adopting back-propagation led to a great expansion in the number of tasks that neural network models could handle and, consequently, in the number of scientists interested in questions answerable with these techniques. The second factor involved the translation of key concepts and mathematical approaches from physics into neuroscience (see chapter 2). For instance, in the 1980s, physicists like John Hopfield and Daniel Amit elegantly showed how a memory model could be further analyzed using statistical techniques originally developed to address theoretical issues related to disordered magnets (Amit, Gutfreund, and Sompolinsky 1985; Hopfield 1982).

Mathematical models, such as those adopted from physics, have clear advantages over more abstract schematics and word descriptors. They force the modeler to be as precise, self-consistent, and as complete as possible in deriving the implications of the model. Such models can be used for different purposes:

- to describe the available data in a concise and synthetic way, possibly unifying different sets of data in the same formalism (i.e., answer the question "what?"—as in, what are the fundamental properties of the phenomenon studied?)
- to link the observed data to possible underlying mechanisms (i.e., answer the question "how?"—as in, how do the necessary and sufficient conditions for a phenomenon emerge?)
- to understand "why" observed behaviors emerge as a consequence of a principle that can be justified theoretically (e.g., through understanding the process of individual optimization under some biological, environmental, or developmental constraints).

In describing the question that a model can answer, it is also common to refer to Marr's levels of analysis (Marr 1982; figure 1.4). Marr proposed that information-processing

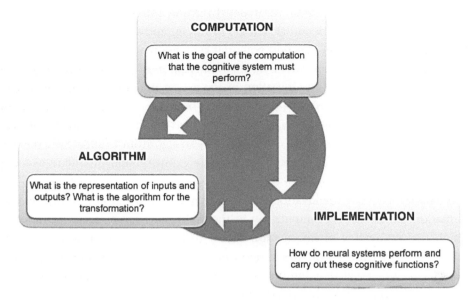

Figure 1.4
Marr's three levels of analyses. Originally introduced to advance the understanding of vision, Marr's approach postulated three distinct ways (computational, algorithmic, implementational) to consider information processing in the context of neuroscience. This distinction has since been used in research across other cognitive domains (e.g., memory, attention, learning), though many have not strictly adopted the classically rigid framework of Marr's hierarchy. Instead, the hierarchy is most commonly used as an organizing principle to highlight distinct conceptual questions at different levels of analysis. Image credit: Debbie Yee and Todd Braver.

systems can be understood at three distinct, complementary levels of analysis: computational, algorithmic, and implementational. The computational level specifies the problem to be solved in terms of some generic input-output mapping (e.g. "list sorting"). The algorithm specifies how the problem can be solved, what representations it uses, and what processes it employs to build and manipulate the representations (e.g., "quick-sort," "bubble-sort"). Implementation is the level of physical parts and their organization (e.g., specific programming language). It describes the physical mechanisms that carry out the algorithm. These levels function mostly independently and can often be described using different mathematical models. The challenge is often to bridge these levels of description and to understand how they might constrain each other.

Computational approaches have dramatically changed how basic neurobiological phenomena are described. Examples of successful and influential theoretical models include Lapicque's integrate-and-fire model (Lapicque 1907; Lapicque 1926), which provides a simple model of neuronal changes in voltage and activity (see section 2.1.5); the Hodgkin–Huxley model of action potential generation and propagation (Hodgkin and Huxley 1952), which provides a detailed description of the dynamics of sodium and potassium channels in the initiation of the action potential; Rall's cable theory (Rall et al. 1977), which provides a description of how the neuronal voltage relates to various morphological properties of neuronal processes (e.g., axons and dendrites); and Hebb's plasticity rules (Hebb 1949), which provide an algorithm to update the strength of neuronal connections within neural networks (e.g., the synaptic plasticity, as a consequence of learning).

Fundamental theoretical advances in neuroscience have also changed how we view information encoding and computation in the brain. This can be seen, for example, through the application of information theory in Barlow's hypothesis of predictive coding (see also section 2.4.6). Horace Barlow (1985), a prominent figure of theoretical neuroscience, suggested that the hierarchic organization of sensory systems reflects two imperatives: (1) to take in a maximum of new information to detect statistical regularities in the environment; and (2) to exploit these learned regularities to construct predictions about the environment. Those predictions are then used to guide adaptive behavior. In other words, he proposed that the brain evolved to efficiently code sensory information by using information-processing strategies optimized to the statistics of the perceptual environment (Olshausen and Field 1997). This framework suggests that the brain functions as a predictive engine rather than a purely reactive sensory organ, using an internal model of the statistics of the world to continuously and automatically infer what environment it is placed in and what best action to take.

More recently, it has been proposed that computational models of cognitive function could be used to explain psychopathology. For example, impairments in the processes involved in predictive coding could explain a variety of observations, ranging from impoverished theory of mind in autism to abnormalities of smooth-pursuit eye movements in schizophrenia (see section 2.4.6 and chapter 6). The development of such ideas marked the birth of the field of "computational psychiatry."

1.2.2 Computational Psychiatry

Simply defined, computational psychiatry consists of applying computational modeling and theoretical approaches to psychiatric questions. Although very young, computational psychiatry is already an extremely diverse field, leveraging concepts from psychiatry, psychology, computer science, neuroscience, electrical and chemical engineering, mathematics, and biophysics. Computational psychiatry seeks to understand how and why the nervous system may process information in dysregulated ways, thereby giving rise to the full spectrum of psychopathological states and behaviors. It seeks to elucidate how psychiatric dysfunctions may mechanistically emerge and be classified, predicted, and clinically addressed. Computational psychiatry models can also be used to connect distinct levels of analysis through biologically grounded theories and rigorous analytical methods.

Integrating computational modeling into psychiatry can aid research in several fundamental ways. First, in a formalized computational model, all assumptions underlying a clinical characterization, moderating factors, and experimental hypotheses must be made explicit. Both manipulated (independent) and measured (dependent) variables can be included as factors in mathematical formulas. The extent to which experimental results match model predictions can qualitatively and quantitatively inform our mechanistic understanding and guide future experiments. In this way, developing and testing computational models provides a clear, iterative approach to increased understanding of psychopathological complexity. Additionally, computational models can explicitly incorporate time, enriching our ability to understand how functional neurocognitive architectures develop and to identify critical temporal windows associated with abnormal developmental trajectories.

Similar to their broader role in computational neuroscience, computational models can help psychiatric researchers answer three fundamental questions regarding the differences in neural information processing that may characterize psychopathology:

- *What* are the main biological components involved in psychopathology and what are the mathematical relationships between these components? Computational approaches require clear and precise definitions of the basic building blocks of cognitive functions and their impairment.

- *How* do dysfunctions in the individual biological units or in their interactions lead to the behavioral changes seen in mental illness? Answers to this question may allow targeted and dynamic manipulations of the system to treat the emotional, cognitive, and behavioral problems associated with psychiatric disorders.

- *Why* have these changes occurred? Understanding etiology in a dynamical system is most challenging, because early, initial changes may have had downstream effects on several nodes. Full investigation therefore requires integrating time into computational models and testing their predictive value using longitudinal designs across various neurodevelopmental trajectories.

This approach, which seeks to bridge the gap between neuroscience and psychopathology, is consistent with the RDoC research framework because it conceptualizes psychopathology with reference to specific neural circuits (what), seeks to understand the relationships between psychological constructs and neurobiological function (how), and explicitly considers the impact of both biological and environmental etiological factors on neurodevelopmental trajectories (why). Progress regarding these questions should open up a range of potential preventative approaches to mental illness.

1.2.3 Data-Driven Approaches

While a wide spectrum of computational approaches exists, computational models in psychiatry can be divided into two broad groups: data-driven models and theory-driven approaches (Huys, Maia, and Frank 2016b). This book focuses on theory-driven models. However, the two approaches are complementary, equally promising, and can be combined.

The data-driven approach to computational psychiatry can be described as the application of machine learning techniques to a vast amount of data related to psychiatric patients, without explicit reference to current psychological or neurobiological theory. The goal is to find new statistical relations between high-dimensional data sets (e.g., genetics, neuroimaging findings, behavioral performances, self-report questionnaires, response to treatment, etc.) that could be meaningful for classification, treatment selection, or prediction of treatment outcome. Here, the assumption is that our understanding of mental illness will improve primarily through improvements in data quality, quantity, and analytics. This "blind" or "brute force" approach may allow researchers to generate new theories based purely on multifaceted clinical data rather than on potentially outmoded historical perspectives (Huys et al. 2016b).

Figure 1.5 illustrates how a data-driven approach might lead to new descriptions and classifications, going beyond traditional symptom-based categories of mental disorder. Consider a population of patients with a range of mood disorders (e.g., major depressive disorder, dysthymia, and bipolar disorder). Machine learning techniques, applied to a range of genetic, physiological, brain activity, and behavioral data and social, cultural, and environmental factors related to those patients, might lead to the discovery of new, unbiasedly derived bio-behavioral clusters. Such clusters might form groups that are more homogeneous than the original *DSM* classification and might connect more directly with the underlying causes of the illness.

1.2.4 Theory-Driven Approaches

Theory-driven models are the focus of this book and can be described as the application of "classical" computational neuroscience approaches to psychiatric questions. In general, these models mathematically describe the relationships between observable

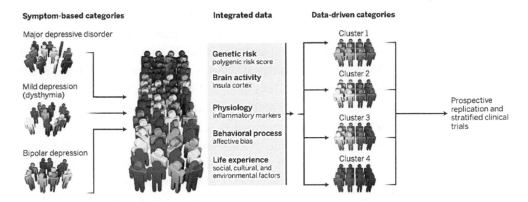

Figure 1.5
Data-driven computational psychiatry. A hypothetical example illustrates how a data-driven approach might lead to new descriptions and classifications, beyond traditional, symptom-based categories of mental disorder. Consider a population of patients suffering from different types of mood disorders and for whom a variety of data has been collected (genetic, brain, physiological data, etc.). New clusters might be found in the data that might connect more directly with mechanisms underlying their symptoms. Such clusters might form groups that are more homogeneous than the original classification, and possibly more relevant in terms of possible treatment. Reproduced from Insel and Cuthbert (2015) with permission.

variables (e.g., behaviors) and theoretically relevant, but potentially unobservable, biological mechanisms. Theory-driven models commonly incorporate known experimental knowledge of brain anatomy and/or physiology, or of higher-level functions for which basic theories have been developed (e.g., perception, learning, or decision making). These models are particularly useful when the cognitive/behavioral function of a neurobiological network is known and/or when accurate and detailed experimental data are available to constrain the model. Theory-driven models can span across multiple levels of analysis and abstraction, from molecules to complex behaviors. They can show whether existent data are sufficient to explain the measured physiological behavior of the circuit; they can also highlight whether unaccounted biological mechanisms could better explain the data, and they can point to gaps in knowledge.

Three representative exemplars of theory-driven models are discussed below: biophysically realistic neural-network models, reinforcement learning models, and Bayesian models (Huys et al. 2016b).

Biophysical models are commonly used to elucidate how biological abnormalities found in mental disorders affect neuro-behavioral dynamics. Biophysical models rely on the theoretical assumption that the essential computations of single neurons and synapses can be captured by sets of first-order differential equations of the type proposed by Hodgkin and Huxley (1952). *Synthetic* computational models recapitulate biophysically realistic properties of neurons and can be used to test the proposed input-output properties of neurophysiological systems in a behavioral context (Wang and Krystal 2014; Ferrante et al. 2016; Huys et al. 2016b; Shay et al. 2016). Biological models are most appropriate when our biological knowledge base is well established and could help identify biological mechanisms that best explain natural variance in patient populations. Biologically realistic models vary in complexity, and the optimal degree of biological detail depends upon the scientific question asked. Simpler models can be more generalizable, while complex models may lose their reductionist appeal as they increase their biological realism. Because biological realism tends to be computationally expensive, these models are most easily implemented when the network is relatively small and/or when the relevant biological parameters are relatively few. A reductionist approach incorporating the fundamental biological features of a complex system can be the simplest possible framework to elucidate the relationship among biological mechanism, neural computations, and functional output. Examples include models of dopamine signals linked to reward-prediction error, working memory internally represented as sustained neural activity, and neural integrators in perceptual decision-making tasks, all of which are relevant to our understanding of some of the cognitive impairments observed in psychiatry (see chapters 2–4). On the other hand, using biologically realistic models might be premature for explaining other psychiatric symptoms, such as psychosis, where a clear neurophysiological characterization at the cellular and systems level is still lacking (Wang and Krystal 2014; see also chapter 6).

Reinforcement learning as a research field lays at the intersection between mathematical psychology, artificial intelligence, and control theory. It addresses how systems of any sort, be they artificial or natural, can learn to gain rewards and avoid punishments in what might be very complicated environments involving states (such as locations in a maze) and transitions between states. They describe how an agent "should" behave under some explicit notion of what that agent is trying to optimize. In that sense, they offer a normative framework to understand behavior.

Reinforcement learning was born from the combination of two long and rich research traditions, which had previously been pursued independently (Sutton and Barto 2018). The first thread concerns optimal control and solutions using value functions and dynamic programming. Optimal control relates to mathematical techniques that deal with the problem of finding a control law for a given system such that a certain optimality criterion is achieved. The second thread concerns learning by trial and error. This thread finds its origin in the psychology of animal learning, particularly in the scientific exploration of Pavlovian (classical) and instrumental (operant) conditioning. Classical conditioning is a form of learning whereby a neutral stimulus (called the *conditioned stimulus*) becomes associated with an unrelated rewarding or punishing stimulus (called the *unconditioned stimulus*) in order to produce a behavioral response (called *conditioned response*). In the famous example studied by Pavlov, the repeated pairing between a bell (the conditioned stimulus) and food (the unconditioned stimulus) would lead to dogs salivating (the conditioned response) when the bell was presented alone. Instrumental conditioning relates to learning associations between actions and outcomes. B. F. Skinner showed that behaviors followed by positive reinforcement are more likely to be repeated, while behaviors followed by negative reinforcement are more likely to be extinguished. Pavlovian conditioning, instrumental conditioning, and subsequent research show that animals and humans naturally learn the associations between objects, actions, and reinforcement contingencies in their environment and use this learning to predict future outcomes. Learning occurs to optimise those predictions (or reduce prediction errors). Interestingly, studies of operant conditioning also form a basis for some modern psychotherapies, particularly behavioral psychotherapies, which offer methods designed to reinforce desired behaviors and eliminate undesired behaviors. As such, such models relate naturally with psychiatry.

Converging evidence from lesion studies, pharmacological manipulations, and electrophysiological recordings in behaving animals, as well as fMRI signals in humans, have provided links between reinforcement learning models and neural structures. In particular, a significant body of literature suggests that the neuromodulator dopamine provides a key reinforcement signal: the temporal-difference reward-prediction error (see sections 2.3 and 5.3). Dopamine-dependent temporal-difference models provide a key link between neuromodulation (often hypothesized to be dysregulated in mental illness), pharmaceutical treatments, substances of abuse, and learning systems.

Finally, a prominent idea in modern computational neuroscience is that the brain maintains and updates internal probabilistic models of the world that serve to interpret the environment and guide our actions. In doing so, it uses calculations akin to the well-known statistical methods of Bayesian inference (see section 2.4). Bayesian inference methods are used to update the probability for a hypothesis, as more evidence or information becomes available. When applied to psychiatry, this approach conceptualizes mental illness as the brain trying to interpret the world through distorted internal probabilistic models, or incorrectly combining such internal models with sensory information, generating maladaptive beliefs.

Bayesian models can be particularly useful in predicting expected behaviors (what would be the optimal thing to do in a given task), quantifying the severity of dysfunctional behavior as the "distance" from optimality, and understanding how maladaptive beliefs can arise. Traditionally, Bayesian inference has been applied primarily to behavioral data, but more recently there has been an effort to integrate behavioral data with neural or fMRI data (Fischer and Peña 2011; Turner et al. 2013).

These main types of theory-driven models—biophysical models, reinforcement learning, predictive coding, and Bayesian models—will be described in more detail in chapter 2.

Of course, theory- and data-driven models are not mutually exclusive. Theory-driven models are often heavily grounded to and validated by experimental data. Similarly, fully unbiased methods of collecting and analyzing data do not exist and often incorporate hypotheses that can be formulated as theories. Both approaches are complementary. Ultimately, they will need to be combined to provide precise diagnostic classifications, predictions, and explanations of mechanistic neurobehavioral trajectories.

A number of initiatives have been created that encourage the development of both types of approaches. As discussed above, NIMH's RDoC initiative encourages psychiatric researchers to study focused aspects of dysfunction that may cut across current diagnostic categories and link mechanistic explanations across different levels of biological analysis. The U.S. Brain Research through Advancing Innovative Neurotechnologies (BRAIN) Initiative has fostered the development of innovative neuro-technologies able to record simultaneously from large numbers of cells and to stimulate brain activity with high spatio-temporal precision. Together, these initiatives are generating large, complex, multimodal data sets that will provide fertile ground for cutting-edge computational modeling.

Computational psychiatry is undoubtedly rising. The first article to use the term computational psychiatry was published in 2007 (Montague 2007). In the following 10 years, the field has rapidly expanded, with 220 publications and several technical books (Parks, Levine, and Long 1998; Sun 2008; Redish and Gordon 2016; Anticevic and Murray 2017; Heinz 2017; Wallace 2017). Groups interested in such questions, as well as summer schools and workshops, have also recently blossomed. However, the field is still in its infancy and comprehensive models able to explain psychopathology at the individual level still need to be implemented. We hope that this book will inspire a new cohort of scientists and help advance a new understanding and treatment of mental illness.

1.3 Structure of the Book

In the next section, we survey the main methods of theory-driven computational psychiatry. We will cover neural networks and connectionist methods, drift-diffusion models, reinforcement learning models, predictive coding, and Bayesian models as well as methods related to fitting computational models to behavioral data.

In the spirit of RDoC (see figure 1.3), the following three chapters describe models relevant to the dimensions of behavioral functioning, focusing on models of healthy function with an emphasis on cognitive systems and positive and negative valence systems. Chapter 3 describes biologically detailed models of working memory and decision making. Chapter 4 describes models of cognitive control. Chapter 5 focuses on reinforcement systems. The following chapters then illustrate the application of computational approaches to schizophrenia (chapter 6), depression (chapter 7), anxiety (chapter 8), addiction (chapter 9), and the example of a tic disorder (Tourette syndrome, chapter 10). In chapter 11, we offer additional pointers on disorders not covered in chapters 5–10 and offer some guidelines for future research.

1.4 Chapter Summary

- The burden of mental health diseases is enormous in terms of suffering, life expectancy, and economic cost.
- There has been stagnation in the discovery of new pharmacological drugs and treatments in recent decades.
- The definition and diagnosis of psychiatric disorders has been problematic for centuries. It is likely that, for most disorders, it will be impossible to pin down a single cause, a single organic substrate, or a single time course. The current categorical classification of mental disorders, known as the *DSM*, has proved to be clinically very valuable, but the heterogeneous phenotypes associated with *DSM*-based diagnoses and the manual's atheoretical structure make it difficult to consider biological mechanisms that could lead to more effective treatments.
- New approaches aim to move from the description of mental illnesses as collections of symptoms toward methods to bridge neuroscience and cognitive modeling with psychopathology. The NIMH RDoC initiative encourages this approach, and computational modeling can provide a useful approach to solve some challenges highlighted by RDoC (e.g., causally linking distinct units of analysis, modeling

temporal trajectories, and dynamic interactions between specific constructs across neurodevelopment).

• Computational approaches are considered central to progress in neuroscience. They could similarly benefit the field of psychiatry.

1.5 Further Study

A historical perspective about the field of psychiatry can be found in Fischer (2012). For reviews describing the emerging field of computational psychiatry, see Montague et al. (2012); Friston et al. (2014); and Stephan and Mathys (2014). To read about the NIMH's RDoC initiative, the reader can consult Kozak and Cuthbert (2016).

2   Methods of Computational Psychiatry: A Brief Survey

Peggy Seriès
University of Edinburgh

"One thing I have learned in a long life: That all our science, measured against reality, is primitive and childlike—and yet it is the most precious thing we have."
—Albert Einstein, *Creator and Rebel*, 1972

The methods that are currently used in computational psychiatry are very diverse, mirroring progress in computational neuroscience and cognitive science and ranging from early connectionist work to reinforcement learning, probabilistic methods, and applied machine learning. This chapter offers a brief survey of these methods, as well as pointers to additional resources for further study.

2.1 Neural Networks and Circuits Approach

The earliest models that aimed at explaining mental computations and disorders are known as "connectionist" models. Donald Hebb introduced the term "connectionism" in the 1940s to describe a set of approaches that models mental or behavioral phenomena as emergent processes in *interconnected networks of simple units* (figure 2.1), a.k.a. "neural networks."

Those simple units, often called "neurons" by analogy with the brain, are described by their value or "output," which can be binary (1/0) or real-valued. The value of each unit is equal to the sum of its inputs, passed through a nonlinear function, called the "activation function." The network connections typically have a "weight" that determines how strongly the units influence each other. The weight can be positive or negative and may change according to a learning procedure. Units may also have a threshold, such that only if the sum of the signals it receives crosses that threshold is the unit activated.

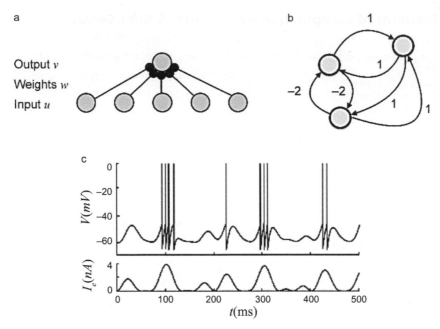

Figure 2.1
Example of neural network models. (a) The perceptron is a feedforward neural network. Here the output unit v receives inputs from all input units v, weighted by weight w. (b) A Hopfield network is a network of binary units connected by recurrent connections. (c) Integrate and fire neuron. This model accounts for the changes in voltage observed when a neuron receives an input current I_e. When the voltage crosses a threshold, the voltage suddenly jumps to 0 and is reset. This models a spike, or action potential.

For example, McCulloch and Pitts (1943) proposed a binary threshold unit as a computational model for an artificial neuron. This neuron computes a weighted sum of its n input signals x_j:

$$y = f\left(\sum_{j=1}^{n} w_j x_j - u\right) \tag{2.1}$$

and generates an output y of 1 if the sum is above a certain threshold u. Otherwise, it outputs 0. Here, f is chosen to be a unit step function, whose value is zero for negative argument and one for positive argument, and w_j is the synapse weight associated with the jth input. Positive weights correspond to excitatory synapses, while negative weights model inhibitory ones. McCulloch and Pitts proved that, in principle, this model could be used to implement any Boolean logic function, such as AND, OR, XOR[1] gates (the latter by combining AND, NOT, and OR units). These logical gates are the building blocks of the digital logic electronic circuits, which modern digital computers are built from. In principle, therefore, such circuits could achieve any type of computation. The McCulloch and Pitts neuron has been generalized in many ways. Different types of activation functions can be used instead of the unit step function; for example, sigmoidal functions such as the logistic function: $f(x) = 1/(1 + \exp(-bx))$, where b is a slope parameter.

2.1.1 Artificial Neural Network Architectures

Typically, artificial neural networks are organized in layers. Neural networks can be feedforward or recurrent. In feedforward networks, the information moves in only one direction—forward from the input nodes through to the intermediate nodes (if any), which are also called "hidden" nodes—and then to the output nodes. The so-called multilayer perceptron, for example, has neurons organized into layers that have unidirectional connections between them. There are no cycles or loops in the network. In recurrent networks, on the contrary, units in the same layer are interconnected. While feedforward networks are static or "memory-less," in the sense that they produce only one set of output values from a given input, recurrent networks can produce sequences of values and rich temporal dynamics and are considered more biologically plausible, since neurons in the brain are also heavily interconnected in circuits that present loops and can generate rich dynamics, such as oscillations.

2.1.2 Learning in Feedforward Networks

Learning in neural networks is viewed as the problem of updating network architecture and connection weights so that the network becomes more efficient at performing a specific task, defined as mapping a desired output to a given input. At a theoretical level, we can distinguish three main learning paradigms: supervised, by reinforcement, and unsupervised. In supervised learning, the network is provided with a correct output for every input pattern in a training data set. Weights are dynamically updated to allow the network to produce answers as close as possible to the known correct answers. This is achieved using learning rules known as error-correction rules. Reinforcement learning is a variant of supervised learning in which the network is provided with only a critique on the correctness of network output (correct/incorrect or reward/punishment), not the correct answers themselves. In contrast, unsupervised learning does not require a correct answer associated with each input pattern in the training data set. It explores the underlying structure in the data, or correlations between patterns in the data, and organizes patterns into categories from these correlations.

The basic principle of error-correction rules is to use the error between the real output of the network and the desired output $(y_{\text{desired}} - y)$ to modify the connection weights so as to gradually reduce this error, using a method known as gradient descent. For example, the perceptron learning rule is based on this error-correction principle. A perceptron consists of a single neuron receiving a number of inputs $x = \{x_1, x_2, \dots, x_n\}$ fed through connections with adjustable weights w_i and threshold u (figure 2.1a). The net input v of the neuron is:

$$v = \sum_i^n w_i x_i - u \tag{2.2}$$

and the output is set to +1 if $v > 0$ and 0 otherwise. The perceptron can be used to classify two classes of inputs: one set of inputs will be trained to lead to an output of 1, while the other set will lead to an output of 0. Rosenblatt (1958) showed that this can be achieved by using the following steps:

1) Initialize the weights and threshold to small random numbers;

2) Present an input vector $x_j = \{x_{j,1}, x_{j,2}, \dots, x_{j,n}\}$ for pattern j and evaluate the output of the neuron y_j;

3) Update the weights according to

$$w_i(t+1) = w_i(t) + \eta\left(d_j - y_j(t)\right)x_{j,i} \tag{2.3}$$

where d_j is the desired output for pattern j, t is the iteration number, and η is the learning rate, which determines how much we adjust the weights in each trial with respect to the loss gradient (the lower it is, the slower we travel along the downward slope of the gradient).

Like most artificial intelligence (AI) researchers, Rosenblatt was very optimistic about the power of neural networks, predicting enthusiastically that the "perceptron may eventually be able to learn, make decisions, and translate languages." However, Minsky and Papert (1969) showed that, as a general result, single-layer perceptron are very limited in what they can do: they can only separate linearly separable patterns. It fails to implement the XOR function, for example. This was perceived as a devastating result concerning what could be achieved with neural networks and played a part to what is known as the "AI winter" in the 1970s and 1980s: a period of reduced funding and interest in artificial intelligence research.

The AI winter came to an end in the mid-1980s, when the work of John Hopfield and David Rumelhart revived interest in neural networks. Rumelhart, Hinton, and Williams (1986) showed that that error-correction rules could be adapted to multilayer networks and provided a method that made neural networks able to approximate any nonlinear function: the back-propagation algorithm. Such networks (and the variants that followed) can be trained to perform sophisticated classification or optimization tasks, such as character recognition and speech recognition. These new results led to a new growth of the field. Neural networks would become commercially successful in the 1990s. Initially limited by the computational power of early computers, this research was leading the way to the current success of deep learning networks, which are based on similar principles.

2.1.3 Recurrent Networks and Attractor Dynamics

Around the same time the back-propagation algorithm was introduced, physicist John Hopfield was able to prove that another form of neural network, now called a Hopfield net, could learn and process information in a completely new way. The units in a Hopfield net are binary threshold units, like in the perceptron, so they take only two different values, usually 1 and –1, depending on whether or not the units' summed input exceeds their threshold (figure 2.1b). The connections in a Hopfield net typically have the following restrictions: i) no unit has a connection with itself: $w_{ii} \neq 0$; and ii) the connections are symmetric: $w_{ij} = w_{ji}$.

Updating one unit in the Hopfield network is performed using the following rule:

$$x_i = \mathrm{Sgn}\left(\sum_{j=1}^{n} w_{ij} x_j - b_i \right) \tag{2.4}$$

where $Sgn(x)$ is the sign function, whose output is 1 or –1; w_{ij} is the weight of the connection from unit j to unit i; x_j is the state of unit j; and b_i is the threshold of unit i.

Updates in the Hopfield network can be performed in two different ways. In an asynchronous update, only one unit is updated at a time. This unit can be picked at random, or a predefined order can be imposed from the very beginning. In a synchronous update, all units are updated at the same time. This requires a central clock to the system in order to maintain synchronization. Importantly, Hopfield found that the network could be described by a quantity that he called energy E (by analogy with the potential energy of spin glass), defined by:

$$E = -\frac{1}{2} \sum_{i,j=1}^{n} w_{ij} x_i x_j - \sum_{i=1}^{n} b_i x_i \tag{2.5}$$

As the network state evolves according to the network dynamics, E always decreases and eventually reaches a local minimum point, called attractor, where the energy stays constant. Hopfield also showed that those energy minima could be set to correspond to particular n-dimensional patterns $\{\varepsilon_1, \varepsilon_2, \dots, \varepsilon_n\}$. This is done by setting the weight from unit j to unit i such that it corresponds to the average (over all patterns) product of the ith and j^{th} elements of each pattern:

$$w_{ij} = \frac{1}{n}\sum_{k=1}^{n} \varepsilon_i^k \varepsilon_j^k \qquad (2.6)$$

where $\varepsilon^k \{\varepsilon_1^k, \varepsilon_2^k, \dots, \varepsilon_n^k\}$ denotes the pattern number k to be encoded. This is called the storage stage. The network can then be used as an associative memory: in the so-called retrieval stage, an input is given to the network to be used as initial state of the network, and the network will evolve according to its dynamics to finally reach an equilibrium that will correspond to the stored pattern that is most similar to the input. For example, if we train a Hopfield net with five units so that the state (1, –1, 1, –1, 1) is an energy minimum, and we give the network the state (1, –1, –1, –1, 1), it will converge to (1, –1, 1, –1, 1).

2.1.4 Application to Psychiatry

The discovery of the back-propagation algorithm and Hopfield networks triggered a strong revival of interest for neural networks. In cognitive science, connectionism—as a movement that hopes to explain intellectual abilities in terms of neural networks—became further inspired by the appearance of *Parallel Distributed Processing* (PDP) in 1986. This is a two-volume collection of papers edited by David E. Rumelhart, psychologist James L. McClelland, and the PDP Group (Rumelhart, McClelland, and PDP Group 1987) that has been particularly influential. Connectionism offered a new theory about cognition, knowledge, and learning—and their impairments. In theory, neural networks can be trained to perform any task (pattern classification, categorization, function approximation, prediction, optimization, content-addressable memory, control) to the level of human participants. The PDP approach led to the idea that possible impairments in cognitive function, such as those observed in mental illness, for example, could be explained by impairments in either the structure or the elements of the underlying neural networks (e.g., the destruction of some connections, or an increase in the noise of some units).

For example, connectionist models have been prominently applied to schizophrenia. Patients with schizophrenia or mania can characteristically display hallucinations and delusions as well as rapidly changing, loose associations in their speech. Early work examined how parameters governing the dynamics of Hopfield networks might reproduce this. An increase in noise can lead to less specific memories, mirroring a broadening of associations in schizophrenia, and less stable, constantly altering memories. Similarly, deletions of connections, mimicking excessive pruning, or overload of the network with memories beyond its capacity, produce the emergence of localized, parasitic attractors, reminiscent of hallucinations or delusions (for a review, see Hoffman and McGlashan 2001).

2.1.5 Biological Networks

More recently, such hypotheses have been explored in the context of neural networks that are much more biologically realistic. Those networks are made of so-called "spiking" neurons that mimic what is known of real neurons: biological neurons use short and sudden increases in voltage, known as action potentials or "spikes," to send information (figure 2.1c). The leaky integrate-and-fire neuron (LIF) is probably the simplest example of a spiking neuron model, but it is still very popular due to the ease with which it can be analyzed and simulated.

The state of the neuron at time t is described by the membrane potential of its soma $v(t)$. The neuron is modeled as a "leaky integrator" of its input $I(t)$:

$$\tau_m \frac{dv(t)}{dt} - v(t) + RI(t) \tag{2.7}$$

Here, τ_m is the membrane time constant and R is the membrane resistance. In electronics terms, this equation describes a simple resistor-capacitor (RC) circuit: the membrane of a neuron can be described as a capacitor because of its ability to store and separate charges. Ion channels allow current to flow in and out of the cell. When more ion channels are open, more ions are able to flow. This represents a decreased resistance, which leads to an increase in conductance.

The dynamics of the spike are not explicitly modeled in the LIF model. Instead, when the membrane potential $v(t)$ reaches a certain threshold v_{th} (spiking threshold), it is instantaneously reset to a lower value v_r (reset potential) and the leaky integration process described by equation (2.7) starts anew with the initial value v_r. To add more realism, it is possible to add an absolute refractory period Δabs immediately after $v(t)$ crosses the threshold v_{th}. During the absolute refractory period, $v(t)$ might be clamped to v_r and the leaky integration process is reinitiated following a delay of Δabs after the spike.

The input current can be constant, or dynamic. If the neuron is modeled as part of the network, the input current will reflect the synaptic inputs coming from other neurons. These in turn can be modeled as weighted inputs, where each connection is given a weight (positive for excitatory neurons or negative for inhibitory neurons), or in a more realistic way as a synaptic conductance that models the dynamics of real synaptic inputs (excitatory post-synaptic potentials, a.k.a. EPSPs, and inhibitory post-synaptic potentials, a.k.a. IPSPs).

More detailed information about modeling individual neurons and networks of bio-logically realistic neurons can be found, for example, in Dayan and Abbott (2000).

Chapter 3 describes applications of such spiking neural networks to understand decision-making and working memory deficits in healthy subjects and schizophrenia. Patients with schizophrenia also show impairments in cognitive flexibility and control tasks that require the inhibition of a pre-potent response. Chapter 4 shows how mod-eling the circuits involved in those tasks might lead to a better understanding of the cognitive control deficits in mental illness.

2.2 Drift-Diffusion Models[2]

Drift-diffusion models (DDM) (Ratcliff 1978) belong to another class of models that are also inspired from physics. Here, the aim is to provide a phenomenological description of a particular psychological process: the performance of animals or humans when they make simple decisions between two choices, without worrying about the underlying possible biological substrate. These models are interesting because, although they were initially proposed only as phenomenological descriptions of psychological processes, it is now clear that they also connect to notions of optimal decision theory as well as observed dynamical processes in real biological neurons.

The DDM is applied to relatively fast decisions (commonly less than 2 seconds) and only to decisions that are a single-stage decision process (as opposed to the multiple-stage processes that might be involved in, for example, reasoning tasks). Such tasks include, for example, perceptual discrimination (are these two objects the same or dif-ferent?), recognition memory (is this image new or was it presented before?), lexical decision (is this a word or a nonword?), and so on. Performance is described in terms of reaction times and accuracy. Such tasks are commonly used in psychiatry to assess how information is processed in different groups—for example, to determine whether anxious or depressed participants process threatening or negative information differ-ently from controls when they have to make simple decisions.

Drift decision models aim at dissecting the different elements that are involved in the decision: in particular, at separating the quality of evidence entering the decision from decision criteria and from other, nondecision, processes such as stimulus encod-ing and response execution.

In these models, decisions are made by accumulating noisy evidence until a thresh-old has been reached, at which point a response is initiated (figure 2.2).

Several mathematical expressions exist for the DDM. A typical equation will be of the form of a Wiener process (one-dimensional Brownian motion). The diffusion pro-cess $x(t)$ evolves dynamically according to:

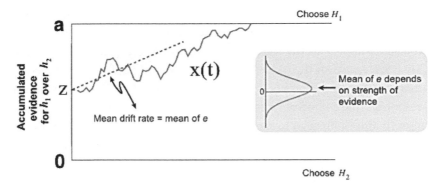

Figure 2.2
The drift-diffusion model (DDM). The decision variable is a noisy cumulative process (blue) composed of the evidence (*e*) with starting point in the middle of [0, a] (no starting bias). The evidence is sampled from a Gaussian distribution whose mean μ depends on the strength of the evidence. The bounds represent the stopping rule, and their separation accounts for accuracy-speed trade-off. Reprinted from Gold and Shadlen (2007) with permission.

$$\frac{dx(t)}{dt} = v + \sigma\eta(t) \tag{2.8}$$

- where v is called the drift rate. It represents the quality of the information evidence from the stimulus. If the stimulus is easily classified, it will have a high rate of drift and approach the correct boundary quickly, leading to fast and accurate responses.
- $\eta(t)$ is a white noise term.
- σ^2 is the variance of the process.

In the model, noisy evidence is accumulated from a starting point, z, to one of two boundaries, *a* or 0. The two boundaries represent the two possible decisions, such as yes/no, word/nonword, etc. Once the process *x(t)* reaches a boundary, the corresponding response is initiated.

Each component of the model—the boundary separation (*a*), drift rate (*v*), starting point (*z*), and nondecision processing (T_{er})—has a straightforward psychological interpretation. The position of the starting point, *z*, indexes response bias. If an individual is biased toward a response (e.g., through different frequencies of each option, or payoffs), their starting point will be closer to the corresponding boundary, meaning that less evidence is required to make that response. This will lead to faster and more probable responses at that boundary compared to the other. The separation *a* between the two boundaries indexes response caution or speed/accuracy settings. A wide boundary separation reflects a cautious response style. In this case, the accumulation process will take longer to reach a boundary, but it is less likely to hit the wrong boundary by mistake, producing slow but accurate responses. One can also add parameters that capture between-trial variability in the starting point, drift rate, and nondecision time. Such variability is necessary for the model to correctly account for the relative speeds of correct and error responses. The model can also be extended to include contaminants—that is, responses that come from some process other than the diffusion decision process (e.g., lapses in attention) so as to account for aberrant responses or outliers in the data.

This model was shown to be a satisfying description of the choice process, since it produces the characteristic right skew of empirical RT distributions. For more mathematical details of the diffusion model, interested readers can consult Ratcliff and Tuerlinckx (2002) or Smith and Ratcliff (2004).

There are several advantages of the diffusion model over traditional analyses of RTs and/or accuracy. First, it allows for the decomposition of behavioral data into processing components. This allows researchers to compare values of response caution, response bias, nondecision time, and stimulus evidence. With this approach, researchers can better identify the source(s) of differences between groups of subjects.

For example, White et al. (2010b) used the diffusion model to study how processing of threatening information might differ in high-anxious individuals. In their lexical decision experiment, participants were shown strings of letters and had to decide if the strings were words or nonwords. Some words were threatening words, while others were neutral. They found a consistent processing advantage for threatening words in high-anxious individuals, even in situations that did not present a competition between different inputs, whereas traditional comparisons showed no significant differences. Specifically, participants with high anxiety had larger drift rates for threatening compared to nonthreatening words whereas participants with low anxiety did not.

Another advantage of this model is that, by fitting RTs and accuracy jointly, it can aid with the identification of different types of bias that are notoriously hard to discriminate: in particular, disentangling discriminability (a change in the quality of evidence from the stimulus) versus response bias (a shift of the decision criterion). Finally, because it uses all the data at once, contrary to classical analyses—which look at RTs or percent correct separately—it is potentially more sensitive to detect differences.

2.2.1 Optimality and Model Extensions

A number of extensions and variants of the DDM have been proposed. The link with optimality theory, on the one hand, and neural studies of decision making, on the other, has led to models in which the decision bounds collapse over time. In this model, less evidence is required to trigger a decision as time passes. Another variant, which has a similar effect, has fixed boundaries but uses an "urgency signal" added to the accumulated evidence.

Recent work has shown that learning effects can be accounted for by integrating the DDM with reinforcement learning models (Pedersen, Frank, and Biele 2017). In such models, reward expectations are computed and dynamically updated for each of the options using a reinforcement learning scheme, while the DDM is the choice mechanism—with the drift rate being dependent on the difference in reward expectation for the two options.

It has also long been known that the random walk of the DDM can be easily related to the sequential probability ratio test (Bogacz et al. 2006), a procedure that makes statistically optimal decisions when evidence is accumulated in time. The strict mathematical equivalence between the DDM and a Bayesian model has recently been explicitly derived (Bitzer et al. 2014). Other extensions have been proposed to account for longer, more complex decisions between more than two options (Roe, Busemeyer, and Townsend 2001).

For a review of DDM models applied to investigation of clinical disorders and individual differences, see White et al. (2010b) and White, Curl, and Sloane (2016).

2.2.2 Accumulation of Evidence in Biological Neurons

Whether the brain uses diffusion-like algorithms is a matter of significant interest and contention. In a pioneering series of studies, Michael Shadlen, Bill Newsome, and collaborators observed that neurons in the lateral intraparietal sulcus of macaque monkeys behaved very similarly to what one would expect if they implemented a diffusion process (Shadlen and Newsome 2001). These researchers used a stochastic motion-discrimination task in which moving stimuli were shown to a monkey, and the monkey had to indicate whether the motion was left or right. The experimenter could control the amount of motion (the "evidence") on a single trial. They found that lateral intraparietal neurons had a mean spike rate that ramped up for choices that result in an eye movement into their response field and ramped down for choices out of their response field. The level to which the neuron's activity ramped up before leading to a saccadic response seemed fixed, mirroring the boundary of diffusion process. Moreover, the slope of the ramp was steeper for easier trials, mirroring the drift rate of the model. Since then, other cortical and subcortical regions have also been found to exhibit possible correlates of a diffusion process. How evidence accumulation is implemented in real neural circuits is still debated, however. This issue has led to great theoretical advances, such as those described in chapter 3.

2.3 Reinforcement Learning Models[3]

In machine learning, reinforcement learning concerns the study of learned optimal control, primarily in multistep (sequential) decision problems. Most classic work on this subject concerns a class of tasks known as Markov decision processes (MDPs). MDPs are formal models of multistep decision tasks, such as navigating in a maze, or games such as Tetris (figure 2.3). The goal of reinforcement learning is typically to learn, by trial and error, to make optimal choices.

Formally, MDPs are expressed in terms of discrete states s, actions a, and numeric rewards r. Informally, states are like situations in a task (e.g., locations in a spatial maze); actions are like behavioral choices (turn left or right); and rewards are a measure of the utility obtained in some state (e.g., a high value for food obtained at some location, if one is hungry, or money).

An MDP consists of a series of discrete time steps in which the agent observes some state s_t of the environment, receives some reward r_t, and chooses some action a_t. The agent's goal is to choose actions at each step so as to maximize the expected cumulative future rewards. Future rewards are usually penalized by how far in the future they would be received (to account for the intuitive idea that a reward obtained in the near future is more attractive than the same reward in the far future). This delay discounting is usually implemented by applying a decay factor $\gamma < 1$: the expected cumulative future rewards is then defined as the sum $r_t + \gamma r_{t+1} + \gamma^2 r_{t+2} + \ldots$ of future rewards. Thus, the goal is to maximize not the immediate reward of an action, but instead the cumulative reward (a.k.a. the "return"), summed over all future time steps. Each action not only

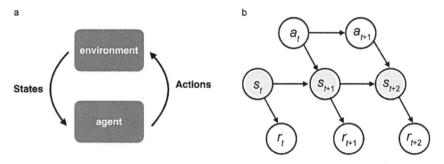

Figure 2.3
Markov decision problems. (a) The setting: an agent interacts with an environment by choosing actions that in turn influence its current state. (b) At each time step, the agent is in some state s and may choose any action available in that state a. This leads to him moving into a new state and giving the decision-maker a corresponding reward r.

affects the current reward but, by affecting the next state, also sets the stage for subsequent rewards. As a consequence, choosing optimally can be quite complicated. What makes these problems nevertheless tractable is the characteristic property of MDPs, the Markov conditional independence property: at any time step t, all future states and rewards depend only on the current state and action. This means that conditional on the present state and action, all future events are independent of all preceding events.

To solve such problem, we can compute the "value" of each state. The state value can be written in terms of the sum of future expected rewards and, thanks to the Markov property, has a recursive mathematical expression:

$$V(s_t) = E\left[r_t + \gamma r_{t+1} + \gamma^2 r_{t+1} + \ldots | s_t\right] = P(r|s_t) + \gamma \sum_{s_{(t+1)}} P(s_{t+1}|s_t) \; V(s_{t+1}) \tag{2.9}$$

Equation (2.9) is a form of the so-called Bellman equation, versions of which underlie most classical reinforcement learning algorithms. Here, it says that the expected future reward in state s_t is given by the sum of two terms: the current reward and the second term, which stands in for all the remaining rewards $r_t + \gamma r_{t+1} + \gamma^2 r_{t+2} + \ldots$. The insight is that this sum is itself just the value V of the subsequent state, averaged over possible successor states, according to their probability. If we manage to learn the values of all the states in the environment (see below), we can choose our actions so as to move toward the most promising ones. The agent will use the value function to select which state to choose at each step, taking the step with the highest value. This is called value-based reinforcement learning.

A common alternative, called policy-based reinforcement learning, is to directly compute the value of taking any action a_t in each state s_t. This is called the state-action value function $Q_\pi(s_t a_t)$ and is the quantity we will want to optimize. This equation has the same form as before:

$$Q_\pi(s_t, a_t) = r_t + \gamma \sum_{s_{(t+1)}} P(s_{t+1}|s_t, a_t) Q_\pi\left(s_{t+1}, \pi(s_{t+1})\right) \tag{2.10}$$

The function $\pi(s_{t+1})$ is called the policy and denotes the way by which the agent choses which action to perform in a given state. It takes the current environment state to return an action. It can be either deterministic or probabilistic.

2.3.1 Learning the V or Q Values

If we can get a good estimate of the V values, we can choose the best action simply by taking steps that will move to the state with highest value. Similarly, if we have an estimate of the Q value function, we can choose the best action simply by comparing Q values across candidate actions. Many reinforcement learning algorithms rely on variations on this basic logic.

How do we learn those values, though? There are two main classes of algorithms for reinforcement learning based on equation (2.9). These classes focus on either the left- or right-hand side of the equal sign in that equation (Gershman and Daw 2017).

The first approach (focusing on the right side of equation [2.9]) is known as model-based reinforcement learning due to its reliance on learning the probabilistic internal model; that is, the one-step reward and state-transition distributions $P(r_t|s_t)$ and $P(s_{t+1}|s_t,a_t)$. Because these transitions concern only immediate events—that is, which rewards or states directly follow other states—they can be learned easily from local experience, essentially by counting. Given these probabilities, it is possible to iteratively expand the right-hand side of equation (2.9) to compute the state-action value for any state and possible action. Algorithms for doing this, such as value iteration, essentially work by simulation: by listing the possible sequences of states that can follow a starting state and action, summing the rewards expected along these sequences, and using the learned model to keep track of their probability. The main advantage of model-based learning is in its simplicity. However, this simplicity comes with a cost of computational complexity, because producing the state-action values depends on extensive computation over many branching possible paths.

The second class of algorithms is called model-free reinforcement learning. These algorithms avoid learning the internal model (the transition and reward probabilities). Instead, they learn a table of state-action values Q (the left-hand side of equation [2.9]) directly from experience and sampling the environment.

The discovery of such algorithms—in particular, the family of temporal-difference learning algorithms (Sutton 1988)—was a major advance in machine learning and continues to provide the foundation for modern applications.

Briefly, these algorithms use experienced states, actions, and rewards to approximate the right-hand side of equation (2.9) and average these to update a table of long-run reward predictions. More precisely, many algorithms are based on a quantity called the reward-prediction error δ_t. This quantity corresponds to the comparison between the value $V(s_t)$ (the predicted reward) and the actual reward plus the prediction computed one time step later:

$$\delta_t = r_t + \gamma V(s_{t+1}) - V(s_t) \tag{2.11}$$

The expression is similar if we are learning the Q values: $\delta_t = r_t + \gamma Q(s_{t+1},a_{t+1}) - Q(s_t,a_t)$. When the value function is well estimated, this difference should on average be zero. If the values are incorrect, however, there will be a discrepancy between the two sides of the equation. In that case, the stored values are updated iteratively to reduce the discrepancy:

$$V_{t+1}(s_t) = V_t(s_t) + \alpha\delta_t = V_t(s_t) + \alpha(r_t + \gamma V(s_{t+1}) - V(s_t)) \tag{2.12}$$

where α is a learning rate between 0 and 1. This is known as the temporal-difference algorithm.

Decisions under model-free models are much simpler than using model-based algorithms because the long-run values are precomputed and need only be compared to find the best action. However, this computational simplicity comes at the cost of inflexibility and less-efficient learning.

Box 10.1 in Chapter 10 can also be consulted for a presentation of commonly used reinforcement learning models and in particular for a comparison between Q-learning and the actor–critic model.

2.3.2 Reinforcement Learning in the Brain

A most-celebrated success of linking theory and neuroscience was the observation that the firing of dopamine neurons in the midbrain of monkeys resembles the reward-prediction error of equation (2.11), when the monkeys are engaged in a reward-learning task. This suggests that the brain uses this signal for reinforcement learning (Montague, Dayan, and Sejnowski 1996). The trial-trial fluctuations in this signal track the model quite precisely and can also be measured in rodents using both physiology and voltammetry. A similar signal can also be measured in the ventral striatum (an important target of the dopamine neurons) in humans using fMRI. Many researchers believe that dopamine drives learning about actions by modulating plasticity at its targets, for example in the striatum. Elicitation and suppression of dopaminergic responses have been shown to modulate learning in tasks specifically designed to isolate error-driven learning.

The link between dopamine and prediction error has important consequences for understanding mental illness and maladaptive behaviors such as addiction. As we will see in chapter 9, for example, drugs of abuse invariably agonize dopamine neurons. This suggests that some aspects of drug abuse and addiction could be understood in terms of the drugs hijacking reinforcement learning processes by interfering with prediction-error signals, giving increasingly higher values to actions leading to the drug.

Boxes 10.1 and 10.2 in chapter 10 give further details about the contributions of tonic and phasic striatal dopamine to action selection and learning.

2.3.3 Evidence for Model-Based and Model-Free Systems

How can we assess whether or when the brain is using model-based or model-free learning?

Although model-free and model-based algorithms both ultimately converge to the optimal value predictions (under various technical assumptions), they differ in the trial-by-trial dynamics by which they approach the solution. Evidence for one or the other model can be shown in experimental tasks that use staged sequences of experience ordered in such a way so as to defeat a model-free learner. For example, in latent learning or "sensory preconditioning" tasks, animals are first preexposed to an environment that does not have any reward (e.g., by exploring a maze). Later, rewards are introduced at particular locations. For a model-based learner, this experience results in them first learning the transition function $P(s_{t+1}|s_t,a_t)$—that is, the map of the maze—and then, subsequently, the reward function $P(r_t|s_t)$, which they will incorporate to their model. However, for a model-free learner, the preexposure stage does not teach them anything useful (only that Q values are zero everywhere). They will not learn a representation of the map of the maze (the state-transition distribution). Because of this, when rewards are introduced, they must relearn the navigation task from scratch.

There is some evidence for model-free learning in animal behavior. As the theory predicts, under certain circumstances, animals fail to integrate information about contingencies and rewards if both types of information have been learned separately. For instance, following overtraining on lever-pressing for food, rodents will press the lever even after being satiated—despite satiation corresponding to a devaluation in the outcome. However, less thoroughly trained animals can successfully adjust. In general, experiments looking at how animals adjust their decisions following changes in reward value (e.g., outcome devaluation) or task contingencies show that their behavior cannot be entirely accounted for with model-free reinforcement learning.

In psychology, these two sorts of behaviors (incapable and capable of integration, respectively) are known as habitual and goal-directed behaviors. The predictions of model-free learning and the prediction-error theories of dopamine are well matched to habitual behavior but fail to account for goal-directed behavior and the ability of organisms to integrate experiences. It is thought that model-based learning operates alongside the model-free system and that both systems compete to control behavioral output (Daw, Niv, and Dayan 2005). Little is known about how the brain determines which of these systems controls behavior at one moment in time. Various models have been proposed to govern arbitration between model-based and model-free values— for instance, according to their relative certainties (which vary with the degree of learning and computational inefficiencies; Daw et al. 2005), or the opportunity cost of the time that it takes to perform model-based calculations (Keramati, Dezfouli, and Piray 2011; Pezzulo, Rigoli, and Chersi 2013). Lee, Shimojo, and O'Doherty (2014), for example, proposed an arbitration mechanism that allocates the degree of control over behavior

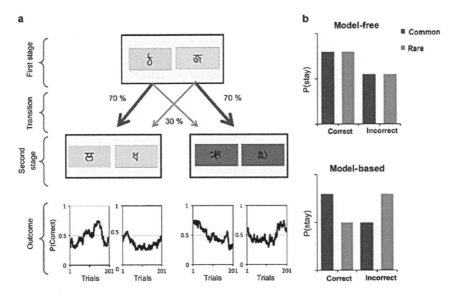

Figure 2.4

Two-step decision-making task. (a) On each trial, choosing between two stimuli leads with fixed probabilities (transition) to one of two pairs of stimuli in stage 2. Each of the four second-stage stimuli is associated with a probabilistic outcome (monetary reward). Those probabilities change slowly and independently across the trials. (b) Model-based and model-free strategies make different predictions about the influence of the outcome obtained after the second stage onto subsequent first-stage choices. They thus predict different choice patterns: in the model-free system, obtaining a reward increases the chance of choosing the same stimulus on the next trial independently of whether the type of transition was rare or common (upper row). In a model-based system, on the contrary, the choices of the stimuli on the next trial integrate the transition type (lower row). Reproduced from Worbe et al. (2015c) with permission.

by model-based and model-free systems as a function of the reliability of their respective predictions (figure 2.4; section 5.2.2 in this volume).

The neural circuits supporting putatively model-based behavior are not well understood. Human neuroimaging suggests that there might be more overlap between neural signals associated with model-based and model-free learning than initially expected.

2.3.4 Implications for Psychiatry

The distinctions between model-based learning and model-free learning appear particularly relevant for psychiatry. It has been proposed, in particular, that addictive and compulsive disorders might involve a shift from model-based to model-free decision making, which would explain inflexible behavior in patients.

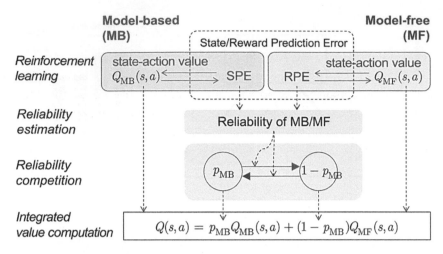

Figure 2.5

Example of a possible arbitration between model-based and model-free learning strategies. Accumulating neural evidence supports the existence of two distinct systems for guiding action selection, a deliberative "model-based" and a reflexive "model-free" system. However, little is known about how the brain determines which of these systems controls behavior at one moment in time. Lee et al. (2014) propose an arbitration mechanism that allocates the degree of control over behavior by model-based and model-free systems as a function of the reliability of their respective predictions. Reliability is computed based on the state prediction error (SPE) in the model-based learning system and based on the reward-prediction error (RPE) in the model-free learning system. The computed reliability functions as a transition rate for the two-state transition model, in which each state represents the probability of choosing the model-based learning strategy (p_{MB}) and the model-free ($1 - p_{MB}$), respectively. The state-action value regulating the actual choice behavior is given by the weighted average of values from the two reinforcement learning systems. Reproduced from Lee et al. (2014) with permission.

Daw et al. (2011) designed a task (figure 2.5) to measure the trade-off between the two types of learning within an individual. This task has since been examined extensively, with some supporting evidence for an association between deficits in goal-directed control and compulsive behavior (Gillan et al. 2016).

More generally, deficits in learning could be at the core of the issues observed in mental illness. Learning and decision making are highly intertwined processes. If learning mechanisms are impaired, maladaptive decisions will be taken, which in turn will influence what will be learned.

The idea that patients with mental illnesses operate with a "wrong" internal model of the world is one that is also central to the Bayesian approach, which we discuss next.

2.4 Bayesian Models and Predictive Coding[4]

2.4.1 Uncertainty and the Bayesian Approach

Bayesian approaches focus on the idea that we live in world of uncertainty. Our environment is often ambiguous or noisy, and our sensory receptors are limited. Often, multiple interpretations are possible. In this context, the best our brain can do is to try to guess what is happening in the world and what best action to take.

This idea of the brain as a "guessing machine" has been formalized in recent years, taking ideas from machine learning and statistics. It is proposed that the brain works by constantly forming hypotheses or "beliefs" about what is present in the world and the actions to take, and by evaluating those hypotheses based on current evidence and prior knowledge. Those hypotheses can be described mathematically as conditional probabilities, denoted $P(\text{hypothesis}|\text{data})$: the probability of the hypothesis given the data, where "data" represents the signals available to our senses. Statisticians have shown that the best way to compute those probabilities is to use Bayes' rule, named after Thomas Bayes (1701–1761):

$$P(\text{hypothesis}|\text{data}) = \frac{P(\text{data}|\text{hypothesis})\,P(\text{hypothesis})}{P(\text{data})} \qquad (2.13)$$

Bayes' rule is of fundamental importance in statistics. Using Bayes' rule to update beliefs is called Bayesian inference. For example, suppose you are trying to figure out whether it is going to rain today. The data available might be the dark clouds that you can observe by the window. Bayes' rule states that we can update our belief, the probability $P(\text{hypothesis}|\text{data})$, which we call the *posterior probability*, by multiplying two other probabilities:

- $P(\text{data}|\text{hypothesis})$: our knowledge about the probability of the data given the hypothesis (e.g., "how probable is it that the clouds look the way they do now, when you actually know it is going to rain?'), which is called the *likelihood*, times

- $P(\text{hypothesis})$: called the *prior* probability, which represents our knowledge about the hypothesis before we collect any new information, here for example the probability that it is going to rain in a day, independently of the shape of the cloud, a number which would be very different whether you live in Edinburgh or Los Angeles.

The denominator, $P(\text{data})$, ensures the resulting probability is between 0 and 1. This posterior becomes our new prior belief and can be further updated based on new sensory input. In a perceptual context, a hypothesis could be about the presence of a given object, or about the value of a given stimulus, while the data consists in the noisy available inputs.

The critical assumptions about Bayesian inference as a model of how the brain works:

- The uncertainty of the environment is taken into account and manipulated in the brain by always keeping track of the probabilities of different possible interpretations.
- The brain has developed (through development and experience) an internal model of the world in the form of prior beliefs and likelihoods that can be consulted to predict and interpret new situations.
- The brain combines new evidence with prior beliefs in a principled way, through the application of Bayes' rule (or an approximation).
- Because currently developed intelligent machines also work in this way—learning from data to make sense of their noisy or ambiguous inputs and updating beliefs—we can get inspiration from machine learning algorithms to understand how this could be implemented in the brain.

2.4.2 Testing Bayesian Predictions Experimentally

Bayesian inference as a model of cognition makes predictions that can be tested using behavioral experiments. This has been the aim of a lot of research in the last 20 years. The first line of research focused on multisensory integration—that is, how the brain combines information coming from different sensory modalities, such as vision and sound. Bayesian inference makes clear predictions about how this should be done: the individual information sources to be integrated should be weighted according to their reliabilities. It also predicts that the combined estimate will then be more reliable than any estimate based on a single one of the sensory cues. For example, if the visual information is much clearer than the auditory information, it should have much more influence on your experience. This can lead to sensory illusions, in situations where there is a conflict between the two modalities and one modality is much more reliable than the other (as observed in the ventriloquism illusion and the McGurk effect). When Bayesian model predictions are compared to experimental data, the general finding is that human behavior is well approximated by Bayesian integration.

The Bayesian model not only predicts how simultaneous signals should optimally be combined, but also how to include prior knowledge. According to Bayes' rule, such knowledge can be represented as a prior probability, which would serve as a summary of all previous experience, and which should be multiplied with the incoming information (the likelihood). An important line of research aims at understanding which priors the brain is using and how such priors impact perception, action, and cognition (see, e.g., Seriès and Seitz 2013). A good way to discover the brain's expectations or assumptions is to study perception or cognition in situations of strong uncertainty or ambiguity—where the current sensory inputs or the "evidence" is very limited. Studying such situations reveals that our brains make automatic assumptions all the time. Sensory illusions have proved particularly important in this field. For example, looking at how the brain interprets shaded objects reveals that the brain assumes that light comes "from above." This makes sense, of course, since light usually comes from the sun above us. Similarly, we seem to expect objects to be symmetrical, to change smoothly in space and time, and orientations to be more frequently horizontal or vertical and angles to look like perpendicular corners. We also expect objects to bulge outward more than inward (i.e., to be convex shapes, like balloons or pears), that background images are colored in a uniform way, that objects move slowly or not at all, that the gaze of other people is directed toward us, and that faces correspond to convex surfaces. Such assumptions have been successfully described using the framework of Bayesian priors.

Techniques have been developed that allow measurement of individual participants' priors based on experiment measurements and performance biases, by fitting Bayesian models to performance (Stocker and Simoncelli 2006). In the sensory domain, it is commonly found that human participants learn quickly, effortlessly, and unconsciously the statistics of the perceptual environment and come to expect the perceptual inputs that are most likely. This can lead to biases in the estimation of sensory features, perceiving the world as being more similar to what is expected than it really is, and sometimes even "hallucinating" expected inputs, even when they are absent (Chalk, Seitz, and Seriès 2010). It has also been shown that the brain can update "long-term" prior beliefs, such as that light comes from above or that objects move slowly, if placed in environments where lights come from below or where objects move quickly (Seriès and Seitz 2013). This shows that the brain constantly revises its assumptions and updates its internal model of the environment.

Many aspects of human cognition, such as language acquisition and processing, action selection, prediction, reasoning, and sensory inference have been modeled as optimal readouts of statistical inference processes.

2.4.3 Decision Theory

Bayes' rule computes beliefs about the state of the world, s, given noisy or ambiguous sensory input D, $P(s|D)$. However, it does not specify how these beliefs are used to generate decisions and actions. Decision theory extends Bayesian inference to deal with the problem of selecting the best decision or action based on our current beliefs and, as such, encompasses the methods of reinforcement learning described above. The difference, of course, is that here we have to infer the states instead of them being given, as commonly assumed in reinforcement learning formalisms. The essence of making the best decisions is, then, to minimize the expected loss (or maximize expected reward/utility) given our beliefs. One simply calculates the expected loss for a given action; that is, the loss averaged across the possible states weighted by the degree of belief in the state, $\sum_s L(a, s)P(s|D)$, and then chooses the action that has the smallest expected loss.

Here, $L(a,s)$ denotes the benefit or loss associated with taking action a in state s, and Σ denotes a summation over all possible states s.

We can also consider domains with temporal dynamics, where $s(t)$ changes over time, with each action evoking its own set of stochastic transitions. Here, it is necessary to determine not an individual optimal action, but rather a sequence of actions in the light of possible transitions.

Bayesian decision theory (BDT) therefore requires two sorts of inference: one is to compute the posteriors to estimate the states as well as possible (using Bayesian inference), and the other is to compute the best action. Both are computationally hard; the latter is particularly difficult when it is necessary to optimize over long trajectories of future actions—and becomes much harder in the face of the first problem. When the state s is known, BDT reduces to common descriptions of reinforcement learning (see section 2.3).

2.4.4 Heuristics and Approximations: Implementation in the Brain

Exact Bayesian inference is thought to be intractable for most everyday problems the brain encounters. An important line of research tries to understand whether human behavior can be described using simple heuristics that might approximate Bayesian inference, without involving complex computations.

While, in theory, it seems feasible for neural circuits to implement (possibly rough) approximations of Bayesian computations, how such computations are actually implemented in the brain and relate to neural activity is still an open question and an active area of research. Whether the Bayesian approach can actually make testable predictions for neurobiology (for example, which parts of the brain would be involved, or how neural activity could represent probabilities) is also debated. It is as yet unclear whether the Bayesian approach is only useful at the "computational" level, to describe the computations performed by the brain overall, or whether it can be also useful at the "implementation level" to constrain and predict how those algorithms might be implemented in the neural tissue.

2.4.5 Application to Psychiatry

Many researchers believe that the Bayesian approach has promising applications for the field of psychiatry. Bayesian models could potentially help quantify differences between different groups (e.g., healthy vs. ill) and identifying whether such differences come from using different internal models, for example different prior beliefs, or from different learning or decision strategies.

A common idea in psychiatry is that the internal models used by patients, in particular their prior beliefs, could be different from those of healthy subjects. In the study of schizophrenia, for example, it has been proposed that "positive symptoms" (hallucination and delusions) could be related to an imbalance between information coming from the senses and prior beliefs or expectations (see chapter 6). In autism, similarly, it has been proposed that the influence of prior expectations might be weaker compared to that of sensory inputs, which could explain why patients feel overwhelmed by a world perceived as being "too real" (see section 11.1).

More generally, it has been proposed that three different classes of failure modes could be at the root of mental illness. They may stem from 1) abnormalities in the framing of problems or tasks that the brain is trying to solve (abnormalities in the priors, likelihood, or utility); 2) from the mechanisms of cognition used to solve the tasks; or 3) from the historical data available from the environment (i.e., abnormal experience such as trauma; Huys et al. 2015b).

2.4.6 Predictive Coding and Bayesian Models Used in Psychiatry

Despite the popularity of these ideas, in practice, only a limited number of studies have tried to compare or fit the behavior of participants with quantitative models. We here describe some of the models that can be found in the literature.

a) Predictive Coding Models Predictive coding became popular as a model of visual processing at the turn of the century (Rao and Ballard 1999). The general idea is to view visual processing as a hierarchical system, composed of a number of levels connected by feedforward and feedback connections. In this system, feedback projections from one level to the lower level are trying to predict the activity of the neurons they target: feedback connections carry predictions of lower-level neural activities, whereas the feedforward connections carry the residual errors between the predictions and the actual lower-level activities. It was shown that this model could explain a number

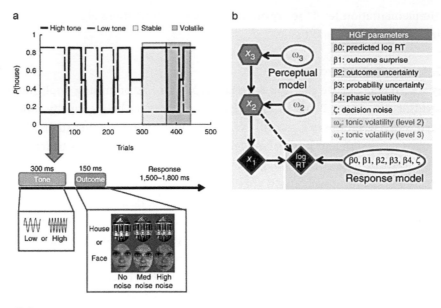

Figure 2.6

(a) Example of the task used by Lawson, Mathys, and Rees (2017). Schematic of the task, showing the volatile environmental structure (top)—for example, the probability of seeing a house (given the preceding high or low tone) across trials. The green area shows a "stable" period of 72 trials in which the probabilities remained fixed, and the violet area shows a "volatile" period of 72 trials in which the outcome probabilities switched three times. A single trial is also seen (bottom) showing example stimuli. (b) Hierarchical Gaussian model (HGM). Schematic depiction of the three-level hierarchical Gaussian filter that was used to model this task. The perceptual model comprises three hierarchical states (x_1, x_2, and x_3). The lowest-level variable, x_1, describes the uncertainty about outcomes—that is, the presence of a house or face; level 2 (x_2) addresses uncertainty about the cue-outcome contingencies; and level 3 (x_3) addresses uncertainty about environmental change—that is, the volatility of the cue-outcome contingencies. Participant-specific free parameters (ovals) are estimated from individual reaction times (log RT) data. Red parameters relate to the perceptual model, whereas black parameters relate to the response model. Diamonds: quantities that change over time (trials); hexagons: quantities that change over time, and that additionally depend on their previous state in time in a Markovian fashion. Reproduced from Lawson et al. (2017) with permission.

of phenomena observed in real neural activities in the visual cortex. The idea that the brain uses some form of predictive coding has become very widespread. There is, however, a debate about how such a scheme would be implemented in neural activities, in particular about whether neural activities in the visual cortex should really be interpreted in terms of prediction errors (as proposed by Rao and Ballard 1999), or whether they would be better understood in terms of the predicted input itself—or maybe whether there would be different categories of neurons representing either the prediction error or the predicted input.

Predictive coding and Bayesian inference are concepts that are often confounded. Although predictive coding and Bayesian inference do not necessarily imply each other (Aitchison and Lengyel 2017), predictive coding is often proposed as an effective way for Bayesian inference to be implemented in the brain: while Bayesian inference would describe the general computation that the brain is trying to perform, predictive coding would describe the algorithm that is being carried out.

Why the two concepts are related can be understood as follows. As explained above, Bayesian inference entails updating our existing belief (the prior distribution) with new information (the likelihood distribution) to form our new belief (the posterior distribution). If we assume those distributions are Gaussian, they can each be represented by their mean μ and their variance, or precision π (where π refers to the inverse variance). It can be shown that the Bayesian sequential updating of beliefs can be expressed as follows (Mathys et al. 2011; Palmer, Lawson, and Hohwy 2017), where x is the new measurement, $\mu_{posterior}$ is the mean of the new posterior, and $\pi_{posterior}$ its precision:

$$\mu_{posterior} = \mu_{prior} + \frac{\pi_{likelihood}}{\pi_{posterior}}\left(x - \mu_{prior}\right) \tag{2.14}$$

where:

$$\pi_{posterior} = \pi_{prior} + \pi_{likelihood} \tag{2.15}$$

This last term of equation (2.14), $\left(x - \mu_{prior}\right)$, can be interpreted as a prediction error: the mean of the prior belief (prior), μ_{prior}, can be considered a prediction about what the new measurement, x, will be. This means that Bayesian inference can be implemented by iteratively updating predictions with the prediction error produced by each new measurement.

The precision of the prior distribution π_{prior} indicates our confidence in our existing prediction, while the precision of the likelihood distribution $\pi_{likelihood}$ represents the ambiguity inherent in the measurement (the noisiness of incoming data). Together, these two parameters give an indication of how reliable or informative prediction errors are expected to be regarding the true (hidden) state of the world. Prediction errors are therefore weighted by the estimated precision of the new information relative to the estimated precision of existing beliefs.

The weighting term $\left(\pi_{\text{likelihood}}/\pi_{\text{posterior}}\right)$ plays the role of a learning rate. A high learning rate means that prediction errors will drive inference about the state of the world to a greater extent. Conversely, a low learning rate means that prior information is given more weight in determining what is inferred. The fact that the learning rate depends on the ratio $\pi_{\text{likelihood}}/\left(\pi_{\text{prior}}+\pi_{\text{likelihood}}\right)$ implies that beliefs are more highly sensitive to new measurements when we know little about the environment (π_{prior} is small) but less sensitive when we have already gathered plenty of information (π_{prior} is large).

Importantly, this update expression—which links Bayesian inference with predictive coding—is not specific to the univariate Gaussian case, but can be shown to be valid much more generally.[5]

b) Hierarchical Gaussian Filter Model   Inference in realistic environments is thought to be hierarchical, involving different levels of predictions described by random variables, which interact with each other. The set of probabilistic steps that can be followed to generate the values of these random variables is known as the generative model. Often, we represent these steps using a graph representation. In such a graphical model, the nodes represent the random variables, and the edges represent condition dependencies (see, e.g., figure 2.6b).

While Bayesian belief updating in such generative models is optimal from the point of view of probability theory, it is difficult to achieve in practice: it requires computing complicated integrals, which are not tractable analytically and difficult to evaluate in real time. For this reason, it is thought that the brain can only achieve approximations of Bayesian inference. Different types of approximations are usually considered, inspired from research in Machine Learning. A popular model recently developed is the hierarchical Gaussian filter.

The hierarchical Gaussian filter model (Mathys et al. 2011; Mathys et al. 2014) describes a hierarchical generative model of the environment and its (in)stability. In this model, all states except the lowest level evolve as coupled Gaussian random walks,[6] such that each state determines the step size of the evolution of the next lower state.

For example, imagine a task where participants have to perform a binary classification of images as either faces or houses, where the images had high, medium, or no noise added (figure 2.6a). A tone preceding each image is highly, weakly, or not predictive of a given outcome, and the associations between images and tones change across time. Such a task can be represented by the graphical model depicted in figure 2.6b, where the lowest-level variable, x_1, describes the uncertainty about outcomes (i.e., the presence of a house or face), level 2 (x_2) addresses uncertainty about the cue-outcome contingencies, and level 3 (x_3) addresses uncertainty about environmental change (i.e., the volatility of the cue-outcome contingencies).

Using the so-called "mean-field" approximation, Chris Mathys and collaborators derived analytic update equations for beliefs at each level, whose form resembles reinforcement learning updates and equation (2.14) above, with dynamic learning rates and precision-weighted prediction errors. The update equations make the model well suited for filtering purposes; that is, they can be used to predict the value of, and the uncertainty about, a hidden and moving quantity based on all information acquired up to a certain point. Importantly, the coupling across levels is controlled by parameters whose values can be fit to each individual participant performing the task.

The hierarchical Gaussian filter model has been used, for example, to investigate how participants with autism learn about changing environments (Lawson et al. 2017). They used the task described above, in which participants performed binary classification of images as either faces or houses. By fitting the model to their data, Lawson et al. could show that participants with autism tended to overestimate the volatility of the sensory environment, at the expense of building stable expectations that would lead them to be surprised when aberrant outcomes arise.

Chapter 6 will provide another example for the use of the hierarchical Gaussian filter in schizophrenia research.

c) Belief Networks and Circular Inference[7] An alternative, very general, powerful, and efficient algorithm to perform inference in generative models is known as belief propagation. Consider, for example, a hierarchical generative model with three nodes: the "leaf" is caused by a "tree," which is caused by a "forest." In belief propagation, sensory information S—for example, the probability that a leaf is present in the image—climbs the hierarchy in a feedforward way and, at the same time, prior information moves downward as feedback. Each node calculates a belief for the underlying variable it represents, equivalent to the posterior; for example, $P(X_{\text{tree}}|S)$, and sends local messages (e.g., $M_{\text{tree}\to\text{leaf}} = P(X_{\text{leaf}}|X_{\text{tree}})$) to all the neighboring nodes. As a result, information, in the form of beliefs, is propagated throughout the system. Assuming binary variables and using the log-ratios of the probabilities, then beliefs and messages can be calculated by the recursive equations of the form:

$$M_{ij}^{t+1} = W_{ij}\left(B_t^t - M_{ij}^t\right) \tag{2.16}$$

$$B_t^{t+1} = \sum_j M_{ji}^{t+1} \tag{2.17}$$

where M_{ij}^t is the message from node i to node j at time t, B_i^t is the belief of node i at time t, and $W_{ij}(B)$ is a sigmoid function of B.

The second equation simply means that each node calculates a belief by summing the messages coming from all its connected neighbors (e.g., the belief about the presence of a tree is equal to the sum of the messages from the forest and the leaf nodes). The first equation, on the other hand, means that the message travelling from node i (here, the forest) to node j (the tree) is a function of the belief of the sending node i after we subtract the effect that the receiving node j has on the sending node i (e.g., here, the message from tree to forest). This latter correction is crucial. Without it, the algorithm would produce loops; that is, reverberations of bottom-up and or top-down information. In such "loopy" belief propagation, the consequences are treated as causes, and vice versa, and the information in the upward and the downward stream can be mixed and overcounted. Jardri and Denève have proposed that such "circular inference" could underlie the symptoms of schizophrenia and may also be present to some extent in the general population (Jardri and Denève 2013; Jardri et al. 2017).

2.5 Model Fitting and Model Comparison

Having provided a brief overview over different modeling techniques, we now turn to a tutorial overview of how these techniques can be used to probe behavior and fit to real data. We mostly focus on the computational methods that use a generative framework, namely reinforcement learning models and Bayesian models. The following uses material from Huys (2018) (see also Wilson and Collins 2019 for related material).

2.5.1 Choosing a Suitable Model

Assessing whether a given model is a suitable description of the data at hand can be tricky. In theory, there will always be many other types of models that could be suitable as well. So how do we choose and validate a particular one? As a rule of thumb for good practice, the modeling should contain three general steps. We first need to build the model. Second, this model should be validated with artificial data. Finally, the model is applied to the real data. These points are detailed below:

1. Clarifying the hypotheses to be tested. The initial choice of the model is usually motivated by the hypotheses that we wish to test. We will usually be guided by an

effort to: i) have a model that is flexible enough to describe the data and relates to previous literature in the field; ii) contains parameters that directly relate to our hypotheses; iii) is as simple as possible given those constraints. There will usually be different possible variants of the model. A reasonable approach is to build a series of models starting from a very simple "null" hypothesis (a "no–interest" model that does not include the element we wish to show the importance of) and then adding in the various features of interest to examine to what extent they contribute toward explaining the data. A probabilistic component will need to be included, so as to account for the variability intrinsic to each individual's performance. The different variants can be tested against each other using model comparison (see below).

2. Validation on artificial data means using the model to generate artificial data, by setting the parameters by hand and exploring the different behaviors exhibited by the model. First, this is a way to check that the data the model generates is actually comparable to the data obtained in the experiment. Second, this can be used to test the fitting procedure: once the parameters have been chosen by hand and the artificial data has been generated, we can try to recover the parameters using our fitting procedure (i.e., inverting the model): can we discover which parameters were used for the model just by looking at the model's performance? This step is called parameter recovery. This is an important step prior to interpreting any parameters. This can be used, as well, to ask whether we can distinguish between the behavior generated by different models, and whether we can recover a particular model reliably. This is called model recovery. It is recommended to attempt to perform these steps prior to collecting the experiment data, since they may suggest changes in experimental parameters, such as the number of trials or the number of subjects to run.

3. Finally, the models need to also be validated on the actual data of interest. One possibility is to compare data generated from the model (with fitted parameters) to the real data. For learning experiments, it is, for instance, often useful to plot learning curves and ask whether the model captures the shape of these curves well. Once the models have been validated in this way, it is meaningful to ask which of the models provides the most parsimonious account of the data. This is the domain of model comparison, where the performances of different models are weighted against their number of free parameters. Model comparison is always relative: even the best amongst a set of models may still be too poor to provide any meaningful information. The interpretation of parameters in the models should only follow

at the end, once one model has been chosen as a satisfactory characterization of the data.

2.5.2 A Toy Example

To illustrate this process, we can consider a very simple learning experiment (Huys 2018). On each trial, participants have to choose one of two squares. The blue square yields small rewards on 80% of trials, and the red square small rewards on 20% of trials. Participants have to discover which of the two squares is best, based on their successive choices. On each trial t, they thus perform a single choice a_t, which yields an immediate reward r_t. This choice does not have any influence on future options.

We can consider two different models. The first model assumes that individuals perform temporal-difference learning to compute the values of the two stimuli in this extremely simple scenario. Taking equation (2.12) and observing that there is no next state, but only immediate rewards, the temporal-difference prediction-error learning takes the simpler form of Rescorla-Wagner learning (Rescorla and Wagner 1972):

$$V_{t+1}^{TD}\left(s_t\right) = V_t^{TD}\left(s_t\right) + \alpha\left(r_t - V_t^{TD}\left(s_t\right)\right) \qquad (2.18)$$

The second model assumes that individuals simply perform averages over the rewards earned for each of the two stimuli. This model is actually the correct inference to perform given how the outcomes are generated.

$$V_{t+1}^{av}\left(s_t\right) = \frac{1}{t}\sum_t^1 r_t \qquad (2.19)$$

It can be easily shown that this equation can also be expressed in this recurrent form:

$$V_{t+1}^{av}\left(s_t\right) = V_t^{av}\left(s_t\right) + \frac{1}{t}\left(r_t - V_t^{av}\left(s_t\right)\right) \qquad (2.20)$$

Comparing these expressions, we see that while the temporal-difference learning rule uses a fixed learning rate α, the average has a decaying term $1 / t$. The temporal-difference rule has one free parameter, α, while the averaging rule has no free parameter. How can we determine which model best accounts for participants' performance?

a) Generating Data   We first start by generating artificial data from both models. To do this, we need to determine a model for the function that maps the values V onto probabilities of choosing one action or the other (here, choosing one square or the other). A frequent choice is the use of a softmax function whereby the probability of choosing stimulus s on trial t (e.g., the blue square) is

$$p\left(a_t = s|V_t\right) = \frac{e^{\beta V_t(s)}}{e^{\beta V_t(s)} + e^{\beta V_t(\bar{s})}} \tag{2.21}$$

where $\bar{s}$ denotes the alternative stimulus (i.e., the green square) and β determines how precisely the choices follow the values; that is, also how noisy the choice process is. This parameter can also be interpreted as controlling exploration versus exploitation.

b) Fitting Models Once we have built a model and generated artificial data from it, we can proceed to the next step: fit the model to the generated data to assess how well we are able to recover the model's parameters. To find the set of parameters that are most compatible with the data, we can use maximum likelihood (ML). To find the ML parameters, for each subject, we look for the parameters θ (in our example, $\theta = \{\alpha, \beta\}$) that maximize the likelihood of all their T actions $a_1, \ldots , a_T$:

$$\hat{\theta}_{ML} = \text{argmax}_\theta \, \log p\left(a_1, a_2, \ldots , a_T|\theta\right) \tag{2.22}$$

On first sight, this calculation may appear difficult, because the choices a_t depend on previous choices. However, since every choice only depends on the value V_t at the time of the choice t, then the probability of observing a sequence of stimulus choices $a_1, \ldots , a_T$ is simply:

$$\log p\left(a_1, a_2, \ldots , a_T|\theta\right) = \log \prod_{t=1}^{T} p\left(a_t|V_t\right) = \sum_{t=1}^{T} \log p\left(a_t|V_t\right) \tag{2.23}$$

That is: once we condition on the values, the choices become independent of the previous choices.

The values can be updated iteratively prior to computing the likelihood of each choice, leading to an algorithm that takes the following general and very simple form.

- Initialize the values V for each stimulus
- foreach trial t do:

    compute log likelihood of choice a_t on trial t given parameters: $l_t = \log p\left(a_t|V_t, \theta\right)$

    update value V_{t+1} given outcomes on trial t

  end

- compute total log likelihood $l_T = \sum_{1}^{T} l_t$.

The total likelihood (a function of α and β) can now be passed to any of a number of optimization tools to solve equation (2.22).

Parameter recovery using ML is, however, often very imperfect. This is particularly true in situations where parameters have overlapping effects and therefore can trade off each other. A very simple, and often very powerful, solution is to impose a soft prior on the parameters and perform maximum a posteriori (MAP) inference rather than ML. This is very simply achieved by replacing equation (2.22) with

$$\hat{\theta}_{MAP} = \text{argmax}_\theta \, \log p(a_1, a_2, \dots, a_T | \theta) p(\theta) \qquad (2.24)$$

The computation of the posterior likelihood is thus just the same as before, but now we also add the log likelihood of the prior to the total log likelihood of the choices. The choice of the prior $p(\theta)$ is not always straightforward. In many situations, it can make sense to infer the prior from the data itself. This is called empirical Bayes. There are a number of techniques available for this, and this is becoming a more common approach. In this toy example, little would be gained over the basic MAP approach, but this would change for larger models (Huys 2018).

c) **Model Comparison**   Having fitted the model to the data, the next step is to assess how well the model can actually account for the data. Simply looking at how closely the model fits the data is not sufficient: a model that is too flexible (has many free parameters) could fit the data perfectly, but would lead to poor prediction of new data. This issue is known as overfitting.

Bayesian model comparison takes into account the trade-off between the flexibility of the model and the fit it provides to the data by using as a measure of fit, not the best possible likelihood, but the average likelihood over all possible parameter settings:

$$P(A|M) = \int d\theta P(A|\theta, M) p(\theta) \qquad (2.25)$$

where A denotes all the behavioral data and M the model.

The Bayes factor, which measures whether model M_1 is more strongly supported by the data under consideration than model M_2, is then defined as

$$BF = \frac{P(A|M_1)}{P(A|M_2)} \qquad (2.26)$$

and is considered substantial if greater than 3, and conclusive if greater than 5. Unfortunately, the integral in equation (2.25) is not always straightforward to evaluate, and there exist a number of approximations to it. A commonly used measure is the Bayesian information criterion, defined as

$$BIC = -2 \, \log p(A|\hat{\theta}_{ML}) + d \, \log(n) \qquad (2.27)$$

where d is the number of parameters in the model and n is the number of data points. Other measures exist, such as the Aikake information criterion, or other related techniques such as using a Laplace approximation for $P(A|M)$; that is, approximating the function being integrated with a Gaussian, for which the integral can then be computed analytically.

d) Group Studies The methods so far have considered individual subjects. However, most studies, particularly in clinical settings, deal with group data. Two simple approaches for model fitting exist in this case. First, we can treat all individuals in one group as using the same parameters; this is called a fixed-effects treatment. Alternatively, we can treat them as having entirely separate parameters. This is called a random-effects treatment. A fixed-effects treatment confounds inter- and intra- individual variability and is therefore not recommended. On the other hand, a random-effects treatment can inflate noise depending on how the parameters are estimated. One solution to this is to consider that individuals in a group tend to be similar, and hence should have similar parameters. For instance, parameters of individuals in a group could cluster around a particular value. To implement this idea, we can follow a hierarchical approach and formulate a model about how the parameters vary across the population.

Another question is whether all individuals use the same generative model to perform the task, which might not always be the case. Here again, we can either employ a random-effects treatment over models, considering that some individuals in a group will behave according to model 1, others according to model 2, and yet others according to model 3, and so on. This implies that different individuals may differ in terms of the internal processes they invoke to perform a given task. Alternatively, one can nest multiple models in a more complex model. This solution corresponds to assuming that individuals use a mixture of strategies, but that this is true across the entire group. Daw (2011) offers a more in-depth treatment of those issues.

2.6 Chapter Summary

A variety of computational tools have been developed that can be applied to psychiatry, either to describe behavior or to try to relate observed behavior to underlying neurobiological differences. The choice of the model will depend on the data to be modeled, the hypothesis that is tested, and the questions to be addressed.

- Connectionist models, or neural networks, can be used to explore the relationship between connectivity, dynamics, and function. In psychiatry, they have, for example, been used to explore how attractor dynamics could be impaired in mental illness (see also chapter 3).

- Drift-diffusion models can be used to dissect the origin of differences in performance and reaction times between groups in tasks involving choices between two alternatives.

- Reinforcement learning models are used to model the dynamics of learning of an environment, where discrete states (or objects) are associated with rewards or punishment. Because of the link between prediction-error signals and dopamine, reinforcement learning models have shown to be very promising tools in understand impairments in learning and decision making in mental illness (see also chapters 5–10).

- Bayesian models account for learning and decision making in terms of statistical inference. They can be used to assess how "optimal" a given performance is and to discover the internal models that participants have learned or use in a particular environment. Because they explicitly model beliefs, they can be used to describe mental illness in terms of maladaptive or broken beliefs and false inference.

- Fitting a particular model to data is usually performed using maximum likelihood or maximum a posteriori. One then needs to verify that the model can account well for the data. Model comparison is used to assess what model describes the data best, taking into account the number of free parameters of each model. Before using them on real data, it is recommended to test the model fitting and comparison techniques on artificial data generated by each model; that is, to perform parameter and model recovery.

2.7 Further Study

Due to space limitations, this chapter could only provide a very quick survey of the methods of computational neuroscience and computational cognitive neuroscience that can be applied to psychiatry. Each section has been the subject of entire books and review articles. A great reference regarding artificial neural networks is Hertz, Krogh, and Palmer (1991). Dayan and Abbott (2000) is also a recommended reference for further study of biological neurons and of neural networks.

For the drift decision model, we recommend reviews by Roger Ratcliff; for example, Ratcliff et al. (2016). The use of drift decision models in psychiatry has been covered, for example, by White, Curl, and Sloane (2016).

For reinforcement learning techniques, the classic reference is Sutton and Barto (1998). More recent developments and their relation to neuroscience have been covered, for example, by Daw and Tobler (2013) and Gold and Shadlen (2007).

Bogacz (2017) provides a tutorial on the free-energy framework for modeling perception developed by K. Friston and collaborators, which extends the predictive coding model of Rao and Ballard (1999).

Wilson and Collins (2019) provide excellent advice regarding computational modeling of behavioral data, in the form of 10 rules to follow so as to make sure that modeling is used with care and yields meaningful insights.

Readers particularly interested in modeling fMRI data can also consult Cohen et al. (2017).

3 Biophysically Based Neural Circuit Modeling of Working Memory and Decision Making, and Related Psychiatric Deficits

Xiao-Jing Wang
Center for Neural Science, New York University

John D. Murray
Department of Psychiatry, Yale University School of Medicine

3.1 Introduction

The brain is not a uniform system made of equal parts. Instead, it is characterized by a modular organization of areas with distinct properties, connection patterns, and specialized functions. In the primate cerebral cortex, certain areas like the prefrontal cortex play a central role in higher cognitive functions, in contrast to early sensory information processing or motor generation. Those areas of the "cognitive type" are the ones commonly implicated in a variety of mental disorders; therefore, understanding such systems is especially relevant to the field of computational psychiatry.

A key property of cognitive-type neural circuits is the presence of strong recurrent connections underlying reverberatory network dynamics. The behavior of any nonlinear system endowed with an abundance of feedback connection loops is difficult to predict by intuition alone. To illustrate our point, consider two identical, mutually inhibitory neurons (Kristan and Katz 2006; figure 3.1a). Given this "connectome," how would the network behave? It turns out that experiments and theory have uncovered multiple dynamical scenarios. First, both neurons may simply stay silent. Second, when driven by inputs, the system may behave as a "switch," with one neuron active while inhibiting the other neuron, or vice versa, and a brief input can switch the system between the two states (figure 3.1b). Third, if neurons are endowed with a slow adaptation, each of the two neurons could take turns being active, and over time eventually stop firing due to "fatigue" when the other neuron takes over, leading to a "half-center" oscillator which is the core of rhythmic central pattern generators (figure 3.1c). Fourth and finally, under certain conditions, the two neurons can be perfectly synchronized, spike by spike: the two neurons fire at the same time, leading to mutual inhibition after a brief delay, and when this inhibition decays away they can fire again together (Wang 2010; figure 3.1d). This simple example illustrates that behavior often

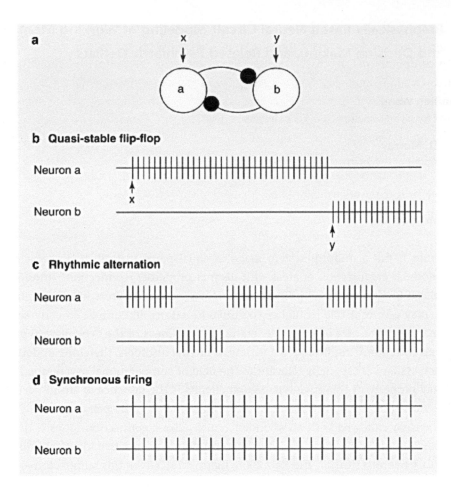

Figure 3.1
Distinct dynamical regimes in a circuit of two reciprocally connected inhibitory neurons. (a) Neurons a and b receive excitatory inputs x and y, respectively. (b–d) Under different conditions of neuronal and synaptic properties, the circuit can exhibit qualitatively distinct dynamical regimes, including quasi-stable flip-flop (b), rhythmic alternation as a "half-center" oscillator (c), and spike-by-spike synchrony (d). Adapted from Kristan and Katz (2006).

cannot be deduced from anatomy in a straightforward fashion; physiology and modeling are important for discovering the dynamical operations of neural circuits.

In computational psychiatry, some researchers are concerned with behavioral performance and its mathematical modeling. For instance, as described later in this book, reinforcement learning models have been applied to addiction, anxiety, and depression (see chapters 7–9). Such models can be used to quantify abnormal sensitivity to motivation and reward in affected subjects. However, they are typically relatively abstract and difficult to relate to specific brain circuits in a concrete manner. Another approach, which is the focus of this chapter, strives to develop neural circuit models that are capable of linking a particular behavior to the biological mechanism responsible for generating neural activity patterns that causally underlie an observed behavioral trait.

This is a tall order. One could argue that, at present, we do not yet adequately understand how a neural system generates complex symptoms of any psychiatric disorder. But that is precisely why biologically realistic neural circuit modeling should be a priority of our field. Ultimately, a central goal of neuropsychiatric research is to explain how symptoms and cognitive deficits arise from neurobiological pathologies. This demands we bridge the stark explanatory gaps between levels of analysis: mechanisms underlying a psychiatric disease occur at the level of neurons and synapses, whereas symptoms are manifested and diagnosed at the level of cognition and behavior, which involve collective computations in brain circuits. Linking these levels is vital for gaining mechanistic insight into mental illness, and for the rational development of pharmacological treatments, which act at the molecular level with physiological impact at the synaptic level. Biophysically based neural circuit modeling is a framework particularly well suited to link synaptic-level disruptions to emergent brain dysfunction.

In the following, we will review a set of studies that use biophysically based neural circuit models to understand how synaptic disruptions may induce cognitive deficits, with particular relevance for schizophrenia (Murray et al. 2014; Starc et al. 2017; Lam et al. 2017).

3.2 What Is Biophysically Based Neural Circuit Modeling?

Biophysically based neural circuit modeling incorporates key physiological properties of neurons and synapses, as well as circuit connectivity. Dynamic neural activity is simulated through systems of differential equations governing the biophysical properties of neurons and synapses (see section 2.1). Emergent patterns of activity in the model can be informed by—and tested with—empirical measures of neural activity. In certain circuit models, neural activity can also be mapped onto a behavioral response, thereby generating model predictions that can be tested with behavioral data from corresponding task paradigms.

It is important to emphasize that biological realism does not mean that the more biological details a model incorporates, the better. We typically first formulate a well-defined question, such as, "what is the microcircuit mechanism of stimulus-selective persistent activity during working memory?" Then we carefully determine the level of complexity of models for single neurons and synapses, as well as network connectivity, that are appropriate for investigating that question. For instance, a single neuron can be modeled in detail with morphologically reconstructed dendrites and axons, or using a few compartments so that dendritic compartments are separated from the soma, or a single compartment described by the Hodgkin–Huxley model or the integrate-and-fire model (see section 2.1.5). Which one to choose depends on the question under study (e.g., which may or may not require distinct dendritic compartments).

Neurons in a network interact with each other through synaptic connections, which are either excitatory (or, respectively, inhibitory) if spiking of a (presynaptic) neuron produces an increase (or, respectively, a decrease) of membrane potential in recipient (postsynaptic) neurons. Synaptic excitation is mediated by AMPA and NMDA receptors that bind with the neurotransmitter glutamate and have different time constants, NMDA being much slower than AMPA. Synaptic inhibition is mainly mediated by the GABA$_A$ receptor, which binds with neurotransmitter GABA. Like single-neuron models, synaptic interactions can be described mathematically with varying degrees of complexity. For the sake of simplicity, even to this day, many recurrent neural network models use "kick synapses," namely a presynaptic spike that induces an instantaneous jump of postsynaptic potential (which is positive for excitation, negative for inhibition). Therefore, no temporal aspects (latency, rise and decay times, summation) are taken into account. However, the basic dynamical properties of synaptic transmission can play a crucial role in shaping the collective behavior of a recurrent neural circuit. As described below, for example, slow NMDA receptors at recurrent excitatory synapses have been found to be crucial for the maintenance of mnemonic persistent activity (Wang 1999), a theoretical prediction that years later was supported by a monkey experiment (Wang et al. 2013). Such a discovery suggests that biologically based modeling has the potential to make predictions at the receptor level that bridge with a cognition function via understanding neural circuit dynamics. This may, in turn, provide opportunities to mechanistically understand how synapse-level disruptions produce aberrant neural activity and deficits in cognition and behavior.

The specific scientific questions under study determine the level of biophysical detail included in a particular model. For instance, questions related to dopaminergic dysregulation (such as are found in schizophrenia; see also chapters 6 and 10) can be addressed in a biophysically based model of an individual synapse that includes subcellular signaling pathways (Qi, Miller, and Voit 2010). In contrast, emergent circuit-level dynamics, such as oscillations or persistent activity, can be simulated in thousands of recurrently connected spiking neurons, whose individual dynamics are simplified to include only certain channels and receptors (Wang 2010, 2008). Modeling systems-level disturbances, such as large-scale connectivity alterations in schizophrenia, may entail coarse-grained mean-field models of local nodes organized in large-scale networks. Such models still contain neurophysiologically interpretable parameters and enable study of questions related to excitatory/inhibitory (E/I) balance (Yang et al. 2014; Yang, Murray, and Wang 2016).

An important area of research in clinical neuroscience is the discovery and characterization of predictive neurophysiological biomarkers for psychiatric disorders; that is, characteristics that can be objectively measured and evaluated as an indicator of pathogenic biological processes.

As one area of modeling progress with relevance to biomarkers, there is a large literature on studying neural oscillations that emerge at the network level in recurrent cortical circuits (Wang 2010). Cortical oscillatory activity is found to be abnormal in a number of neuropsychiatric disorders. In particular, schizophrenia is associated with alterations in oscillatory activity in the gamma (30–80 Hz) range (Gonzalez-Burgos and Lewis 2012; Uhlhaas 2013). Computational models, in conjunction with physiological findings, support the idea that neocortical gamma oscillations arise from a feedback loop in a microcircuit of pyramidal cells reciprocally connected with perisomatic-targeting, parvalbumin-expressing interneurons (Buzsáki and Wang 2012). These models of gamma oscillations can be used to explore the dynamical effects of putative synaptic perturbations associated with schizophrenia, including reduced production of GABA and parvalbumin[1] in inhibitory interneurons (Vierling-Claassen et al. 2008; Spencer 2009; Volman, Behrens, and Sejnowski 2011; Rotaru et al. 2011). In each case, the models provide specific hypotheses for how systems-level dynamics, which can be measured in humans through techniques such as electroencephalography or magneto-encephalography, may be altered as a result of synaptic- or cellular-level changes.

Below, we focus on how circuit models of cognitive functions can be applied to understand cognitive deficits resulting from synaptic disruptions associated with schizophrenia. For some core cognitive computations, we have knowledge of the neural circuit basis underlying these processes, which typically involve contributions from animal studies. For these cases, detailed circuit models can be developed rigorously to provide the link from synaptic disruptions to behavior (e.g., cognitive deficits discussed below). In other cases, psychiatric symptoms relate to complex cognitive functions for which we lack understanding of the underlying neuronal representations or circuit mechanisms. At present, these circuit models are limited and cannot be applied to complex behavioral tasks, for which we lack understanding of neural circuit correlates. We now turn to the conditions in which circuit models may be best suited to study cognitive deficits in psychiatric disorders.

3.3 Linking Propositions for Cognitive Processes

A major goal in computational psychiatry research is for biophysically based neural circuit models to explain mechanistically how synaptic-level disruptions induce cognitive-level deficits. For this approach to be most effective, the circuit model should be grounded in a well-supported relationship between neuronal activity and a given cognitive process. Such relationships have been formalized by the concept of a *linking proposition*, which states the nature of a statistical correspondence between a given neural state and a cognitive state. Related to the concept of the linking proposition is that of a *bridge locus*, which is the set of neurons for which this linking proposition holds (Teller 1984). Convergent evidence supporting a linking proportion comes from a number of experimental methodologies applied to animal models, especially to the behaving nonhuman primate, given the strong homologies of areas in the human and nonhuman primate brains (Schall 2004). Single-neuron recordings can relate neuronal activity to computations posited in psychological processes. Further evidence can come from perturbative techniques such as micro-stimulation or inactivation.

As an exemplary application of this perspective to a nonsensory function, Schall (2004) considered the neural underpinnings of the preparation of saccadic eye movements. In the case of saccade preparation, a well-supported candidate for the bridge locus is a distributed network of cortical and subcortical areas, including the frontal eye field and superior colliculus. During saccade preparation, so-called "movement" neurons in these areas exhibit a location-selective ramping of their firing rates, and a saccade is initiated when their firing rates reach a threshold level. At the level of mental processes, a leading psychological model for response preparation is accumulation of a signal until reaching a fixed threshold level that triggers the response. In such accumulator models, sequential sampling of a stochastic signal generates variability in the rate of rise to the fixed threshold, which can explain the observed variability in saccade reaction times. The linking proposition between a neural state (movement cell-firing rates) and a psychological state (level of an accumulator) provides a framework for detailed hypothesis generation and experimental examination of psychological models.

What linking propositions do we have for core cognitive functions, and specifically for working memory and decision making? The neural correlates of working memory have been studied extensively through single-neuron recordings from monkeys performing tasks in which the identity of a transient sensory stimulus must be maintained in working memory across a seconds-long mnemonic delay to guide a future response. For instance, in one well-studied experimental paradigm, the oculomotor delayed-response task, the subject is shown a visual cue appearing in one of eight possible locations. The cue disappears during a delay period of a couple of seconds, and the subject needs to maintain the position in working memory. The subject is then trained to perform a saccadic eye movement to the location of the cue so as to receive a reward (Funahashi, Bruce, and Goldman-Rakic 1989). These studies revealed that a key neural correlate of working memory is stimulus-selective persistent activity—that is, stable elevated firing rates in a subset of neurons—that spans the mnemonic delay (Goldman-Rakic 1995; Wang 2001). These neuronal activity patterns are observed across a distributed network of interconnected brain areas, with prefrontal cortex as a key locus. In the oculomotor delayed-response task, for example, during the mnemonic delay, a subset of prefrontal neurons exhibit tuned persistent activity patterns, with single neurons firing at elevated rates for a preferred spatial location (figure 3.2). These neurophysiological findings have grounded the leading hypothesis that working memory is supported by stable persistent activity patterns in prefrontal cortex that bridge the temporal gap between stimulus and response epochs.

The neural computations underlying decision making have been most studied in task paradigms in which a categorical choice is based on the accumulation of perceptual evidence over time. In one highly influential task paradigm, the subject must decide the net direction of random-dot motion stimuli, which encourages decision making based on the temporal integration of momentary perceptual evidence (Roitman and Shadlen 2002). Behavior can be well captured by psychological process models of evidence accumulation to a threshold. This is, for example, the idea behind the drift-diffusion model described in section 2.2. Single-neuron recordings have found possible correlates of such an evidence-accumulation process in association cortex, such as the lateral intraparietal area (LIP): choice-selective ramping of neuronal firing rates reflects accumulated perceptual evidence, with activity crossing a threshold level reflecting the decision commitment (Gold and Shadlen 2007). This is illustrated in figure 3.3. These neural correlates reflect two key computations needed for perceptual decision making: accumulation of evidence and formation of categorical choice.

Conceptually, a neural circuit model can instantiate a linking proposition for a cognitive process and propose circuit mechanisms underlying the computations. If

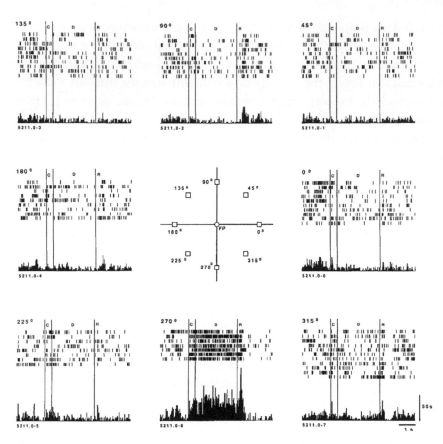

Figure 3.2
Example of directional delay-period activity of a principal sulcus neuron during the oculomotor delayed-response task. In this seminal experiment described by Funahashi et al. (1989), monkeys were trained to fixate a central spot during a brief presentation of a peripheral cue and throughout a subsequent delay period (3 seconds) and then, upon the extinction of the fixation target, to make a saccadic eye movement to where the cue had been presented. Visual cues were randomly presented at one of the eight locations indicated in the center diagram. The neuron shown in this example had strongly directional delay-period activity responding only when the cue had been presented at the bottom location. It was suppressed during the delay when the cue was presented in the upper visual field. Reproduced from Funahashi et al. (1989) with permission.

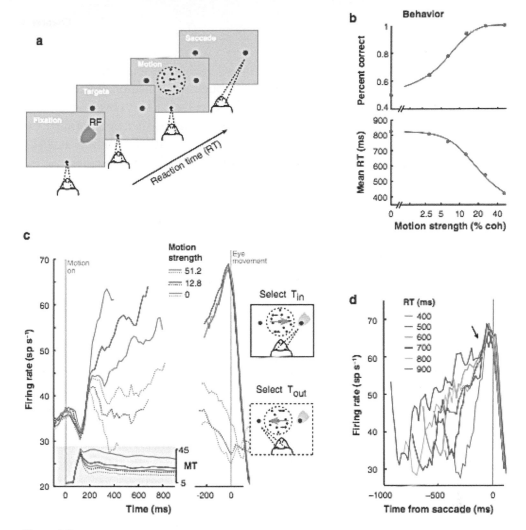

Figure 3.3

Neural mechanism of a decision about direction of motion. (a) The subject views a patch of dynamic random dots and is requested to indicate, whenever they are ready, which net direction they perceived for the motion (left or right). They need to indicate their decision by making an eye movement to a peripheral target. The gray patch shows the location of the response field (RF) of a LIP neuron. One of the choice targets (T_{in}) is in the RF of the LIP neuron; the other target (T_{out})—as well as the motion stimulus itself—lies outside the neuron's RF. (b) Effect of stimulus difficulty on accuracy and decision time. (c) Response of LIP neurons during decision formation. Average firing rate from 54 LIP neurons is shown for three levels of difficulty. Responses are grouped by motion strength and direction of choice, as indicated. Left: The responses are aligned to the onset of the random-dot motion. Shaded insert shows average responses from direction-selective neurons in area MT to motion in the preferred and antipreferred directions. After a transient period, MT responds at a nearly constant rate. Right: The responses are aligned to the eye movement. The LIP firing rates ramp up or down, approximating the integral of a difference in firing rate between MT neurons with opposite direction preferences. (d) Responses grouped by reaction time. Only T_{in} choices are shown. All trials reach a stereotyped firing rate ~70 milliseconds before saccade initiation (arrow). Adapted with permission from Gold and Shadlen (2007).

associated with a hypothesized bridge locus, model predictions for these circuit mechanisms can be experimentally tested, such as through single-neuron recordings. For instance, in the case of working memory, experiments have tested how focal antagonism of specific synaptic receptors affects persistent activity, thereby informing the neuronal and synaptic mechanisms supporting the computations (Wang et al. 2013; Rao, Williams, and Goldman-Rakic 2000). The stronger these links are among (i) the synaptic and neuronal processes in circuit mechanisms, (ii) neural activity, and (iii) the cognitive function, the better the model is validated. Once established, the model can then make rigorous predictions for the consequences of alterations in those circuit mechanisms. In this way, circuit models can iteratively contribute to our understanding of these links across levels of analysis and leverage them to study dysfunction in neuropsychiatric disorders.

3.4 Attractor Network Models for Core Cognitive Computations in Recurrent Cortical Circuits

Biophysically based neural circuit modeling has provided mechanistic hypotheses for how working memory and decision-making computations can be performed in recurrent cortical circuits. As noted above, a key neurophysiological correlate of working memory is stimulus-selective, persistent neuronal activity across the mnemonic delay in association cortical areas. Delays in working memory tasks (a few seconds) are longer than the typical time scales of neuronal or synaptic responses (10–100 milliseconds). Similarly, perceptual decision making demands categorical selection and benefits from temporal integration of evidence over long time scales (hundreds of milliseconds). Both of these computations therefore implicate circuit mechanisms.

Motivated by experimental observations of stable persistent activity in single neurons, a leading theoretical framework proposes that working memory–related persistent activity states are dynamical attractors; that is, stable states in network activity. In the mathematical formalism of dynamical systems, an attractor state is an activity pattern that is stable in time, so that, following a small transient perturbation away from this state, the network will converge back to the attractor state. A class of neural circuit models called "attractor networks" has been applied to explain the mechanisms that allow a recurrent network of spiking neurons to maintain persistent activity during working memory (Amit 1995; Wang 2001). An attractor network typically possesses multiple attractor states: a low-firing baseline state and multiple memory states in which a stimulus-selective subset of neurons is persistently active. Because the memory state is an attractor state, it is self-reinforcing and resistant to noise or perturbation by distractors, allowing the stimulus-selective memory to be stably maintained over time (Brunel and Wang 2001; Compte et al. 2000).

In a typical attractor network, subpopulations of excitatory neurons are selective to different stimuli. Recurrent excitatory synaptic connectivity exhibits a "Hebbian" pattern such that neurons of similar selectivity have stronger connections between them (figure 3.4a). When the strength of recurrent excitatory connections is strong enough, the circuit can support stimulus-selective attractor states that can subserve working memory (figure 3.4b). Strong recurrent excitation thereby provides the positive feedback that sustains persistent activity. Wang (1999) found that incorporating physiologically realistic synaptic dynamics poses constraints on the synaptic mechanisms supporting this positive feedback. Strong positive feedback is prone to generate large-amplitude oscillations that can destabilize persistent states and can drive firing rates beyond physiologically plausible ranges. It was found that both of these problems can be solved if recurrent excitation is primarily mediated by slow NMDA receptors.

Critically, recurrent excitation must be balanced by strong feedback[2] inhibition mediated by GABAergic interneurons. Feedback inhibition stabilizes the low-activity baseline state (Amit and Brunel 1997; Wang 1999). In a persistent activity memory state, recurrent inhibition also enforces selectivity of the working memory representation, preventing the spread of excitation to the entire neuronal population (Murray et al. 2014). Attractor dynamics supporting working memory are thereby supported by recurrent excitation and inhibition that are strong and balanced.

These circuit models make predictions for the relationship between synaptic mechanisms and working memory activity. These predictions have been confirmed through experiments with simultaneous single-neuron recording from and pharmacological manipulation of prefrontal cortex: locally blocking excitation mediated by NMDA receptors attenuates persistent activity for the preferred stimulus (Wang et al. 2013). Similarly, locally blocking inhibition mediated by $GABA_A$ receptors reduces stimulus selectivity of delay activity by elevating responses to nonpreferred stimuli (Rao et al. 2000).

In addition to working memory computations, strong recurrent excitatory and inhibitory connections in cortical attractor networks provide a circuit mechanism for decision making, supporting temporal integration of evidence and categorical choice (Wang 2002; Wong and Wang 2006; Wang 2008). In this model, choice-selective neuronal populations receive external inputs corresponding to sensory information (figure 3.4c). Reverberating excitation enables temporal accumulation of evidence through slow ramping of neural activity over time (figure 3.4d). This property highlights that attractor networks not only support multiple stable states (representing categorical

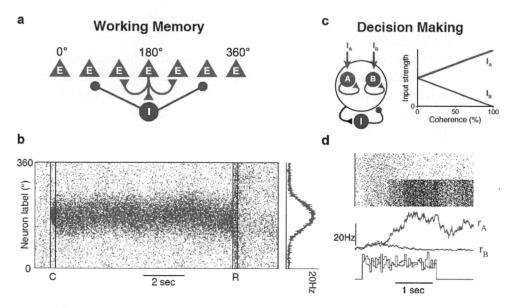

Figure 3.4

Biophysically based cortical-circuit models of working memory and decision-making computations. (a) Schematic of the network architecture for a model of spatial working memory. The
model consists of recurrently connected excitatory pyramidal cells (*E*) and inhibitory interneurons (*I*). Pyramidal cells are labeled by the angular location they encode (0–360°). Excitatory-to-
excitatory connections are structured, such that neurons with similar preferred angles are more
strongly connected. Connections between pyramidal cells and interneurons are unstructured and
mediate feedback inhibition. (b) Spatiotemporal raster plot showing a bump-attractor state in an
example trial. A stimulus is presented at 180° during the brief cue epoch (denoted *C*) and during
the subsequent delay, and the stimulus location is encoded by persistent activity throughout the
working memory delay until the response epoch (denoted *R*). At right is shown the firing rate
profile of the working memory bump-attractor state. (c) Schematic of the network architecture for
a model of perceptual decision making. The circuit contains two populations of pyramidal neurons, which are each selective to one of the two stimuli (*A* and *B*). Within each pyramidal neuron
population there is strong recurrent excitation, and the two populations compete via feedback
inhibition mediated by interneurons (*I*). Right: The selective populations receive sensory-related
inputs determined by the stimulus coherence. (d) Example neuronal activity in a single trial for a
zero-coherence stimulus. Top: Spatiotemporal raster plot for the two selective populations. Middle: Population firing rates r_A and r_B. Bottom: Stochastic sensory-related inputs. During decision
making, the circuit exhibits an initial slow ramping, related to temporal integration of evidence,
which leads to categorical choice (for *A* in this trial). Panels (b) and (d) adapted from Compte et
al. (2000) and Wang (2002), respectively.

choices), but also support slow transient dynamics that can instantiate computations such as temporal integration. In these models, temporal integration via recurrent excitation benefits from the slow biophysical time scale of NMDA receptors (Wang 2002). Feedback and lateral inhibition mediated by GABAergic interneurons mediates competition among neuronal populations underlying the formation of a categorical choice. Irregular neuronal firing, a ubiquitous feature of cortex, contributes to stochastic choice behavior across trials, even when presented with identical stimulus inputs.

These computational modeling studies demonstrate that an association cortical microcircuit model can support working memory and decision-making computations through attractor dynamics. This therefore suggests a shared "cognitive-type" circuit mechanism for these functions, which may furthermore provide components upon which more complex cognitive processes may be built (Wang 2013). Because these functions rely on strong recurrent excitation and inhibition, they are particularly well suited to study how cognitive deficits may arise from alterations in synaptic function, which are implicated in neuropsychiatric disorders.

3.5 Altered Excitation–Inhibition Balance as a Model of Cognitive Deficits

Cortical attractor network models of working memory and decision-making function can be applied to characterize the impact of altered E/I balance in association cortex. Alteration of cortical E/I balance is implicated in multiple neuropsychiatric disorders, including schizophrenia, autism spectrum disorder, and major depression. A key strength of these circuit models is that they make explicit predictions not just for neural activity but also for behavior, which can be tested experimentally in clinical populations or after causal perturbation.

In schizophrenia, cortical microcircuit alterations are complex, with observed dysfunction in both glutamatergic excitation and GABAergic inhibition. Postmortem investigations of prefrontal cortex in schizophrenia find reductions in spines on layer-3 pyramidal cells, which potentially reflect reduced recurrent excitation. Such studies also have revealed multiple impairments in inhibitory interneurons, which potentially reflect reduced feedback inhibition. Pharmacological models of schizophrenia provide complementary evidence. One such approach is to use NMDA-receptor antagonists such as ketamine, which transiently, safely, and reversibly induce cardinal symptoms of schizophrenia in healthy subjects (Krystal et al. 2003). A leading hypothesis regarding ketamine's effects on neural function is that the drug leads to a state of cortical disinhibition, potentially via preferential blockade of NMDA receptors on GABAergic interneurons (Greene 2001; Homayoun and Moghaddam 2007; Kotermanski and Johnson

2009). However, many questions remain regarding the neural effects of ketamine, such as which NMDA-receptor subunits and neuronal cell types may be the preferential sites of action (Khlestova et al. 2016; Zorumski, Izumi, and Mennerick 2016).

Mechanistic links between altered E/I ratio and cognitive impairment remain tenuous, however. To address this issue, the aim of the modeling studies described below is to formulate dissociable behavioral predictions for distinct sites of synaptic perturbation. In particular, they have looked at perturbations of the E/I ratio via hypofunction of NMDA receptors at two recurrent synaptic sites: i) on inhibitory interneurons, which elevates E/I ratio via disinhibition; or ii) on excitatory pyramidal neurons, which on the contrary lowers E/I ratio (figure 3.5a).

3.5.1 Working Memory Models

Working memory function is a promising candidate in clinical neuroscience as an endophenotype—that is, as a quantitatively measurable core trait that is intermediate between genetic risk factors and a psychiatric disorder (Insel and Cuthbert 2009).

_____→

Figure 3.5
Effects of altered excitation–inhibition (E/I) balance in cortical-circuit models of working memory and decision making. (a) E/I ratio was perturbed bidirectionally via hypofunction of NMDA receptors at two recurrent synaptic sites: on inhibitory interneurons, which elevates E/I ratio via disinhibition; or on excitatory pyramidal neurons, which lowers E/I ratio. (b) For the working memory circuit, the firing rate profile of the "bump" attractor activity pattern during working memory maintenance. Elevated E/I ratio via disinhibition results in a broadened working memory representation. (c) Disinhibition impairs the network's ability to filter out intervening distractors. Top: Spatiotemporal plot of network activity in response to a distractor presented during the delay at a distance of 90° from the target. Bottom: Deviation of the read-out report as a function of the angular distance between the distractor and the target. The "distractibility window" is widened by disinhibition. (d) In the decision-making circuit, performance as quantified by the psychometric function; that is, the proportion of correct choices as a function of stimulus coherence. Both perturbations—elevated and lowered E/I ratio—can comparably degrade performance relative to the control circuit. (e) A perceptual decision-making task paradigm that characterizes the time course of evidence accumulation can test dissociable behavioral predictions from elevated versus lowered E/I ratio. Top: The pulse paradigm uses a brief pulse of additional perceptual evidence at different onset times. This pulse induces a shift in the psychometric function, which quantifies the sensitivity of the choice on evidence presented at that time point. Bottom: Shift in the psychometric function, as a function of pulse onset time, for the three E/I regimes. Relative to control, in the elevated-E/I circuit the pulse has a stronger impact at early onset times, but less impact at later onset times. The lowered-E/I circuit shows a flattened profile of the shift, with greater impact at late onset times.

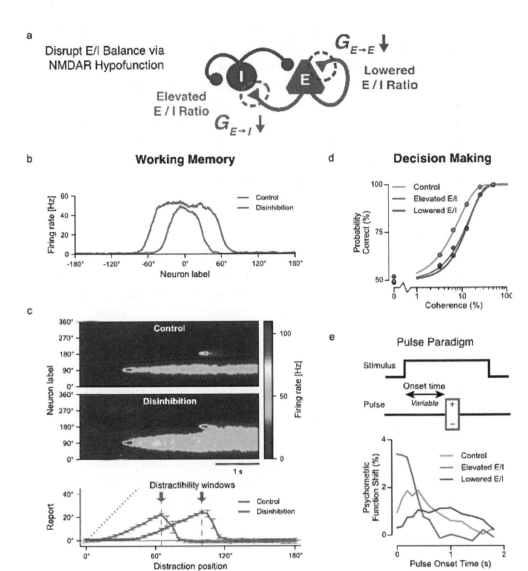

Working memory function involves different component processes: encoding of the memory, maintenance, robustness to distraction, precision, and capacity. Ongoing work in clinical cognitive neuroscience aims at resolving how these processes are impaired. Many studies have found a deficit in working memory encoding in patients with schizophrenia; that is, a deficit that is observed even when the delay is set to zero seconds (Lee and Park 2005). For visuospatial working memory, patients with schizophrenia exhibit deficits not only in encoding but also in maintenance, which results in a graded loss of precision (Badcock et al. 2008; Starc et al. 2017). Other visual paradigms find reduced capacity of working memory but not necessarily precision (Gold et al. 2010).

Murray et al. (2014) examined the effects of altered E/I balance in a cortical-circuit model of visuospatial working memory. Disinhibition, which results in an elevated E/I ratio, was implemented through antagonism of NMDA receptors preferentially onto interneurons. In this model, disinhibition leads to a broadening in the neural-activity patterns in the mnemonic attractor states (figure 3.5b). This neural change induced specific cognitive deficits. During maintenance, the mnemonic activity pattern undergoes random drift, which leads to decreased precision of responses. Disinhibition increased the rate of this drift, thereby inducing a specific deficit in mnemonic precision during working memory maintenance.

Additionally, Murray et al. (2014) found that broadened neural representations make working memory more vulnerable to intervening distractors. In the model, distractors correspond to additional distracting inputs, modeled identically to the initial cues, with the same intensity and duration, but with a different stimulus location. A distractor is more likely to "attract" the working memory activity toward it if the two representations overlap. Distractibility therefore depends on the similarity between the representations of the memory target and the intervening distractor. Consistent with this model behavior, it has been found empirically that in visuospatial working memory, a distractor can attract the memory report toward its location, but only if the distractor appears within a "distractibility (spatial) window" around the target location (Herwig, Beisert, and Schneider 2010). Because disinhibition broadens the mnemonic activity patterns, this model predicts an increased range of distractors that can disrupt working memory for patients with schizophrenia.

To test the model prediction of broadened working memory representations under disinhibition, Murray et al. (2014) analyzed behavior from healthy humans administered ketamine during a spatial delayed match-to-sample task (Anticevic et al. 2012). In this task, subjects must retain the position of a cue in working memory. Subjects are then presented with a probe stimulus corresponding to different locations, and they must indicate if these probes are a "match" to the initial cue, or not. The model predicted a pattern of errors that is dependent on whether the probe is similar to the target held in working memory (a.k.a. the "memorandum"). Analysis of the behavioral data under ketamine versus control conditions revealed a specific pattern of errors that was similar to that predicted by the computational model. Consistent with model predictions, ketamine increased the rate of errors specifically for probes that would overlap with a broadened mnemonic representation. A similar pattern of errors has been observed in schizophrenia, with a selective increase in false alarms for "near" nontarget probes but not for "far" nontarget probes (Mayer and Park 2012). In contrast to the model predictions arising from disinhibition, insufficient recurrent excitation in the model leads to a collapse of persistent activity, which would induce an error pattern of misses and spatially random errors.

To more directly test model predictions for patients with schizophrenia, Starc et al. (2017) designed a working memory task to be explicitly aligned with the model and with the primate electrophysiology task paradigms for which the model was developed. Such an alignment between the clinical study, basic neurophysiology findings, and computational modeling allows stronger inferences and testing of hypotheses. In the working memory task of Starc et al. (2017), the memorandum is a single visuospatial location, and the response is a direct report of the remembered location, which provides a continuous measure of mnemonic coding. To test the model prediction of increased drift during working memory maintenance, the duration of the mnemonic delay is varied. To test the model prediction of increased distractibility dependent on target–distractor similarity, a set of trials included a distractor during the delay with a variable distance from the target. Starc et al. (2017) found that the experimental results largely followed model predictions, whereby patients exhibited increased variance and less working memory precision relative to healthy controls as the delay period increased. Schizophrenia patients also exhibited increased working memory distractibility, with reports biased toward distractors at specific spatial locations. This study illustrates a productive computational psychiatry approach in which predictions from biophysically based neural circuit models of cognition can be translated into experiments in clinical populations.

3.5.2 Decision-Making Models

Broadly, decision-making function is impaired in multiple psychiatric disorders (Lee 2013). To study dysfunction in neural circuit models, we focus on perceptual decision making in task paradigms similar to those studied via electrophysiology in nonhuman primates. As reviewed above, cortical attractor network models have been developed to capture behavior and neuronal activity from association cortex during random-dot motion paradigms (Wang 2002; Furman and Wang 2008). In these two-alternative forced-choice tasks, a random-dot motion stimulus is presented, and the subject must report the net direction of motion (e.g., left vs. right). The coherence of the random-dot pattern can be parametrically varied to control the strength of perceptual evidence and thereby task difficulty. The psychometric function, giving the percent correct as a function of coherence, defines the discrimination threshold as the coherence eliciting a certain level of accuracy.

Random-dot motion paradigms have been applied to clinical populations and have revealed impaired perceptual discrimination in schizophrenia, as measured by a higher discrimination threshold (Chen et al. 2003, 2004; Chen, Bidwell, and Holzman 2005). Similar impairments in the discrimination threshold have also been observed in patients with autism spectrum disorder (Milne et al. 2002; Koldewyn, Whitney, and Rivera 2010). These impairments are typically interpreted as evidence of neural dysfunction in sensory representations (Butler, Silverstein, and Dakin 2008). However, it is possible that such impairments may also result from dysfunction in evidence accumulation downstream from early sensory areas, within association cortical circuits.

To explore this issue, Lam et al. (2017) studied the effects of altered E/I balance in the association cortical-circuit model of decision making developed by Wang (2002). The E/I ratio was perturbed bidirectionally to compare the impact of elevated versus lowered E/I ratio, via NMDA-receptor hypofunction, on inhibitory versus excitatory neurons, respectively. Interestingly, Lam et al. (2017) found that the disruption of E/I balance in either direction can similarly impair decision making as assessed by psychometric performance; that is, the dependence of performance on the E/I ratio is U-shaped, being degraded for both decreased or increased E/I ratio (figure 3.5d). Therefore, the standard psychophysical measurements from clinical populations cannot dissociate among distinct circuit-level alterations: elevated E/I ratio, lowered E/I ratio, or an upstream sensory-coding deficit.

Nonetheless, Lam et al. (2017) found that these regimes make dissociable predictions for the time course of evidence accumulation. The random-dot motion task promotes a strategy of evidence accumulation across the duration of the stimulus presentation. In these settings, it is generally assumed that subjects continuously accumulate information during the stimulus presentation and only commit to a choice at the end of the stimulus stream. Contrary to these assumptions, however, it can be shown that how information is integrated is not uniform in time, and sometimes the decision is actually made long before the stimulus presentation ends. Multiple task paradigms have been developed to characterize the time course of evidence accumulation. For instance, in the "pulse" task paradigm (Huk and Shadlen 2005; Wong et al. 2007), a brief pulse of additional coherence is inserted at a variable onset time during the otherwise constant-coherence stimulus (figure 3.5e). This pulse induces a shift of the psychometric function according to pulse coherence. The dependence of this shift on pulse onset time reflects the weight of that time point on choice.

The pulse paradigm, as well as other paradigms, was able to dissociate distinct decision-making impairments under altered E/I ratio (figure 3.5e). Under elevated E/I ratio, decision is impulsive: perceptual evidence presented early in time is weighted much more than late evidence. In contrast, under lowered E/I ratio, decision making is indecisive: evidence integration and winner-take-all competition between options are weakened. These effects can qualitatively be captured using a modification of the drift-diffusion model, which is a widely used abstract model for decision making from mathematical psychology (described in section 2.2). The standard drift-diffusion model assumes perfect integration with an infinite time constant for memory. Lowered E/I ratio in the circuit model can be captured by "leaky" integration with finite time constant for memory. In contrast, elevated E/I ratio can be captured by "unstable" integration, which has an intrinsic tendency to diverge toward the decision threshold. This study demonstrates the potential to link synaptic-level perturbations in neural circuit models to measurable cognitive behavior, as well as to more abstract models from mathematical psychology.

3.5.3 State Diagram for the Role of Excitatory/Inhibitory Balance in Cognitive Function

As described in the previous section, neural circuit models of cognitive functions can generate dissociable predictions for how distinct synaptic perturbations impact behavior under various task paradigms. Biophysically based models can also suggest what aspects of neural activity or behavior may be differentially sensitive or robust to particular manipulations by pathology, compensation, or treatment. Changes in certain network parameters, or the combinations of parameters, may have much stronger impact on model behavior than changes in other parameter combinations. A "sloppy" axis in parameter space is one along which the model response is relatively insensitive to perturbations in that parameter combination, whereas a "stiff" axis is one in which the model response is highly sensitive to perturbations (Gutenkunst et al. 2007).

Murray et al. (2014) and Lam et al. (2017) characterized function in these neural circuit models under parametric variation in E/I ratio. Specifically, they explored the parameter space of reductions of NMDA-receptor conductances onto both inhibitory interneurons (elevating E/I ratio) and onto excitatory pyramidal neurons (reducing E/I ratio; figure 3.6). For the working memory model, circuit function is determined by the width of the mnemonic persistent activity pattern. For the decision-making model, circuit function can be measured through the discrimination sensitivity (inverse of the discrimination threshold). In both circuit models, E/I ratio was found to be a key parameter for optimal network function. Following relatively small perturbations, circuit function is robust as long as E/I balance is preserved. Preserved E/I ratio therefore corresponds to a "sloppy" axis in this parameter space. In contrast, even subtle changes to E/I ratio (along a "stiff" axis) have a strong impact on model function.

If the imbalance is substantial, either elevated or lowered, the circuit can lose multistability. If disinhibition is too strong (via elevated E/I ratio), then the spontaneous state is no longer stable. Conversely, if recurrent excitation is too weak (via lowered E/I ratio), then the circuit cannot support persistent activity. Collectively, these analyses reveal that E/I balance is vital for optimal cognitive performance in these cortical-circuit models. This suggests that, despite the complexity of synaptic alterations in a disorder such as schizophrenia, the impact on cognitive function in neural circuits may be understandable in terms of their "net effect" on effective parameters, such as E/I ratio, to which the circuit is preferentially sensitive.

3.6 Future Directions

In this chapter, we have primarily reviewed two studies leveraging biophysically based neural circuit models to explore the effects of altered E/I balance on the core cognitive functions of working memory and decision making. These studies revealed that E/I ratio is a critical property for proper cognitive function in cortical circuits. Furthermore, they provide a test bed for computational psychiatry demonstrating that neural circuit models can play a translational role between basic neurophysiology and clinical applications. Here we turn to some areas to be addressed in future modeling studies.

3.6.1 Integrating Cognitive Function with Neurophysiological Biomarkers

As noted above, biophysically based circuit models are well positioned to explore the mechanisms through which synaptic-level perturbations may be associated with neurodynamical biomarkers. In the context of schizophrenia, for example, circuit models have been applied to studying mechanisms of disrupted gamma-band oscillations (Vierling-Claassen et al. 2008; Spencer 2009; Volman et al. 2011; Rotaru et al. 2011),

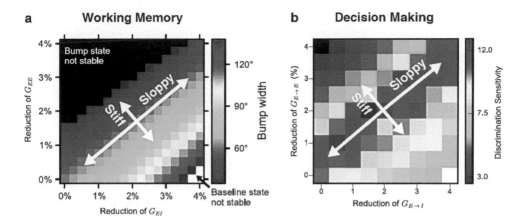

Figure 3.6

Dependence of circuit function on synaptic parameters: a critical role of excitation–inhibition (E/I) balance in both working memory and decision making. The plots illustrate a parameter space of reductions of two recurrent NMDA-receptor conductance strengths from excitatory pyramidal neurons: onto inhibitory interneurons (G_{EI}) or onto excitatory pyramidal neurons (G_{EE}). This analysis characterizes the sensitivity of model function to joint perturbations of these two parameters. (a) For the working memory circuit, we measured the width of the working memory bump-attractor state. Bump width affects mnemonic precision and distractibility during working memory maintenance. (b) For the decision-making circuit, we measured the discrimination sensitivity, which is defined as the inverse of the discrimination threshold (i.e., coherence that yields 81.6% correct). A higher sensitivity corresponds to better performance. For both working memory and decision-making circuits, within this range of perturbation, if G_{EI} and G_{EE} are reduced together in a certain proportion, circuit performance is essentially unaltered because E/I balance is maintained. E/I balance defines a "sloppy" axis in parameter space along which the function is insensitive. In contrast, the function is highly sensitive to small orthogonal perturbations along a "stiff" axis (Gutenkunst et al. 2007). Reduction of G_{EI} in greater proportion elevates E/I ratio and can degrade performance: for working memory, due to broadened mnemonic representations; for decision making, due to highly unstable integration leading to impulsive selection. In contrast, reduction of G_{EE} in greater proportion lowers E/I ratio and can degrade performance: for working memory, due to loss of the bump-attractor state; for decision making, due to indecisive selection. These findings indicate that E/I ratio is a crucial effective parameter for cognitive function in these circuits, with an "inverted-U" dependence of function on E/I ratio. Panels (a) and (b) adapted from Murray et al. (2014) and Lam et al. (2017), respectively, with permission.

which can be related to electroencephalography/magnetoencephalography data from patients (Uhlhaas and Singer 2010). At very different spatiotemporal scales, circuit models of large-scale disconnectivity can be related to resting-state BOLD data (Yang et al. 2014, 2015). At the moment, such biomarker-related models do not directly relate to cognitive function or behavior. Future modeling work is needed in the integration of cognitive function with neurophysiological biomarkers across multiple scales of analysis.

3.6.2 Incorporating Further Neurobiological Detail

To address increasingly complex and detailed questions about neural circuit dysfunction, future models will need to incorporate further elements of known neurobiology, which can be constrained and tested with experiments. One notable limitation in the current models is that they usually contain a single type of inhibitory interneuron, and therefore they are not able to speak to important questions regarding preferential disruptions in specific interneuron cell types. There are key differences between parvalbumin-expressing and somatostatin-expressing interneurons, which have differences in their synaptic connectivity and functional responses (Gonzalez-Burgos and Lewis 2008). Microcircuit models that propose a division of labor among interneuron classes (Wang et al. 2004; Yang et al. 2016 have the potential to make dissociable predictions for dysfunction in distinct cell types. Another avenue for model extension is to take into account the laminar structure observed in cortex (Mejias et al. 2016), which may relate to mechanistic hypotheses of impaired predictive coding (Bastos et al. 2012). Beyond the level of local microcircuitry, further work is needed on distributed cognitive computations across brain areas (Chaudhuri et al. 2015; Murray et al. 2017), and their integration in models of alterations in large-scale network dynamics in psychiatric disorders (Yang et al. 2014, 2015).

3.6.3 Informing Task Designs

These modeling studies offer important considerations for the design of cognitive tasks applied to computational psychiatry. In each model, multiple distinct cortical disruptions (e.g., elevated vs. lowered E/I ratio vs. upstream sensory-coding deficit) can impair performance. Standard performance analyses in common task paradigms (e.g., error rates in working memory, or psychometric threshold in decision making) may be insufficient to resolve dissociable predictions. Fine-grained analyses of task behavior should distinguish different types of errors or deficits, rather than simply measuring overall impaired performance, which could be due to deficits in distinct cognitive subprocesses (e.g., encoding vs. maintenance for working memory) or opposing deficits in a single subprocess (e.g., leaky vs. unstable integration in decision making). Circuit modeling can provide insight into the variety of potential "failure modes" in a cognitive function, and into which task designs can reveal them. In turn, alignment of a task design with a circuit model allows for generation of mechanistic neurophysiological hypotheses from behavioral measurements.

3.6.4 Studying Compensations and Treatments

Finally, of utmost relevance to psychiatry, biophysically based circuit modeling has the potential to provide a method for simulating possible effects of treatments that act at the level of ion channels and receptors. As a proof of principle example of this, Murray et al. (2014) examined in the working memory circuit model how E/I balance can be restored through compensations acting on multiple parameters; for instance, elevated E/I ratio due to disinhibition can be compensated for by a treatment that strengthens inhibition or by one that attenuates excitation. In turn, restoration of E/I balance ameliorated the associated deficits in working memory behavior. However, further development and refinement of biophysically based models is needed to go beyond proof of principle. Future development in this area will benefit from the other directions noted above. Incorporation of more detailed micro-circuitry and receptors will be needed to better capture pharmacological effects. Integration of biomarkers and behavior in the models will allow refinement through more direct testing with empirical data from pharmacological manipulations in animal models and humans.

3.6.5 Distributed Cognitive Process in a Large-Scale Brain System

In this chapter, we focused on local circuit modeling, but cognitive processes involve multiple cortical and subcortical regions. Researchers have begun to consider abnormalities of the global brain connectivity and dynamics in mental illness (Rubinov and Bullmore 2013; Yang et al. 2015), but this area of research is still in its infancy. In particular, persistent activity during working memory has been observed in a number of brain areas (Christophel et al. 2017). What are the general principles for such distributed persistent activity patterns? What determines whether a given brain area does or does not display persistent activity? For an area engaged in persistent activity, what does it store in working memory, and what role does it play in contributing to, or controlling (i.e., as a network hub), the global persistent activity pattern? Time is ripe to seriously tackle these questions. Human brain connectomics and functional imaging are rapidly developing. At the same time, in animal research it is becoming possible to physiologically record from neurons in multiple brain areas during a working memory task, and biologically based large-scale modeling now can be built on quantitative mesoscopic connectivity data (Chaudhuri et al. 2015; Mejias et al. 2016; Wang and Kennedy 2016).

Advances in all these directions hold exciting promise of rationally guiding treatment development in psychiatry, grounded in basic neuroscience.

3.7 Chapter Summary

Research based on biophysically based neural circuit modeling has led to insights into neural circuits involved in cognitive processes in areas such as the prefrontal cortex. Working memory is thought to be dependent on persistent neural activity during the delay period in areas such as the prefrontal cortex. Such persistent activity is usually modeled using attractor models. Decision making is thought to correspond to ramping neural activity during the decision period, corresponding to an "accumulation of evidence." In simulations, excitatory reverberation and maintenance of sustained activity during working memory and accumulation of evidence during decision making was found to require slow synapses, and particularly NMDA receptors. This theoretical prediction was verified experimentally and is meaningful for research in psychiatry: NMDA impairments have indeed been observed in schizophrenia and other psychiatric illness. Computational models can explain how changes in the balance of synaptic excitation and inhibition (through NMDA impairments) give rise to specific impairments in working memory and decision making. Such local circuit models could provide basic building blocks in the development of more sophisticated models and large-scale brain circuit models in the emerging field of computational psychiatry.

3.8 Further Study

Shall (2004) discusses linking propositions and correspondence between mental states and brain states. An approach to relating attractor models and schizophrenia, which is related to the one described here, can be found in the work of Rolls and Deco (2011).

Durstewitz, Huys, and Koppe (2018) provides a more general dynamical systems perspective on psychiatric symptoms and disease and discusses its potential implications for diagnosis, prognosis, and treatment.

On the physiological side, a recent review of the neural mechanisms that may underlie memory-associated persistent activity can be found in Zylberberg and Strowbridge (2019).

O'Connell et al. (2018) offers a recent description of neural and computational viewpoints on perceptual decision making.

3.9 Acknowledgments

XJW was partly supported by the NIH grant R01 MH062349, STCSM grant 15JC1400104. A version of this chapter appeared in *Computational Psychiatry: Mathematical Modeling of Mental Illness*, 2017, edited by A. Anticevic and J. Murray, Elsevier Press.

4 Computational Models of Cognitive Control: Past and Current Approaches

Debbie M. Yee and Todd S. Braver
Washington University in St. Louis

4.1. Introduction

A core challenge of cognitive, computational, and systems neuroscience research is to provide a satisfying answer to the following question: how does cognition arise from neural systems? Although researchers have spent decades using a variety of tools (e.g., magnetic resonance imaging, electroencephalography, single-unit recordings) to investigate this question, we have only begun to scratch its surface in terms of understanding how neural substrates work together in synchrony to give rise to complex cognitive processes.

To provide an analogy, imagine listening to a concerto performed by a symphony orchestra. Perhaps you are interested in understanding how the orchestra can blend together so many different sounds from vastly different instruments to give rise to this beautiful masterpiece. In the initial hearing, the piece sounds clearly melodic, lyrical, and filled with multiple complex musical layers that sound cohesive when in concert. However, upon closer examination, it becomes evident that even such complex musical layers can be deconstructed into the contributions from different instruments within the entire ensemble. One approach for understanding the concerto may be simply to listen to one instrument or one section (e.g., attending to a violin solo or the entire violin section when playing the same melody); however, that would only provide a small window into how that specific instrument contributes to the entire piece. Another approach would be to parse out all of the sounds in the piece by instrument, which provides a structural division of the different sounds that comprise the concerto, but neglects the temporal ordering of when the instruments are played, an important aspect of the composition. Perhaps the most insidious problem is that even if we are able to understand the structural and temporal aspects of how each instrument contributes to this specific concerto, the same instruments in this symphony orchestra can also perform a wide variety of other compositions (e.g., other concertos, sonatas, ballads) at other periods in time! Thus, the characterization of the violin's contribution to the current concerto may not be applicable when considering other musical performances, which makes this type of analysis effort not quite as generalizable as one might have hoped.

4.1.1 The Homunculus Problem of Cognitive Control

The challenge of this problem and the "orchestra concerto" metaphor becomes particularly salient when considering one of the most compelling mysteries of human cognition: how the brain enables human beings to plan, implement, and accomplish the types of controlled, complex, and temporally extended goal-directed behaviors that make up much of modern daily life (e.g., preparing a multi-course meal, constructing IKEA furniture from an instruction manual, writing a computer program, solving a Sudoku puzzle, or figuring out how to successfully complete an MD or PhD). In the orchestra metaphor, it would be akin to understanding how the conductor guides the ensemble to put together a beautiful-sounding and cohesive concerto performance. This mystery has often been posed as the "homunculus problem," which presents the following conundrum: if control over thoughts and action emerges from brain function, then are there special neurobiological and computational properties that differentiate the components that should be labeled as "controller" from the components that are "controlled"? Does the controller/controlled distinction even make sense? And if not, how are we ever going to understand the emergence of intelligent, goal-directed behavior in neurobiological terms?

Within psychology and neuroscience, researchers have often taken a primarily localizationist approach, studying individual brain regions in terms of their associated cognitive functions (Poldrack 2007). At the other extreme is the integrationist perspective, which focuses on the entire brain, parsing it into networks that may be structurally or functionally related (Eliasmith et al. 2012). However, neither of these approaches has yet provided a fully satisfying answer to the fundamental problem of cognitive control. Indeed, as this discussion hopefully makes clear, properly addressing the seemingly intractable homunculus problem likely requires a computational modeling approach. Computational approaches can be utilized in both a reductionist and emergentist manner: deconstructing the mysterious intelligence of the homunculus into hopefully more understandable "dumb" neural subcomponents, while at the same time making clear how complex control functions can emerge from the dynamic interactions among these multiple, simpler subcomponents of cognitive control.

Computational modeling approaches to cognitive control are uniquely powerful, relative to other neuroscience techniques, in that they provide the researcher with a means of generating specific and concrete hypotheses, along with explicit experimental predictions regarding generative and causally efficacious control mechanisms and their influence on brain activity and behavior (Botvinick and Cohen 2014; O'Reilly 2006; O'Reilly, Herd, and Pauli 2010). More broadly, within the cognitive sciences, the utility of modeling approaches has long been established and appreciated (Newell and Simon 1961). Over thirty years ago, and as described in chapter 1 and figure 1.4, David Marr attempted to formalize these approaches by articulating an influential proposal for decomposing and investigating complex cognitive systems across three levels of analysis: the *computational*, the *algorithmic*, and the *implementational* (Marr 1982; Bechtel 1994). These levels of analyses were initially introduced to tackle computational questions in vision, and have been criticized by various researchers as potentially being too rigid to be universally applicable (Dayan 2006). Yet the Marr framework can be fruitfully applied when considering complementary questions about the neural and computational mechanisms that underlie more complex temporally extended goal-directed behavior, such as: What computational goal is accomplished by a putative control function? What is the algorithm that encodes this function? Can we identify the neural systems and mechanisms that implement the algorithm? Consequently, we will make use of the Marr framework in this chapter, in order to provide a general intuition for how various computational models attempt to address specific questions about cognitive control function.

4.1.2 Why Cognitive Control?

The current chapter highlights past and current computational models of cognitive control, and the purpose is twofold. First, cognitive control is a well-known psychological construct, with a long history of researchers using computational modeling approaches to attempt to explain its underlying cognitive mechanisms (Newell and Simon 1972; Rumelhart et al. 1986; Cohen, Dunbar, and McClelland 1990; Braver and Cohen 2000; Anderson et al. 2008). Second, cognitive control ability is disrupted across a wide range of mental disorders, with a vast body of literature now supporting the hypothesis that cognitive control impairments are prominent in many such disorders, including schizophrenia, depression, obsessive-compulsive disorder, ADHD, addiction, Alzheimer's disease, and Parkinson's disease (Lesh et al. 2011; Fales et al. 2008; Halari et al. 2009; Greisberg and McKay 2003; van Meel et al. 2007; Vaidya et al. 2005; Belleville, Chertkow, and Gauthier 2007; Brown and Marsden 1990; Wylie et al. 2010; Snyder, Miyake, and Hankin 2015). Indeed, it may not be an exaggeration to argue that an impairment of cognitive control, in one form or another, is the defining feature of many forms of mental illness. Thus, understanding the mechanisms that underlie cognitive control function can provide a crucial window into psychopathology.

Cognitive control is operationalized as the ability to perform task-relevant processing in the face of distractions or in the absence of environmental support, specifically by active maintenance and flexible updating of task representations over time, in order to pursue task-relevant objectives and behavioral goals (Engle and Kane 2004; Braver 2012; O'Reilly, Braver, and Cohen 1999). A core tenet of cognitive control is the distinction between controlled and automatic processing (Posner and Snyder 1975; Shiffrin and Schneider 1977; Norman and Shallice 1986). It is now generally appreciated that a fundamental tradeoff exists between recruiting and directing cognitive resources to deliberately perform a demanding task versus carrying out less effortful and habitual responses that may require fewer attentional resources, but that also may be less flexible. Typically, the allocation of control depends on the amount of cognitive effort or mental demand required. In other words, the control of behavior arises from the cognitive demands imposed by the requirement to successfully perform a task, and effort allocation arises from the dynamic recruitment of available cognitive processes that can appropriately meet these demands during task performance (Botvinick and Cohen 2014). Some have proposed various computational models and frameworks to understand this tradeoff between effort and automaticity in controlled behavior (Cohen, Dunbar, and McClelland 1990; Schneider and Chein 2003), whereas others have hypothesized that humans perform cost-benefit analyses between expected payoff and cognitive effort to determine the optimal allocation of cognitive control (Shenhav et al. 2017; Dixon and Christoff 2012; Kool and Botvinick 2014; Westbrook and Braver 2015). All in all, there still remain many unanswered questions regarding the computational and neural mechanisms that underlie cognitive control; we argue these can be more adequately addressed with computational modeling approaches.

As a brief aside, we wish to acknowledge that such computational modeling approaches have been prevalent and successful in advancing understanding for other related, but potentially more specialized higher cognitive processes, such as attention (Gershman, Cohen, and Niv 2010), learning (Tenenbaum, Griffiths, and Kemp 2006), semantic knowledge (Rogers and McClelland 2004), and memory (Polyn, Norman, and Kahana 2009). Thus, while this chapter will focus primarily on cognitive control, we hope that the reader may extrapolate these principles to obtain a broader perspective for how computational models can be used to study other cognitive systems.

4.1.3 Roadmap to This Chapter

This chapter contains two main sections. First, we will provide a brief review of several key computational models that have been influential in advancing understanding of cognitive control mechanisms. This review of such models is not meant to be comprehensive but will hopefully provide a useful primer for readers to become familiar with classical and current computational models of cognitive control, with the understanding that the principles behind these models can be extended to other related models. Next, we discuss key features of computational models that make them particularly useful and generative in guiding further research efforts (i.e., what "tests" can we run to determine whether a computational model can make accurate and generalized predictions about controlled behavior?). The chapter concludes with a concrete example of how such modeling frameworks can be used to make predictions in mental illness, with some speculation about how cognitive control function breaks down in schizophrenia, a psychiatric disorder hypothesized to be strongly associated with cognitive control impairment.

4.2 Past and Current Models of Cognitive Control

A broad range of computational models have played a prominent role in the development and understanding of cognitive control theory and its underlying mechanisms, including those that have primarily arisen from symbolic modeling traditions, such as those involving production system architectures (ACT-R, Anderson 1996; EPIC, Kieras and Meyer 1997). At the other end of the spectrum are models arising from the computational neuroscience tradition (Wang 2013), similar to those covered in chapter 3. Here, we focus on four contemporary models that address challenging and unique computational problems integral to cognitive control function, and which have also played an influential role in advancing research within this domain:

1. How do we determine when to actively maintain versus rapidly update contextual information in working memory?
2. How is the demand for cognitive control evaluated, and what is the computational role of the anterior cingulate cortex?
3. How do contextual representations guide action selection during hierarchically organized task goals, and what is the computational role of the prefrontal cortex (PFC)?
4. How are task sets learned and organized during behavioral performance, and when do they generalize to novel contexts?

4.2.1 How Do We Determine When to Actively Maintain versus Rapidly Update Contextual Information in Working Memory?

A key cognitive control challenge is in determining what information is relevant to be maintained (i.e., in working memory) during the pursuit of task goals, and when this information should be updated with newer task-relevant information. A potentially useful analogy for visualizing this issue is the concept of a "mental blackboard," which describes the dilemma of deciding between when learned information in working memory should be kept, or instead erased and overwritten (Baddeley 1986). Early computational models attempted to use attractor models to understand the mechanisms that underlie robust active maintenance of working memory against irrelevant distractors (Changeux and Dehaene 1989; Zipser et al. 1993; Cohen, Braver, and O'Reilly 1996; Compte et al. 2000; Durstewitz, Seamans, and Sejnowski 2000; Deco and Rolls 2003). However, a major limitation of these models is their lack of a mechanism for precisely updating working memory when newer, task-relevant information is introduced. This tension between these two working memory functions is difficult to reconcile, as they inherently contradict each other—active maintenance increases resistance to distractors, whereas flexible updating makes the system more vulnerable to distraction. Thus, the computational challenge lies in building a model that can explain how a system regulates the fundamental trade-off between learning when to actively maintain context representations (i.e., task-relevant information that is internally represented) to achieve controlled processing versus rapidly updating new information into working memory, a core problem of cognitive control (O'Reilly, Braver, and Cohen 1999; Braver and Cohen 2000).

One approach toward understanding the computational mechanisms that underlie this trade-off comes from the "parallel-distributed-processing" approach (also dubbed "connectionist" or "neural network" models in the literature; see section 2.1). These models view control as arising from the interaction of multiple relatively simple elements (e.g., neurons or neural assemblies that perform local processes within a single brain system or unit). Thus, the models emphasize how cognitive control functions emerge from a network of brain regions activated interactively and in parallel, rather than the more historical modular approach of localizing cognitive function to a single brain region (Hinton 1984; O'Reilly 2006).

A well-established model from within the connectionist tradition is the PFC and basal ganglia (PBWM) model developed by Frank, O'Reilly, and their colleagues (Frank, Loughry, and O'Reilly 2001; O'Reilly and Frank 2006; Hazy, Frank, and O'Reilly 2007). In the PBWM model, the PFC and basal ganglia (BG) interact to solve the maintenance versus updating problem by implementing a flexible working memory system with an adaptive gating mechanism. This represents an elegant algorithmic solution for resolving this computational question, as it provides two separate modes of working memory that optimize active maintenance and flexible updating, respectively (figure 4.1a). Specifically, working memory is insulated from distractor signals (i.e., irrelevant sensory input) when the gating mechanism is closed, but is receptive to utilizing information from such sensory signals when gating mechanisms are open. However, the introduction of this gating mechanism then begs the following question: how does the brain know when to open or close the gate? In other words, who or what controls the gate?

At the biological (i.e., implementational) level, the PBWM model proposes that the PFC facilitates the active maintenance mechanisms for sustaining task-relevant information, whereas the BG provides the selective gating mechanism, which independently switches between updating versus maintenance of information in PFC. Specifically, the key component of PBWM is that the BG performs this selective dynamic gating via disinhibition and, moreover, that this dynamic gating functionality depends upon the dopaminergic system (DA, see figure 4.1b). In this framework, dopaminergic "Go" neurons in dorsal striatum fire to disinhibit PFC to enable updating of working memory representations in PFC, while "NoGo" neurons counteract this effect to support robust maintenance of PFC working memory representations and resistance to distractions.

Notably, other computational models have proposed similar gating mechanisms that regulate flexible updating and maintenance of task-relevant representations during working memory, but driven primarily by direct dopamine (DA) projections to PFC (Braver and Cohen 1999, 2000). However, a criticism of the global DA-firing hypothesis is that this mechanism would not fully explain more complex cognitive tasks in which individuals would need to maintain and update different task representations simultaneously, such as when there is a hierarchical structure to working memory (e.g., remembering to press a button for a specific stimulus only during context A, but not context B).

Taken together, the PBWM leverages the gating mechanism as an algorithmic solution to the computational problem of switching between active maintenance and flexible updating within working memory mechanisms. This model suggests that the PFC implements active maintenance of task-relevant information, whereas the BG contains selective gating mechanisms which switch between "robust maintenance" and "selective updating" of information held in PFC during working memory. Midbrain DA release is hypothesized to modulate this gating mechanism. However, exactly how, when, and where DA firing drives these working memory functions (e.g., only in the BG or also directly in PFC), is a question that remains to be fully explored.

4.2.2 How Is the Demand for Cognitive Control Evaluated, and What Is the Computational Role of the Anterior Cingulate Cortex?

Another core computational challenge within the domain of cognitive control is the following: how is the current demand for control evaluated, and in what form is this

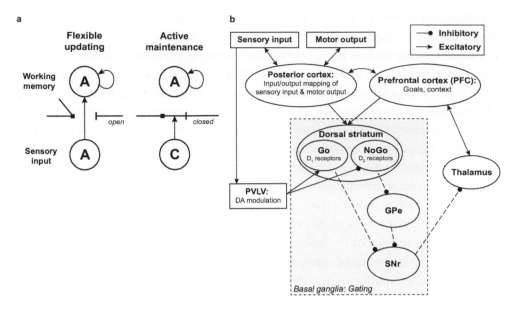

Figure 4.1
A) Gating mechanism from Frank and O'Reilly's prefrontal basal ganglia and working memory (PBWM) model (Frank, Loughry, and O'Reilly 2001). At the algorithmic level, this connectionist computational model features a gating function, which switches between active maintenance and flexible updating of working memory to incorporate task-relevant information, two core functions of cognitive control. B) Neural network model implementation of the PBWM. Here, sensory inputs are mapped onto motor outputs via posterior ("hidden") layers. The PFC contextualizes this information and encodes relevant prior information and goals. The basal ganglia (BG) updates the PFC via dynamic gating, which is driven by dopaminergic modulation from a separate "PVLV" (primary value and learned value learning algorithm) system (O'Reilly et al. 2007). Specifically, dopamine (DA) is excitatory onto the Go neurons via D_1 receptors and inhibitory onto NoGo neurons via D_2 receptors. Thus, increased DA firing will inhibit SNr (substantia nigra pars reticulata) and disinhibit PFC to facilitate flexible updating of working memory representations in PFC. Decreased DA firing, on the other hand, counteracts this effect and facilitates active maintenance of current working memory representations in PFC.

evaluative signal transmitted? In other words, how does the brain determine which situations or task conditions require more mental resources (than are currently available) to successfully pursue task goals, and what is the necessary relevant information that underlies this evaluation? This type of question is difficult to address from a purely theoretical perspective, as "cognitive demand" is an elusive construct that appears to arise under a wide variety of mentally challenging tasks. Thus, a prerequisite for building a computational solution is understanding which experimental conditions demand and elicit greater cognitive control, along with identifying relevant behavioral measures as empirical evidence for increased cognitive effort (note that in the literature, the terms cognitive effort and mental effort are used interchangeably).

A plethora of work has identified tasks with behavioral measures that demonstrate selective recruitment of cognitive control (Botvinick, Cohen, and Carter 2004; Ridderinkhof et al. 2004; Braver and Ruge 2006). For example, in the Stroop task, cognitive control is required to override the prepotent response to read a word, in order to perform the correct task of reading the color ink of the word. In the N-back, cognitive control is required to respond selectively to N-back matches (e.g., in a two-back task, a target response should be given only if the current stimulus matches the one presented two stimuli ago) rather than based on simple familiarity. In the stop-signal (or change-signal) task, cognitive control is required to cancel an already initiated behavioral response if a stop signal (or change cue) is presented. In the Erikson flanker task, cognitive control is required to respond selectively to a centrally presented stimulus and ignore the flanker stimuli, particularly when these are distracting and incongruent with the central stimulus. Critically, all of these tasks contain experimental conditions that reliably increase cognitive control demands in a transient, trial-by-trial manner (i.e., the cognitive system monitors ongoing responses and adjusts to the level of cognitive control needed on the current trial). Likewise, they are indexed by specific behavioral measures that reflect this enhanced cognitive control demand (e.g., Stroop interference effect, stop-signal reaction time).

A well-established finding is that canonical control tasks, such as the ones listed above, consistently co-activate the dorsolateral PFC (dlPFC) and the dorsomedial PFC (Egner 2009; Duverne and Koechlin 2017), a brain region that spans the dorsal anterior cingulate cortex (ACC) and presupplementary motor area (Duncan and Owen 2000; Duncan 2010). The dlPFC is thought to play a primary role in actively maintaining representations of task goals and the associated actions (or behavioral rules) needed to achieve them. In contrast, the ACC is thought to be involved in signaling when more control should be implemented by the dlPFC to accomplish these goals. It is generally accepted that the interaction between these two brain regions is important for dynamically adjusting cognitive control. Many have argued for the ACC as an important locus of cognitive control (Holroyd et al. 2004; Kerns 2004), although there remains much controversy over what actual information is represented by the ACC and signaled to the dlPFC to indicate that cognitive control is needed during tasks.

Several prominent theoretical accounts of ACC's computational role in cognitive control have arisen in recent years, including the detection of error signals (Gehring et al. 1993; Holroyd et al. 2005), reinforcement learning (Holroyd and Coles 2002), conflict monitoring (Botvinick et al. 2001; Botvinick, Cohen, and Carter 2004), error likelihood (Carter et al. 1998; Brown and Braver 2005), cost-benefit analyses of implementing control (Shenhav, Botvinick, and Cohen 2013), and even uncertainty in the environment (Behrens et al. 2007). An account developed to reconcile and unify these divergent perspectives is the predicted response-outcome (PRO) model (figure 4.2; Alexander and Brown 2011, 2014). The PRO model contains two components. One component of the model learns to predict multiple likely outcomes of various chosen actions, regardless of whether these outcomes are good or bad (i.e., response-outcome learning). A second component of the model detects discrepancies between actual and predicted outcomes and uses this prediction-error signal (i.e., actual outcomes minus expected outcomes) to update and refine subsequent predictions. Moreover, a key aspect of the prediction-error signal is that it also indicates "negative surprise," when an expected outcome does not occur. This form of negative surprise signal can indicate not only when an unexpected error occurs, but also when the response is slower than expected or when the correct action is more ambiguous (which is likely to happen on trials associated with high response conflict).

At the implementational level, the PRO model postulates that separate neural signals within ACC represent outcome prediction and prediction error (negative surprise), respectively. Specifically, the model suggests that the prediction signal should reliably increase immediately prior to when the most likely outcome will occur (i.e., a pre-response anticipatory signal). The negative surprise signal, on the other hand, will reliably activate after the action that produces an unpredicted outcome has occurred (i.e., a post-response evaluative signal). Critically, these hypotheses have been tested empirically across multiple tasks (e.g., change-signal task, Erikson flanker), as well as across different types of neural data (e.g., fMRI activity, event-related potentials, monkey single-unit neurophysiology). This validation of the PRO model across such a wide range of neural data demonstrates that it provides a useful generalizable computational algorithm by which the ACC can signal an increased need for cognitive control. Recent

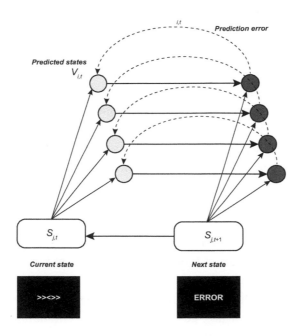

Figure 4.2
Schematic of the predicted response-outcome (PRO) model by Alexander and Brown (2011, 2014). First, the PRO model learns predictions of multiple possible future outcomes of various chosen actions (indicated by $V_{i,t}$), using an error-likelihood signal. Thus, activity in the PRO model reflects a temporally discounted prediction of such outcomes, which are proportionate to their likelihood of occurrence. Second, the PRO detects discrepancies between predicted and observed outcomes, and then uses their prediction-error signal (δ) to update and improve subsequent predictions. S refers to the representation of the stimulus (e.g., conflicting arrows from the Erikson flanker task) or task-related feedback (e.g., a screen indicating an error was made). Thus, the PRO model continually learns and updates associations between task-related cues and feedback in cognitive tasks.

efforts have attempted to expand this account to include hierarchical representation within ACC and dlPFC (Alexander and Brown 2015), a topic relevant to the next section. Other recent efforts have attempted to link ACC signals with more affective/motivational quantities (Vassena, Holroyd, and Alexander 2017). These include the expected value of control (EVC; Shenhav, Botvinick, and Cohen 2013) and related accounts (Holroyd and McClure 2015; Westbrook and Braver 2016), which postulate that ACC regulates the allocation and persistence of cognitive effort based on signals indicating the current subjective motivational (and/or hedonic) value of task and goal outcomes.

4.2.3. How Do Contextual Representations Guide Action Selection toward Hierarchically Organized Task Goals, and What Is the Computational Role of the Prefrontal Cortex?

A third computational question of control relates to the issue of abstraction. How can a "high-level" goal constrain and implement a "lower-level" goal? As an example, imagine the following scenario: you hear a nearby phone ring, and you have an instinctive impulse to answer it. However, context plays an important role in your action plan, so while you might automatically answer a nearby phone in your own home, you would inhibit this tendency to answer a ringing phone at your friend's home. Yet you might switch your action plan if your preoccupied friend asks you to answer the ringing phone on their behalf (e.g., when they are busy with a task). This example articulates a fundamental computational challenge of implementing task goals—specifically, how do humans utilize contextual representations and higher-level goals to guide action selection during pursuit of lower-level goals, and how does the brain implement this type of hierarchical control?

One promising algorithmic solution for this perplexing question is the concept of hierarchical organization of task–goal representations. The notion of applying hierarchical structure to parse complex systems into subordinate and interrelated subsystems has long been established, with subsystems being further subdivided into "elementary" units (Simon 1962). Similarly, some theorists have argued that control signals used to guide behavioral actions, based on internal plans and goals, can also be subdivided into sensorimotor, contextual, and episodic levels of control (Koechlin, Ody, and Kouneiher 2003; Koechlin and Summerfield 2007; figure 4.3). Critically, this information-theoretic model (i.e., based on principles from information theory; Shannon 1948), which has also been termed the "cascade model," postulates that the hierarchical division occurs according to a temporal dimension; that is, when in time control is implemented. Specifically, according to the model, actions selected based on temporally proximal stimuli would be lower on the hierarchy, whereas actions selected based on past information that is actively maintained in conjunction with the recent stimulus would be higher on the hierarchy. According to this framework, greater demand for cognitive control can also be formalized as the amount of information required to be actively maintained over longer time periods to enable successful behavioral action selection. As a brief aside, it is worth noting that earlier models also utilized hierarchical frameworks to understand temporal abstraction in behavior (Cooper and Shallice 2006), but the primary thrust of the cascade model and related variants has been to use reinforcement learning to subdivide temporally abstract complex action plans (i.e., "options") into simpler behaviors, an adaptive and efficient

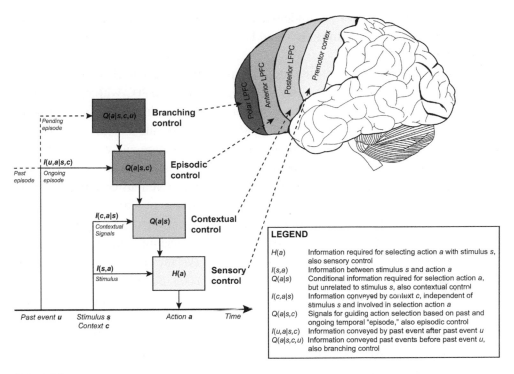

Figure 4.3

Model of hierarchical cognitive control by Koechlin and colleagues (2003, 2007). This information-theoretic model posits that cognitive control operates according to three nested levels of control processes (branching, episodic, contextual), which are implemented as a cascade from anterior to posterior prefrontal regions. $H(a)$ represents sensory control, the information required to select an action (a) to appropriate incoming stimuli, and is the sum of two control terms: bottom-up information conveyed by the stimulus (s) regarding the appropriate action [$I(s, a)$] and top-down information processed in the posterior lateral PFC [$Q(a|s)$]. The Q(a|s) term represents contextual control, the incoming signals congruent with the subject's response, and is the sum of two control terms: bottom-up information from the contextual (c) signals and stimulus [$I(c, a|s)$, $I(s, a)$], and top-down information processed in anterior lateral PFC [$Q(a|s,c)$]. The $Q(a|s,c)$ term represents episodic control, neural signals that guide actions based on information retrieved from past events stored in episodic memory (i.e., tonically maintained over a longer temporal interval), which is the sum of bottom-up information from past event u [$I(u,a|s,c)$] and top-down information processed in the polar lateral PFC [$Q(a|s,c,u)$]. The branching control term [$Q(a|s,c,u)$] relates to information conveyed by events prior to event u, and are maintained until the current episode or trial is complete. Thus, this computational model parses different levels of control based on how much information must be internally represented and actively maintained in order to select and perform a correct action.

encoding strategy relevant for understanding structured abstract action representations (Botvinick 2008; Botvinick, Niv, and Barto 2009; Solway et al. 2014; Holroyd and Yeung 2011).

At the neural level, the cascade model implements hierarchical cognitive control along the anterior-posterior (i.e., rostral–caudal) axis of lateral PFC, with control signals higher up in the hierarchy represented in more anterior prefrontal regions (Koechlin, Ody, and Kouneiher 2003; Badre 2008; Badre and D'Esposito 2009). Although it is well accepted that PFC subserves high-level cognitive function and cognitive control, researchers have only recently attempted to build a parcellation scheme of this large brain region according to a functional organizing principle (Fuster 2001). Evidence from human neuroimaging studies supports the hypothesis of hierarchical representation, with more anterior regions of lateral PFC being activated when cognitive control is implemented for past information, and posterior regions being activated during action selection from more immediate information (Velanova et al. 2003; Braver and Bongiolatti 2002; Braver, Reynolds, and Donaldson 2003; Badre and D'Esposito 2007; Nee and Brown 2013). Additionally, single-unit studies in nonhuman primates are supportive of the idea that PFC is functionally organized according to the rostral–caudal axis: whereas caudal regions are involved in direct sensorimotor mappings, more rostral regions are involved in higher-order control processes that regulate action selection among multiple competing responses and stimuli (Petrides 2005; Shima et al. 2007). Thus, the hierarchical organization of PFC appears to be central to performing the neural computations underlying task–goal abstraction and action selection. Active research efforts focus on understanding how these divisions in the hierarchy are initially learned (Reynolds and O'Reilly 2009; Frank and Badre 2012), and whether the hierarchical structure is primarily anatomic or dynamic (Reynolds et al. 2012; Nee and D'Esposito 2016).

4.2.4 How Are Task Sets Learned during Behavioral Performance, and When Are They Applied to Novel Contexts?

The fourth and final computational question in this chapter relates to the interaction of cognitive control and learning. In daily life, humans are faced with the challenge of learning a set of actions, sometimes simple or complex, in order to complete a specific task (i.e., a task set). A related challenge is discerning between knowing when task-set rules that are learned in one context can be applied to a novel context (i.e., they generalize), or instead when a new task set needs to be constructed. For example, when searching for the restroom at a shopping mall, one may learn a rule to look for signs that contain the text "Bathroom" with arrows pointing to a particular location. However, while this task-set rule may be pertinent when navigating malls in the United States, the same strategy may not be effective when searching for a restroom in other countries (e.g., United Kingdom), since the signs may read "W.C." instead of "Bathroom." Broadly speaking, creating a set of behavioral tools not tied to the context in which they were learned is useful, as this strategy enables flexible and efficient learning of task-set rules that can be generalized to novel contexts. However, the neural computations that underlie how cognitive control is deployed to learn task sets are less well understood. Thus, the main motivating computational question is the following: in a new context requiring representation of tasks and task-set rules, is it more effective and efficient to generalize from an existing task-set representation (presumably stably encoded in long-term memory), or to instead build a new representation that is more optimized for the current context?

In the last decade, many accounts of cognitive control looked to algorithms and approaches from the reinforcement learning literature for inspiration in how task-set and goal representations might be acquired (Botvinick, Niv, and Barto 2009; Dayan 2012c). A recent model that directly targeted this learning question is the context-task-set (C-TS) model, which aims to approximate how humans create, build, and cluster task-set structures (Collins and Frank 2013; figure 4.4). The model's algorithm harnesses the power of both reinforcement learning and Bayesian generative processes that can infer the presence of latent states. Specifically, the model is designed to accomplish three goals: 1) create representations of task sets and their parameters; 2) infer at each trial or time point which task set is relevant in order to guide action selection; and 3) discover hidden task-set rules not already in its repertoire. A key element that drives the learning process is context—here defined as a higher-order factor associated with a lower-level stimulus—which influences which action/motor plan would be selected. When the model is exposed to a novel context, the likelihood of selecting an existing task set is based on the popularity of that task set; that is, its relevance across multiple other contexts. Conversely, the probability of creating a new task set is set to be inversely proportional to a parameter indicating conservativeness; that is, the prior probability that the stimulus-action relationship would be governed by an existing rule rather than a new one. Further, if a new task set is created, the model must learn predicted reward outcomes following action selection in response to the current stimulus, as well as determine if the task set is valid for the given context. If a selected action leads to a rewarding outcome, the model then updates the parameters to strengthen the association between a context and a specific task set. Thus, the C-TS model provides

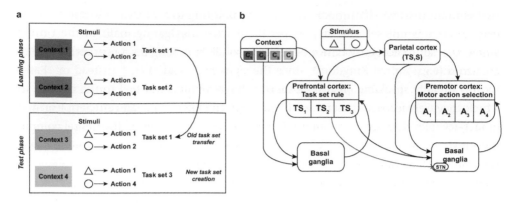

Figure 4.4

(a) Context-task-set (C-TS) model by Collins and Frank (2013). This model solves the problem of how to learn hidden task-set rules (i.e., when in a given state and presented with sensory input, which action should be taken in order to maximize reward). The C-TS model posits that states are determined hierarchically; that is, an agent will consider some input dimension to act as a higher-order context (C), which indicates a task set (TS) and other dimensions to act as lower-level stimuli (S), in determining which motor actions (A) to produce. Here, the color context determines a latent task set that facilitates learning of shape stimulus–action associations in the learning phase (e.g., C_1 is associated with TS_1). In the test phase, C_3 maps onto the same shape stimulus-action association as C_1, so the C_3 context is transferred to TS_1, whereas C_4 should be assigned to a new task set. Critically, the model predicts that it should be faster to transfer a task set than learn a new task set. (b) Schematic of two-loop corticostriatal-gating neural network model. These two loops are nested hierarchically, such that one loop learns to gate an abstract task set (and will group together the contexts that are associated with the same task sets), whereas the other loop learns to gate a motor action response conditioned on the task set and perceptual stimulus. Here, color context (c) serves as the input for learning to select the correct task set in the PFC loop. This information is multiplexed with the shape stimulus in parietal cortex to modulate the motor loop and select the correct motor actions. These two loops accomplish two objectives: 1) constrain motor actions until a task set is selected; and 2) allow conflict at the level of task-set selection to delay responding in the motor loop, preventing premature action selection until a valid task set is selected. Taken together, both algorithmic and neural network models similarly and accurately predict behavioral task performance. The synergism of different modeling levels provides an account of how humans engage cognitive control and learning to produce structured abstract representations that enable generalization in the long term, even if it may be costly in the short term.

a computationally tractable algorithm for task-set learning and clustering that not only feasibly links multiple contexts to the same task set, but also discerns when to build a new task set to accommodate a novel context. This process has been since dubbed "structure learning."

This structure-learning process also has an implementational solution, simulated in a biologically plausible neural network model (in the same PDP tradition as the PBWM model), which provides a specific hypothesis about how structure learning occurs in the brain. In particular, the model formalizes how higher- and lower-level task-set structures and stimulus-action relationships are learned analogously within a distributed brain network involving interactions between PFC and BG. The key functional components of the model are two corticostriatal circuits arranged hierarchically with independent gating mechanisms. The higher-order loop involves anterior regions of PFC and striatum, which learn to gate an abstract task set and cluster contexts associated with the same task set. The lower-order loop between posterior PFC and striatum also projects to the subthalamic nucleus, which provides the capability of gating motor responses based on the selected task set and perceptual stimulus. Thus, the execution of viable motor responses is constrained by task-set selection, and conflict that occurs at the level of task-set selection delays the motor response, thus preventing premature action selection until a valid task set is verified.

Both the algorithmic C-TS and the neural network model lead to similar predictions in human behavior. The convergence between these modeling approaches makes clear their joint utility as explanatory tools for understanding the processes that underlie structure learning. Specifically, together these models make an important claim: that humans have a bias toward structure learning, even when it is costly, because such learning enables longer-term benefits in generalization and overall flexibility in novel situations (Collins 2017).

From a broader perspective, a unique strength of using multiple computational modeling approaches is the ability to provide complementary insight into the cognitive and neural processes that result from the interaction of cognitive control and learning functions. These two variants of the C-TS model provide an admirable exemplar for how to integrate computational, algorithmic, and implemental analysis levels, and thus formalize a theoretical account that can approximate human implementation of cognitive control processing and structure learning. Thus, while the C-TS specifically targets understanding key mechanisms of cognitive control, the multilevel approach adopted to investigate these mechanisms provides excellent scaffolding for future computational investigation in other cognitive research domains.

4.3 Discussion: Evaluating Models of Cognitive Control

Next, we address two relevant issues in evaluating computational models of cognitive control: 1) what are good metrics for determining whether a model provides a useful contribution to our understanding of cognitive control mechanisms? And 2) how can models in this domain be successfully applied to understand the nature of cognitive control deficits in psychiatric disorders?

4.3.1 Model Evaluation: Determining Whether a Computational Model is Useful

A famous adage by the British statistician George E. P. Box states the following—"all models are bad; some models are useful." It is generally accepted that most computational models are limited in their ability to account for all observed behavior, and at best typically encompass the critical data variability within a certain limited cognitive domain (e.g., cognitive control phenomena related to standard experimental response-conflict tasks), but do not generalize well beyond this limited domain, such as to novel tasks or contexts. Another common critique of algorithmic approaches, in particular, is that these computations may not necessarily accurately reflect how cognitive processes are implemented on the biological level. For example, while a model may provide a sufficient hypothesis of cognitive control function and account for the key behavioral variance in a task, it is possible that the brain-behavior relationship may arise from a completely different computational or neural process altogether in the brain. Thus, an important step in this approach is model evaluation; that is, deciding whether a model has utility. In other words, what makes a model useful for advancing cognitive research? Here we describe two complementary metrics for determining the utility of computational models—specifically, examining whether they are descriptive or predictive.

A computational model is *descriptive* if it provides a detailed explanation that accounts for significant variability of observed data (i.e., how well the model fits the data). Since models provide hypotheses about the data-generating process, a descriptive computational model should provide insight into the mechanisms that give rise to the observed behavioral or neural responses in a given task. For example, an indisputable strength of Alexander and Brown's (2011, 2014) PRO model is its ability to account for a diverse range of empirical results, related to evaluation of demands for cognitive control, that span across both human and primate studies. Since the PRO model successfully models diverse neural and behavioral data from multiple cognitive control studies, it consequently provides compelling evidence for the hypothesis that predictive neural computation relating actions to outcomes implemented in the

ACC and associated medial frontal regions may be a useful signal linked to the engagement of cognitive control. However, although the PRO model formalizes one potential algorithmic explanation for the generative process underlying extant data, it may neither reflect the actual neural computations that occur in the brain, nor necessarily accurately predict data outcomes in future studies. Thus, a limitation of this evaluation metric is that while a model with high explanatory power may explain prior data, the proposed mechanism may not be able to explain new data.

Conversely, a computational model is *predictive* if it describes a generative process that accurately forecasts and extrapolates to novel tasks or contexts. A predictive model contains a specific hypothesis about the neural computations that generate relevant data from one task or context and incorporates theory to reliably estimate behavioral and neural outcomes in a novel task/context. Collins and Frank's (2013) convergent C-TS and neural network models provide excellent examples of predictive modeling, as both models make accurate predictions of behavioral outcomes in novel tasks/contexts. Critically, a theoretical assumption guiding development of these models is that humans spontaneously build task-set structure in learning problems. This structure-learning assumption was tested in empirical studies, validating that the model could generalize to task contexts not previously learned. To summarize the key distinction put forth here, both "descriptive" and "predictive" computational models provide process mechanisms for how data are generated, but the former describes how well the model may fit extant data, whereas the latter describes how well the model generalizes to unseen data.

More broadly and generally, a computational model can serve a very useful function if it is explicitly specified to the degree that it can provide a focal point to drive and rejuvenate new research efforts. For example, while there is much controversy over ACC function, computational models have helped to elucidate potentially relevant cognitive mechanisms by providing specific testable hypotheses for empirical study (Botvinick and Cohen 2014; Vassena, Holroyd, and Alexander 2017). Moreover, although models may not always be accurate, they can highlight limitations of existing theory (e.g., what can and cannot be predicted by the model) and provide insight into how the theory should be revised in future iterations. The computational models described in this chapter are theory-driven approaches that attempt to describe how the brain implements cognitive control in an explicit way, in contrast to more vague descriptions by conceptual or verbal models. Thus, by attempting to spell out the exact mechanism for how cognitive control systems can be realized, the models described here provide explicit answers to the mysterious "homunculus" problem of cognitive control. Furthermore, our hope is that such models will eventually be directly useful for elucidating how and why abnormal psychological and neurological processes arise in mental illness.

4.3.2 Cognitive Control Impairments in Schizophrenia

As an example of the point made above, we conclude this chapter with an example in which computational models of cognitive control have already been directly applied to a psychiatric disorder: specifically, to investigate the etiology of cognitive impairments in schizophrenia. A large literature on cognitive function in schizophrenia has reliably established that patients with this illness demonstrate impairments in attention, working memory, episodic memory, and executive functions (Snitz, MacDonald, and Carter 2006). More specifically, an influential hypothesis is that schizophrenia is characterized by disrupted cognitive control, specifically a disturbance in the ability to internally represent and maintain contextual or task–goal information in the service of exerting control over one's actions or thoughts (Cohen and Servan-Schreiber 1992; Barch and Ceaser 2012; Lesh et al. 2011; Barch, Culbreth, and Sheffield 2018). A key feature of the account is that such disruptions in cognitive control and context representation are directly linked to dysfunction of the DA neuromodulation in PFC, which has long been suggested to be a primary mechanism of pathophysiology in schizophrenia (Meltzer and Stahl 1976; Snyder 1976; Seeman 1987; Toda and Abi-Dargham 2007; Rolls et al. 2008; Valton et al. 2017). In particular, a common view is that at least some of the cognitive impairments observed in schizophrenia putatively are related to reduced dysfunctional DA signaling in striatum and PFC, as well as increased "noise" potentially resulting from increased tonic DA activity or aberrant phasic DA activity (Braver, Barch, and Cohen 1999; Rolls and Grabenhorst 2008; Maia and Frank 2017).

As a direct test for this hypothesis of dysregulated cognitive control and its relationship to DA and PFC, Braver and colleagues modified an extant computational model of PFC function and context processing. Specifically, the goal was to make explicit predictions about behavioral and brain activity patterns that would be observed in schizophrenia patients performing the AX Continuous Performance Task, or AX-CPT, an experimental paradigm designed to distill key aspects of cognitive control and context/goal maintenance (Braver and Cohen 1999; Braver, Barch, and Cohen 1999; Braver, Cohen, and Barch 2002). A key feature of this connectionist model, similar to the PBWM model discussed earlier by Frank and colleagues, is that contextual/goal representations are actively maintained in dorsolateral PFC, via mechanisms of recurrent connectivity and lateral inhibition. Most importantly, in this model, DA serves a joint neuromodulatory function within PFC, both gating representations into active maintenance (via phasic signals) and also regulating the persistence of maintenance (via tonic signals; Braver, Barch, and Cohen 1999; Cohen, Braver, and Brown 2002). Model simulations with this DA neuromodulatory mechanism in PFC bolstered this hypothesis, providing evidence that context-dependent task performance, a key deficit in schizophrenia, is impaired with a noisy DA system (for more specific details, see Braver, Barch, and Cohen 1999). In particular, the model predicted very particular patterns of behavioral deficit in the AX-CPT task in participants with schizophrenia, as well as disruptions in the temporal dynamics of dorsolateral PFC activity, which were later confirmed experimentally (Barch et al. 2001; Braver, Cohen, and Barch 2002). Nevertheless, it has been difficult to demonstrate direct evidence that such deficits are specifically linked to DA neuromodulatory mechanisms, though recent advances in fMRI techniques have allowed researchers to more precisely measure dopaminergic phasic signals within the brainstem (D'Ardenne et al. 2012).

Evidence for a related account of contextual/goal representation deficits in schizophrenia was shown by Chambon et al. (2008). Here, the goal was to test the cascade model of hierarchical cognitive control in PFC proposed by Koechlin, Ody and Kouneiher (2003) to see whether it could account for particular patterns of behavioral impairment in individuals with schizophrenia. Interestingly, Chambon et al observed that sensory and episodic dimensions of cognitive control were preserved in patients with schizophrenia, whereas contextual control was impaired compared to matched healthy controls. In the study, patients generated significantly greater errors in tasks that required the ability to maintain context representations, and these impairments were highly correlated with disorganization score (e.g., a measure of disordered thought and behavior). Thus, the evidence is so far consistent with the hypothesis that in schizophrenia the ability to represent and actively maintain contextual or task–goal information is disrupted. In future investigations, it will be important to more directly test the claims of the cascade model that these deficits map appropriately along the rostro-caudal axis of PFC among individuals with schizophrenia.

4.4 Chapter Summary

This chapter highlighted several computational models that have played a seminal role in guiding theoretical accounts of cognitive control. We have selected these models because they provide promising testable hypotheses that have already stimulated a great deal of current experimental research, and which are likely to guide future investigations seeking to further elucidate the core neurocomputational mechanisms that underlie cognitive control. Furthermore, we hope that these models can be a useful primer for understanding computational approaches to cognitive processes more broadly, as well as how these processes may be disrupted in mental illness. Although computational modeling approaches have played a central role in understanding normative cognitive function (e.g., memory, attention), many of these models have not yet been explicitly tested in psychiatric populations. Thus, we argue that developing accurate mechanistic models of normative cognitive functions can, in principle and in practice, facilitate greater insight into the etiology of psychopathology.

4.5 Further Study

Rumelhart et al. (1987) and O'Reilly & Munakata (2000) are seminal textbooks, both of which provide an in-depth introduction to connectionist computational models. The second book incorporates more biologically realistic algorithms and architectures, and explicitly accounts for extant cognitive neuroscience data. The authors have updated this work with more recent, free electronic editions, which include a chapter on executive function/cognitive control, available at https://grey.colorado.edu/CompCogNeuro/index.php/CCNBook/Book/.

For a review of the main scientific questions of cognitive control, and computational approaches that have been proposed to address these questions, see also O'Reilly et al. (2010) and Botvinick and Cohen (2014). An example of how different modeling levels can be utilized to provide converging evidence for cognitive control mechanisms can be found in Collins and Frank (2013). An example of how a computational model of cognitive control can be applied to make predictions about psychiatric disorder, specifically schizophrenia, is offered by Braver et al. (1999).

5 The Value of Almost Everything: Models of the Positive and Negative Valence Systems and Their Relevance to Psychiatry

Peter Dayan
Max Planck Institute for Biological Cybernetics

5.1 Introduction

Humans and other animals are sufficiently competent at making choices capable of increasing their long-run expected rewards and decreasing their long-run expected punishments that they can survive in a complex, threat-prone, and changing environment. Bodies of formal theory in economics, statistics, operations research, computer science, and control engineering provide a foundation for understanding how systems of any sort can learn to perform well under such circumstances.

As is richly apparent in the present book, this understanding has been progressively rendered into the modern discipline of reinforcement learning (RL; Sutton and Barto 1998), which provides close links to the ethology, psychology, and neuroscience of adaptive behavior. Further, it is perhaps the central leitmotif of computational psychiatry that dysfunctional behavior can be understood in terms of flaws, inefficiencies, or miscalibration of RL mechanisms (Huys et al. 2015b, Huys et al. 2016b; Maia and Frank 2011; Montague et al. 2012).

In this chapter, we consider one substantial aspect of these treatments, namely the notion of value—in both its definition and use. Conventionally, in RL, immediate utilities quantify the rewards or punishments (such as a pellet of food) provided upon doing a particular action (such as pressing a lever) when the world is in a given state (for instance, if a particular light is shining). These are weighted and summed or averaged over the long run to give rise to values. Since the long-run rewards depend on the long-run policy (i.e., the systematic choice of actions at states), various different sorts of values are often considered depending on aspects of these policies.

We here ask about the source and nature of actual and imaginary utilities, the calculations leading to value, and the influences of utilities and values on action.

In particular, we discuss topics phrased at Marr's computational level (as defined in section 1.2.1) and relevant to computational psychiatry that arise over both the shorter and longer term. Shorter-term issues include risk sensitivity (when utilities may be combined in a sub- or superadditive manner), and, in social contexts, other-regarding preferences (Fehr and Schmidt 1999), which arise when the utility that one agent derives depends on the returns that other agents achieve.

In the longer term, it turns out to be possible to formalize the drive for exploration as a form of optimism in the face of uncertainty. This amounts to a fictitious or virtual reinforcement (Gittins 1979; sometimes known as an exploration bonus) for actions about which there remains ignorance. Separately, we can quantify the opportunity cost of passage of time as arising from rewards that are foregone (Niv et al. 2007).

Finally, we also note the algorithmic problems posed by calculations of long-run expected value. These are addressed by the use of multiple mechanisms, each of which works well in a different regime of the amount of learning, and the time available for making a choice (Daw et al. 2005; Dolan and Dayan 2013; Doya 1999; Keramati et al. 2011; Pezzulo et al. 2013).

These ideas provide the lens through which we then view psychological and neural aspects of utility and value. We discuss three substantive ways in which this is not transparent. The first concerns the very definition of utility and its ties to emotion and affect (Bach and Dayan 2017; Buck 2014; Lindquist and Barrett 2012; Russell and Barrett 1999). The second is to consider asymmetries in the representation and effect of positive and negative values, along with associated notions of opponency (Boureau and Dayan 2010; Daw, Kakade, and Dayan 2002; Dayan and Huys 2009; Deakin and Graeff 1991). Third, we view various apparent flaws in the way that we make choices in terms of heuristics that are tied to values (i.e., Pavlovian programming; Breland and Breland 1961; Dayan et al. 2006). Finally, we suggest some outline links to psychiatric dysfunction.

It is regrettably impossible to provide a complete account of such a rich and complex topic as value in a short and didactic chapter. The references should be consulted for a fuller picture.

5.2. Utility and Value in Decision Theory

5.2.1 Utility
As we have seen in section 2.3, one of the core concepts in RL is the positive or negative immediate scalar utility, r_t, associated with states or states and actions. This quantity describes that the experience of the state or result of the action can be more or less profitable for the agent. For instance, an agent moving in a maze might be penalized ($r_t < 0$) for the cost of every move, and also suffer particular costs for being at a location

in the maze that is very muddy or wet. Utilities are typically treated as being part of the description of the problem (or perhaps the environment)—they are an input to the algorithms we will consider.[1]

Although utilities are basic, they are not necessarily simple. Two complexities that are important from the perspective of computational psychiatry are their dependence on the state of the self or of others.

In terms of the self: utilities depend critically on one's current circumstances; failing to take this into account can readily lead to apparently dysfunctional decision making. For instance, it seems obvious that food should have greater immediate utility when food-deprived; disruptions in this could have an obvious association with eating disorders. Similarly, there is some evidence that the marginal utility of leisure time also decreases as total leisure time increases (Niyogi et al. 2014); breakdown in this can lead to over- or underactivity. Unfortunately, the relevant calculations for all these are not necessarily straightforward—and, as we will see, this problem is exacerbated for the case of distal rewards. The latter is particularly important for quantities such as money, whose immediate utility is questionable. Again, decreasing marginal utility with increasing wealth has been suggested as underpinning phenomena such as risk aversion; that is, the reluctance to accept risky monetary prospects even when they involve an expected gain (but see Rabin and Thaler 2001 for a discussion about the plausibility of this explanation).

Utilities can also depend on other, more psychological issues such as counterfactual (i.e., imaginary or potential) reinforcement (Breiter et al. 2001; Camille et al. 2004; Lohrenz et al. 2007). These can generate emotions such as regret (Bell 1982; Loomes and Sugden 1982).

In terms of the other: most conventional applications of RL pit a single subject against the vicissitudes of an uncaring stochastic environment. However, it is often the case that psychiatric contexts involve the cooperation and competition of multiple intentional agents. Characterizing this requires taking considerations from game theory; that is, mathematical models of strategic interaction between rational decision-makers, into account (Camerer 2003). Such contexts typically imply a second dimension of complexity to immediate utilities—namely, components that depend on the relative outcomes of the various players. For instance, consider two players (A and B) sharing a fixed amount of money. The utility that player A derives from a split might be decreased if she wins too much more than player B (a form of guilt) or not enough more than player B (a form of envy; Fehr and Schmidt 1999). Such other-regarding utilities can then underpin strategies that seem beneficent or malign to other players (who then may engage in recursive modeling of each other's utility function in order to optimize their own utilities; Camerer, Ho, and Chong 2004; Costa-Gomes, Crawford, and Broseta 2001).

5.2.2 Value

With immediate utility as a basic concept in RL, the essential computational step for all decision-making algorithms is to compute either the value of a state $(V(s_t))$, or that of a state-action pair $(Q(s_t, a_t))$ under either a given policy or the optimal policy. These values are defined as long-run summed or averaged utilities expected to accumulate over whole trajectories of interaction between a subject and the environment (potentially including other subjects). The expectations are taken over states and actions (i.e., over the transitions that govern state occupancy) and outcomes or utilities, if these are stochastic. There are different ways of quantifying the present value of multiple future utilities—the two most common are to use a form of exponential or hyperbolic temporal discounting (Ainslie 1992, 2001; Kable and Glimcher 2010; Myerson and Green 1995; Samuelson 1937; figure 9.2, this volume), or to consider the long-run average rate of the delivery of utility (Kacelnik 1997; Mahadevan 1996; Stephens and Krebs 1986). Oddities of the calibration of this discounting are an obvious route to impulsivity in conditions such as attention deficit hyperactivity disorder, for instance (Williams and Dayan 2005). The more general observation that hyperbolic discounting leads to temporally inconsistent preferences has been of great importance in understanding a variety of behavioral anomalies (Ainslie 1992, 2001).

Temporal discounting also animates a different aspect of choice—namely when, or perhaps how vigorously, to perform a selected action. In some cases, the environment itself mandates an appropriate speed (when, for instance, it is necessary to perform an action by a certain time to avoid a punishment; Dayan 2012a). In other cases, the passage of time is penalized because the next, and indeed all subsequent, contributions to the long-run utility are postponed when acting slowly. In other words, waiting to act will result in not receiving potential, or indeed certain, future rewards sooner. This leads to a form of opportunity cost (Niv et al. 2007). If it is also expensive to be quick—for instance, because of the energetic cost of a fast movement (Shadmehr et al. 2010), then the optimal choice of speed of action arises as a balance between these two costs (Niv et al. 2007; Niyogi, Schizgal, and Dayan 2014).

One prominent symptom of neurological disorders (e.g. Parkinson's; Mazzoni et al. 2007) and psychiatric diseases (e.g. depression; Huys et al. 2015a) is a sloth or reluctance to act. For depression, this could arise because the opportunity cost of time is incorrectly perceived to be low (for one of a variety of psychological and neural reasons).

Estimating long-run values is a substantial challenge as trajectories become extended. As explained in section 2.3.1, two classes of methods have considerable currency in RL. Model-based (MB) calculations start from a characterization or cognitive map (Tolman 1948) of the environment and calculate forward to estimate the value. These calculations could involve building and exploring a tree, as in Monte Carlo tree search (Kocsis and Szepesvári 2006). Alternatively, they could involve something closer to the methods of dynamic programming, such as value or policy iteration (Bellman 1952; Puterman 2005). MB methods turn out to be statistically efficient, since cognitive maps are straightforward to learn, but computationally challenging, since long-run estimates are necessary and require long-run or recursive calculations.

One of the most important aspects of MB methods is that they allow the calculation of scalar utilities by combining predictions about what outcomes are imminent with information about the current motivational state (Dickinson 1985; Dickinson and Balleine 2002). The resulting sensitivity to occurrent changes in motivation (for instance, refusing to do work to attain an outcome, such as water, that is not currently valuable, such as when not thirsty) is an important form of flexibility.

Note, though, that making present choices that are sensitive to the motivational state that will pertain in the future—that is, anticipating how we will feel when the outcome will actually arrive—is apparently hard for us (Loewenstein 2000), though it is not necessarily for all organisms (Raby et al. 2007).

The second class of methods is model-free (MF). These involve *caching* the results of observed (or imagined; Sutton 1990) transitions, typically by the bootstrapping method of enforcing sequential consistency in successive value estimates along trajectories (Samuel 1959; Sutton 1988; Watkins 1989). Q-learning MF methods (Watkins 1989) choose actions based on these values: $Q(s_t, a_t)$ reports the benefit of performing action a_t. By contrast, actor–critic methods (Barto, Sutton, and Anderson 1983; see box 10.1 in chapter 10) exploit learned values $V(s_t)$ to criticize, and thereby occasion improvement to, a policy, which is the systematic specification of what to do at each state. The dependence on value in actor–critic methods is thus subtly different. Indeed, one should remember that, as in classical economics, it is the policy that ultimately matters; the values are a means to the end of defining an appropriate policy. Multiple different values might even be consistent with a given policy.

MF methods have the opposite characteristics to MB—they are statistically inefficient, since enforcing consistency allows inaccuracies to persist for long periods. On the other hand, they are computationally efficient (since one only needs to retrieve the value from the cache). However, this efficiency depends on their foundation on scalar utilities. This means that any sensitivity to motivational state has to be explicitly learned based on experiencing the utility of an outcome in that state (perhaps as a consequence of a relevant action), rather than being inferred, as for MB values. There is evidence for an excess influence of MF decision making in diseases involving inflexible compulsions (Gillan et al. 2016; Voon et al. 2015).

Various rationales have been suggested to govern arbitration between MB and MF values (see, e.g., figure 2.5 in this volume)—for instance, according to their relative certainties (which vary with the degree of learning and computational inefficiencies; Daw, Niv, and Dayan 2005), or the opportunity cost of the time that it takes to perform MB calculations (Keramati et al. 2011; Pezzulo et al. 2013). There are also possible ways in which the MB and MF systems could interact—for instance, MB generation of imagined or simulated samples could train MF values or policies (Sutton 1990; Mattar and Daw 2018), MF values could be incorporated into calculations primarily involving MB reasoning (Keramati et al. 2016; Pezzulo et al. 2013), and MB methods could influence the way that MF systems assign credit for long-run rewards to actions or states (Moran et al. 2019).

One particular facet of optimization over trajectories is the influence of ignorance or uncertainty about the environment (or about one's compatriots). This ignorance increases if the environment undergoes change; however, it decreases with observations. Since taking optimal advantage of environments requires knowing enough about them, there is a form of trade-off between exploration and exploitation. Exploration is necessary to be able to exploit; however, if every choice counts, then the possibility that the exploratory choice is bad instead of good (a possibility that must exist for exploration to be worthwhile in the first place) implies that there is a conflict between the two. One approach to addressing the exploration/exploitation tradeoff that has both formal and informal underpinnings (Dayan 2012b; Gittins 1979; Ng, Harada, and Russell 1999; Sutton 1990; Szita and Lőrincz 2008) is by incorporating an exploration bonus. This is an internally awarded addition to the current expected utilities associated with only partly known actions and states. It is justified on the grounds that if, when explored, actions appear to be good, then they can be employed repeatedly in the future.

Exploration is particularly complicated in game-theoretic interactions with other intentional agents. An important formalism suggested by Harsanyi (1967) involves thinking of agents as having types, which determine their utility functions. One example would be their degree of guilt or envy (Fehr and Schmidt 1999). Agents know their *own* type, but can only engage in (Bayesian) inference about the unknown type of their partner. The fact that the players can model each other, and indeed model the other player's model of them, and so on, leads to a structure known as a cognitive hierarchy

(Camerer et al. 2004; Nagel 1995). In combination with the uncertainty about their partner's type, this can be represented as what is called an interactive partially observable Markov decision process (I-POMDP; Gmytrasiewicz and Doshi 2005). This framework generalizes POMDPs to the presence of other, incompletely known, intentional agents. In I-POMDPs, it is necessary to worry that the probing, exploratory actions that one does to gain information about a partially known environment risk convincing other players that one's own utility function is different from its actual form (e.g., that one is more envious and less guilty than is true). One's inferences about the types of other players based on their actions have similarly to be tempered (Hula, Montague, and Dayan 2015).

Other, arguably more heuristic, additions to utilities associated with curiosity and intrinsic motivation are also popular (Oudeyer, Kaplan, and Hafner 2007; Schmidhuber 2010; Singh et al. 2005). These offer rewards for such things as reducing uncertainty or improving one's model of the environment.

However, some forms of ignorance and uncertainty appear to generate negative rather than positive value or utility. This is true in the case of ambiguity (or second-order probability) aversion (Ellsberg 1961; Fox and Tversky 1995), when subjects apparently unreasonably devalue gambles whose outcomes are imperfectly known. It is also seen in the fact that subjects are willing to incur costs to resolve uncertainty early (Bromberg-Martin and Hikosaka 2009; Dinsmoor 1983; Gottlieb and Balan 2010; Kreps and Porteus 1978)—think of how much it would be worth knowing your exam results early, even if you can't change them, and so not experience extended dread (Loewenstein 1987).

5.3 Utility and Value in Behavior and the Brain

In the previous section, we discussed the abstractions of utility and valence that underpin the formal theory of optimizing control. We also saw some of the relevant complexities of both constructs in circumstances relevant to computational psychiatry. In this section, we consider further aspects of their realization in psychological and neuroscience terms.

5.3.1 Utility

Our first concern is the provenance of utility—that is, what determines the degree to which a given outcome or circumstance is rewarding or punishing. This is less straightforward than it may seem, for at least three reasons. First, evolution operates on the macroscopic time scale of reproductive success rather than the microscopic one of, for

instance, slaking one's thirst or sating one's hunger. Our ability to procreate will ultimately depend on our survival and ability to maintain internal states, such as body temperature and blood sugar levels, within narrowly defined ranges, despite being subject to
constantly changing external forces. Thus, there are attempts to define utility in terms
of change in state relative to a point of homeostatic grace (Keramati and Gutkin 2014).
Homeostasis involves maintaining a constant internal environment (e.g., suitable hydra-
tion) in the face of external challenges. Deviations from such a set-point can be dangerous, so reducing such deviations is rewarding. This therefore provides a conventional
reward for drinking while thirsty, for instance. Nevertheless, the difference in time scale
mentioned above suggests that these many, apparently obvious components of utility
are secondary to a primary aim, rather in the way that money, which clearly affords no
direct benefit of its own, has become a central secondary target for modern humans.

One consequence of this is that it becomes compelling to see utility as a pawn in a
(micro-economic) game between competing or cooperating systems, and so detached
from hedonic notions such as "liking" (Berridge and Robinson 2003). That is, if the
architecture of control is such that behavior becomes optimized in order to increase
notional utility, then these utility functions become surrogate means for how systems
attempt to achieve ends. In other words, one system can seize control over behavioral
output indirectly, by manipulating utility, rather than directly, by determining motor
output. One possible illustration of the sort of behavioral anomalies that can result is
anhedonia in chronic mild stress (CMS; Willner 2017). Anhedonia is generally defined
as the inability to feel pleasure in normally pleasurable activities (and is one of the core
symptoms of certain types of depression, as discussed in chapter 7). CMS is a protocol,
typically for rodents, that involves multiple different and unpredictable irritations such
as changing or wetting their bedding, tilting their home cages, exposing them to white
noise, reversing the light/dark cycle, and so on. Rodents subject to this regime exhibit
reduced preference for sweetened, over neutral, fluids. From a conventional utility perspective, this might seem puzzling, since although CMS might reasonably lead the
animals to conclude that the environment contains threats and even lacks opportunities, it seems implausible that sugar should be less immediately valuable. However, if
one sees the utility associated with the sweetness as motivating vigorous behavior (as
it might for a control animal), then decreasing it might be appropriate in CMS, as it
will prevent the animals embarking on potentially dangerous quests in a poor-quality
environment. One could imagine that anhedonia in depression might arise in a similar
manner (Huys et al. 2015a, 2013).

A second, and related, complexity attached to the provenance of utility is the way it
might arise as part of a mechanism of arbitration between separate emotional systems

(Bach and Dayan 2017). By treating utility as a primitive, we have tacitly adopted a dimensional or, with some caveats, constructionist view of emotions (Lindquist and Barrett 2012; Russell and Barrett 1999). These theories view subjectively experienced emotions as constructed representations of more basic psychological components such as valence (positive or negative affectivity—the component of particular relevance to utility) and arousal (how calming or exciting the information is). However, there are also many adherents of an alternative view, according to which there are multiple separate emotional systems that are individually optimized to respond to particular challenges or opportunities in the environment (Buck 2014). Given that more than one such system might be active simultaneously, as for instance in conflicts between approach and avoidance, the brain has to have some form of arbitration. What Bach and Dayan (2017) discussed as virtual or "as-if" utilities can arise as an intrinsic part of the mechanism of arbitration, as studied in design economics (Roth 2002). This is another utilitarian notion of utility, detached from any strong bond to "liking" (Berridge and Robinson 2003).

One might have hoped for a neural resolution to the nature of primary utility. For instance, dopamine neurons are deeply involved in RL (as we discuss below; Montague et al. 1996; Schultz, Dayan, and Montague 1997). Amongst other things, their activity reports a signal that includes information about at least positive utility. Thus, one might hope that an analysis of the activity of their inputs might provide unambiguous information about these utilities. Further, a common assumption had been that at least the positive aspects of utility could be associated with nuclei in the lateral hypothalamus, which are known to be involved in functions such as reward-seeking in the context of food (see, e.g., Berridge 1996; Kelley, Baldo, and Pratt 2005). There is also some direct electrophysiological evidence for reward-sensitivity in neurons in this structure (Nakamura and Ono 1986). Unfortunately, investigations of the activity of those lateral hypothalamus neurons that specifically project to dopamine neurons significantly complicate this view (Tian et al. 2016).

A third, psychological, complexity associated with utility is the influence of counterfactual outcomes. Counterfactual reasoning captures the process in which humans think about potential or imaginary events and consequences that are alternatives to what actually occurred. Regret is the emotion experienced upon discovering that an option not chosen would have been more valuable than the one that was (rejoicing being the positive alternative). This has an important impact in economic choice (Bell 1982; Loomes and Sugden 1982), including as part of algorithms for game-theoretic performance (Camerer and Ho 1999), and has also been frequently examined in psychological and neuroimaging studies (e.g., Coricelli, Dolan, and Sirigu 2007; Kishida et al. 2016; Lohrenz et al. 2007). The prospect of future regret plays an important role in certain choice environments; that is, there can be a substantial contribution to the present value of an option from the future disappointment to which it might lead.

5.3.2 Value

We have argued that it is mostly values—of both states and actions at states—that determine behavior. Indeed, "true" utility is only assessable after the fact—in some cases long after. One famous example of this involves a comparison between nutritive and nonnutritive sweeteners such as glucose and saccharine, respectively. An initial preference can develop for both; but then reverse for the latter, presumably as subjects discover that they have no nutritional value (e.g., Warwick and Weingarten 1994; see also the discussion in McCutcheon 2015). This implies that any immediate report on instant palatability (i.e., the sweet taste) might be best thought of as a prediction that something of actual biological relevance (sugar) has been delivered. More generally, it is the structure of predictions of future outcomes, and their net worth, that determines many aspects of behavior.

5.3.3 Evaluation

There is by now a huge wealth of information about the construction and competition of MB and MF predictions, at least in the appetitive case (Adams and Dickinson 1981; Balleine 2005; Daw et al. 2005; Daw and Dayan 2014; Daw et al. 2011; Dayan and Berridge 2014; Dickinson 1985; Dickinson and Balleine 2002; Dolan and Dayan 2013; Doya 1999; Hikosaka et al. 1999; Killcross and Coutureau 2003; Lee et al. 2014; Montague et al. 1996; Schultz et al. 1997). As noted above, MF predictions typically arise by measuring the inconsistency between successive estimates of long-run value in the form of a temporal-difference prediction error (Sutton 1988), and using this to update predictions.

There is evidence that this prediction error is broadcast via the phasic activity of dopamine neurons (Cohen et al. 2012; Eshel, Tian, and Uchida 2013; Montague et al. 1996; Schultz et al. 1997) to key target structures, notably the striatum (Hart et al. 2014; Kishida et al. 2016), the amygdala, and beyond. Much is known about sources of this prediction error (e.g., Matsumoto and Hikosaka 2007; Tian et al. 2016), although the loci where state or state-action values, or even the actor portion of the actor–critic, are stored is less clear. One prominent idea is that successive "twists" of a helically spiraling connection between the dorsolateral striatum and the dopamine system (Haber, Fudge, and McFarland 2000; Haruno and Kawato 2006; Joel and Weiner 2000) are implicated in forms of MF control (Balleine 2005) that go from being related to state-action values (Samejima 2005) toward being simpler and actor-based (Li and Daw 2011).

This arrangement has various implications. For instance, one of many routes to drug addiction involves substances seizing control of this prediction error, allowing them to masquerade as having substantial value (Redish, Jensen, and Johnson 2008; see also chapter 9). This can then dramatically retune the behavioral direction of the subject toward increased acquisition and consumption of these substances. Subsequent neural changes, such as adaptation, can then cement the malign assessments, making them hard to change.

MB values are constructed on the fly via a process of planning, for instance through a form of constraint satisfaction (Friedrich and Lengyel 2016; Solway and Botvinick 2012) or Monte Carlo tree search (Kocsis and Szepesvári 2006). One account of the latter is episodic future thinking (Schacter et al. 2012); that is, using memory for specific happenings in one's personal past to imagine the future, an operation that involves the hippocampus. Other structures implicated in MB evaluation include regions of the prefrontal cortex and the dorsomedial striatum (Balleine 2005), and there is evidence that parietal regions are involved in the construction and maintenance of the model (Gläscher et al. 2010). Evidence for MB decision making can be found in devaluation paradigms (Dickinson and Balleine 2002). In such experiments, the outcome values are changed suddenly. The change could be internal, for example through selective satiation of the animal, or external, for example, if the previously pleasurable reward is then poisoned. Immediate choice adaptation to this change (before any learning can occur) is evidence for MB (or goal-directed) control, since the MF (habitual) system would require learning about reward experience before it can alter behavior accordingly.

Other sorts of MB sensitivity have also been reported. For instance, aspects of the expected values associated with potential future food rewards appear to be reported in the ventromedial prefrontal cortex in human subjects (Hare et al. 2008). These representations are modulated by apparent top-down goals (potentially via connections with other regions of the prefrontal cortex) such as healthy eating (Hare, Camerer, and Rangel 2009; Hare, Malmaud, and Rangel 2011). Something similar is apparently true for other forms of top-down modulation, as in charitable giving (Hare et al. 2010) or even remunerated sadism (Crockett et al. 2017). As with the observations above about the malleability of primary utilities, this shows how value may also be a pawn in battles over choice.

When salient outcomes are modestly distant in time, their expectation appears also to have direct consequences for value, by generating what are known as anticipatory utilities (Loewenstein 1987). Appetitive prospects generate savoring, which grows as the time of acquisition nears (albeit also then lasting, and so accumulating, for a shorter period of time); aversive prospects generate dread. It has been argued (Iigaya et al. 2016) that such anticipation accounts for the value contributions associated with observing, generating the preference for the early resolution of uncertainty mentioned above (Bromberg-Martin and Hikosaka 2009; Dinsmoor 1983).

5.3.4 Aversive Values and Opponency

We have so far mostly considered appetitive values. However, aversion, punishment, and even the cost of effort are also critical—as is the integration between all these factors. One possibility is that utility and value are signaled by a single system whose neurons enjoy an elevated baseline firing rate, so that positive and negative values could be equally represented by above- and below-baseline activity, respectively (or vice versa). There is some evidence for this (Hart et al. 2014); and indeed, the dopaminergic architecture of the striatum has been argued to be exquisitely tailored to this job, with direct and indirect pathways associated with choosing and suppressing actions and associated with different dopamine receptors, and chiefly sensitive to increases and decreases in dopamine (Collins and Frank 2014; Frank and Claus 2006; Frank, Seeberger, and O'Reilly 2004). However, there is evidence for asymmetric signaling in dopamine activity (Niv et al. 2005), and also for heterogeneity, with particular dopamine neurons responding in aversive circumstances (Brischoux et al. 2009; de Jong et al. 2019; Lammel, Lim, and Malenka 2014; Lammel et al. 2012; Matsumoto and Hikosaka 2009; Mirenowicz and Schultz 1996; but see Fiorillo 2013). There are findings that dopamine concentrations barely reflect effort at all (Gan, Walton, and Phillips 2010; Hollon et al. 2014), along with known associations between this neuromodulator and vigor (Beierholm et al. 2013; Hamid et al. 2016; Niv et al. 2007; Salamone et al. 2016). There are, instead, substantial, albeit controversial, suggestions for opponent representations of reward and punishment (Boureau and Dayan 2010; Daw et al. 2002; Deakin and Graeff 1991; Deakin 1983) involving two interacting systems. It has been argued that these are consistent with what is known as a two-factor account of aversion (Johnson et al. 2001 Maia 2010; Moutoussis et al. 2008; Mowrer 1947), in which actions that cancel predictions of potential negative outcomes (for instance, by leading to signals for safety; Fernando et al. 2014) are themselves reinforced. To put it another way, a unitary mode of reinforcement of choices comes from outcomes being better than expected, rather than good (Dayan 2012a; Lloyd and Dayan 2016).

We noted above that one could justify exploration in the face of ignorance by the benefit that would accrue if one thereby discovers facets of the environment that can be exploited (Dayan 2012b). This benefit only exists if the environment presents a suitable degree of controllability, such that, for instance, actions have reliable consequences (Huys and Dayan 2009). Dual to this beneficial effect of uncertainty are aversive assessments that amount to forms of predictive anxiety: ignorance can be dangerous if bad outcomes are legion (which might perhaps underpin ambiguity aversion; Ellsberg 1961); similarly, change can be expensive, if hard-won knowledge about how to exploit the environment effectively expires. One interpretation of the neuromodulator norepinephrine is that it reports on forms of unexpected uncertainty—induced by unpredictable change (Devauges and Sara 1990; Yu and Dayan 2005); there is indeed evidence of a close association between norepinephrine, stress, and anxiety (Itoi and Sugimoto 2010).

5.3.5 Instrumental and Pavlovian Use of Values

Given some of the various ways that state and state-action values may be determined and learned, we next consider their effect. It is here that the differences between Pavlovian and instrumental behavior become critical (Mackintosh 1983). State-action values [such as $Q(s_t, a_t)$], which estimate the long-run future value that is expected to accrue starting from state s_t, choosing action a_t, and then following a conventional policy thereafter, are part of an instrumental control structure. These values are learned or inferred based on the contingency between actions and outcomes; thus, choice is similarly contingent. The same is true when values just of states $V(s_t)$ are used to train a policy (i.e., in an actor–critic method; Barto et al. 1983), based on the changes in these values contingent on the actions. However, animals are also equipped with forms of preparatory Pavlovian control (Mackintosh 1983). In this, stimuli (signifying states) associated with appetitive or aversive values—that is, predictions of (net) future gain or loss, respectively—elicit actions without regard to the actual contingent consequences of those actions. Appetitive predictions lead to active, vigorous engagement and approach. By contrast, aversive predictions lead to withdrawal, inhibition, suppression, and freezing. Thus, for instance, pigeons will peck at lights that have been turned on just before food is delivered, even if this pecking has no contingent consequence at all. These behaviors are presumably evolutionarily appropriate and have the benefit of not needing to be learned. However, the lack of contingency implies that the actions are elicited even if they paradoxically actually make less likely the outcomes that support the underlying predictions (Breland and Breland 1961; Dayan et al. 2006; Guitart-Masip et al. 2014). For instance, pecking can still be observed in omission schedules, that is, when the pigeons do not actually receive food in any trial in which they peck at an illuminated light (Williams and Williams 1969).

Pavlovian influences interact with instrumental behavior in at least two further ways. One is by modulating the vigor of ongoing instrumentally directed responses, in the form of what is known as Pavlovian-instrumental transfer (PIT; Cartoni, Balleine, and Baldassarre 2016; Estes 1943; Murschall and Hauber 2006; Rescorla and Solomon 1967). PIT is defined as the phenomenon that occurs when a conditioned stimulus (CS) that has been associated with rewarding or aversive stimuli via Pavlovian/classical conditioning alters motivational salience and operant behavior. PIT comes in two flavors: specific and general. Specific PIT happens when a CS associated with a reward enhances an instrumental response directed to the same reward. For example, a rat is trained to associate a sound (CS) with the delivery of a particular food. Later, the rat undergoes an instrumental training where it learns to press a lever to get that particular food (without the sound being present). Finally, the rat is presented again with the opportunity to press the lever, this time both in the presence and absence of the sound. The results show that the rat will press the lever more in the presence of the sound than without, even if the sound has not been previously paired with lever-pressing. The Pavlovian sound-food association learned in the first phase has somehow transferred to the instrumental situation, hence the name, Pavlovian–instrumental transfer. Under general PIT, instead, the CS enhances a response directed to a different reward (e.g., water). The difference between these flavors is analogous to that between the MF and MB predictions that may underpin them.

The anatomical basis of preparatory appetitive and aversive Pavlovian actions and PIT is not completely clear, although there is evidence for the involvement of various regions. One is the ventral striatum (Reynolds and Berridge 2001, 2002, 2008). Another is dopaminergic neuromodulation (Faure et al. 2008; Murschall and Hauber 2006), which is important for active responses in appetitive and aversive domains, and serotonergic neuromodulation, which plays a particular part in aversive contexts (Faulkner and Deakin 2014), underlying its role as the putative opponent to dopamine (Boureau and Dayan 2010; Daw et al. 2002; Deakin and Graeff 1991; Deakin1983). Specific and general PIT depend on distinct circuits linking central and basal nuclei of the amygdala to the core and shell compartments of the ventral striatum, respectively (Balleine 2005; Corbit and Balleine 2011; Corbit, Fischbach, and Janak 2016).

A second interaction between Pavlovian and instrumental behavior is more restricted. As we noted, one process underlying MB evaluation of states or actions at states is thought to be building and traversing a tree of prospective future states—that is, chains of episodic future thinking (Schacter et al. 2012). In planning series of actions in this way, it is usually infeasible to consider all potential future sequences; instead, one must cut the expanding decision tree down to a computationally manageable size.

There is evidence that Pavlovian predictions can be involved in this process of pruning, being reflexively evoked by large losses and persisting even when disadvantageous
(Huys et al. 2012). This is an internal analogue of aversion-induced behavioral inhibition; that is, the tendency to withdraw from unfamiliar situations, people, or environments in the face of expected aversive outcomes. For a more concrete example, imagine
planning chess moves by considering future board positions. A variation in which a
queen was lost might be pruned away in this manner, even if this variation would ultimately have led to an advantageous checkmate.

Both instrumental and Pavlovian predictions can themselves be MB or MF. We
already pointed to this in the instrumental case—apparent, for instance, in the wealth
of devaluation paradigms (Adams and Dickinson 1981; Dickinson 1985; Dickinson and
Balleine 2002). There has perhaps been less focus on this in Pavlovian circumstances,
although we noted that evidence of both specific and general PIT can be interpreted in
this manner; and there are also some direct observations about preparatory Pavlovian
actions along with modulation of instrumental ones (Dayan and Berridge 2014; Robinson and Berridge 2013). Furthermore, the form of the preparatory Pavlovian response
can be influenced by the nature of the outcome as well as that of the predictor (Davey,
Phillips, and Witty 1989). For, instance pigeons exhibit distinct food- and water-directed
pecks and apply them specifically to lit keys that predict food and water, respectively
(Jenkins and Moore 1973). There are also clear individual differences. For instance, during Pavlovian conditioning, individuals vary widely in their propensity to engage with
conditioned stimuli (called sign tracking) or the sites of eventual reward (goal tracking)
in circumstances under which these differ. Sign- and goal-tracking subjects appear to
rely more on MF and MB systems, respectively (Robinson and Flagel 2009).

Along with preparatory Pavlovian responses are consummatory ones that are typically elicited by the presence of the biologically significant outcomes that inspire consumption or defense (rather than by values). There is a particularly rich and complex
set of defensive responses that are specific to the species concerned (Bolles 1970),
and sensitive to subtle aspects of the relationship between the subject and the threat
(McNaughton and Corr 2004). This is apparently controlled in rodents (Blanchard and
Blanchard 1988; Keay and Bandler 2001) and humans (Mobbs et al. 2007) via a structure called the periaqueductal gray.

5.4 Discussion

In this chapter, we have discussed issues of utility and value, which are the engines
underlying choice. We saw some of the many complexities of the definition and

determinants of utility, and then the computational issues that arise with either learning (in a MF manner) or inferring online (in a MB manner) the long-run predicted values of states or states along with actions. We noted additional factors such as information, risk, ambiguity, and motivational state that can change or influence utility and value, along with the behavioral impact of values in terms of mandatory preparatory Pavlovian behaviors such as approach and withdrawal. We also noted that values should optimally influence the alacrity or vigor of action.

We observed that many different neural systems are involved in the assessment and effects of both appetitive and aversive utility and value. Evidence is unfortunately currently somewhat patchy as to how they all fit together, and indeed the many opportunities that each, and their combinations, afford for supporting benign and malign individual differences. Some foundational questions remain to be answered, such as whether there is opponency between systems associated with each valence.

One theoretical approach to computational psychiatry starts from some of the different sources of dysfunctional decision making: the latter can result from the brain trying to solve the wrong computational problem, solving the correct problem incorrectly, and solving the correct problem, correctly, but calibrated to an incorrect environment (Huys et al. 2015b). Although utility and value influence all of these in various ways, in terms of the current chapter, it is most straightforward to consider incorrect utilities ("solving the wrong problem") and inefficient or ineffective calculations (the correct problem "solved incorrectly").

It seems obvious that utilities actually define optimal choices—however, we noted that utilities are not primary and impenetrable, but rather are contextually determined and what one might call meta-adaptive. This affords attractive flexibility, but it is also a clear point of vulnerability: utilities might be influenced by early insult, or incorrect or outdated priors. For instance, following seemingly random aversive events, a person could develop a prior that the world is not very controllable, with actions having highly stochastic consequences. This would come with the implication that there is little point exerting effort trying to explore it, since the information gained would not be expected to be exploitable (Huys and Dayan 2009). As in our description of chronic mild stress, one way for the brain to inhibit exploration would be to dial down the subjective utility of outcomes. This would be pernicious, since failing to explore may entail failing to find out that the prior no longer pertains. We have argued that various such failings of the prior can lead to forms of depression (Huys et al. 2015a), but they can readily extend to addiction and beyond.

Incorrect calculations, leading to incorrect acquisition or calculation of long-run values, are another substantial source of problems. Some particular cases have been studied. One case concerns the automaticity of the Pavlovian pruning of the internal search used to calculate expected future values, such as when encountering losses; this has been considered a point of vulnerability that could be relevant to mood disorders (Huys et al. 2012). Another case concerns the underweighting of MB over MF choice observed in some participants (Voon et al. 2015). This leads to behavior that is inflexible in the face of change and fails to reflect information that the subject can be shown to possess. On the surface, many psychiatric conditions share this characteristic; a deeper investigation using comparisons with factor analytical summaries of answers to structured questionnaires showed that it is actually most closely associated with measures of compulsivity (Gillan et al. 2016). A second set of issues with calculation arises from Pavlovian influences over actions. For instance, we see people as being impulsive (Evenden 1999) when they have apparently chosen immediate, short-term, positive outcomes. One of many possible sources of this is a form of Pavlovian misbehavior (Dayan et al. 2006) approach in the face of predictions of future positive valence irrespective of the contingent consequences.

5.5 Chapter Summary

In sum, although it might seem that nothing could be simpler than learning to favor actions that lead to positive outcomes, there are actually many richly complicating factors. These factors can achieve important ends—including tailoring behavior to long-run goals; adapting those goals in the light of particular contexts; and accommodating prior expectations over the brutishness and brevity afforded by evolutionary contexts by using hard-wiring and heuristics to avoid as much of the cost and danger of learning as possible. These factors leave an architecture of choice replete with readily exposable flaws and vulnerability to the sort of psychiatric disorder on which this book concentrates.

5.6 Further Study

Bach and Dayan (2017) offer a computational perspective on emotion that analyses its relationship with various aspects of appetitive and aversive utility.

Berridge and Robinson (2003) create part of a long series of arguments that there is an important separation between "liking" (the hedonic components of reward) and "wanting" (the motivational and learning force associated with reward that influences choice).

Hare et al. (2008) is an early paper using fMRI in humans to dissociate various different signals related to value.

Keramati and Gutkin (2014) argue that movements of the internal state relative to homeostatic optimality generate internal rewards.

5.7 Acknowledgments

I am grateful to the Gatsby Charitable Foundation for support and to Peggy Seriès for comments.

6 Psychosis and Schizophrenia from a Computational Perspective

Rick A. Adams
University College London

6.1 Introduction

Schizophrenia is a psychiatric disorder that affects around 0.5% of the population worldwide. While it is less common than anxiety and depression, it can have more devastating effects: from its onset, usually around 18–30 years, it can transform a person from being a university student to someone chronically unwell and dependent on social support for the rest of his/her life. It also carries the same risk of suicide as major depression. It is a "psychotic" disorder, meaning that its sufferers' experience of reality departs from others' experience of reality in important and characteristic ways. Its diagnostic symptoms form three broad clusters, known as "positive," "negative" and "disorganized."

Positive symptoms include delusions and hallucinations; in schizophrenia, the former are commonly beliefs about being persecuted or surveilled, or beliefs that people or events refer to you or communicate messages to you in some way, or beliefs that one is controlling or controlled by other people or events, although there can be numerous other themes. Hallucinations can occur in any modality, but the commonest in psychosis are auditory and verbal (i.e., voices). Although voice-hearing is not uncommon in the general population, voices referring to the subject in the third (rather than second) person, for example commenting on them or discussing them, especially in unpleasant ways, are more characteristic of schizophrenia. Symptoms of "thought interference" are a group of experiences partway between hallucinations (i.e., abnormal sensory experiences) and delusions: for example, that others are inserting thoughts into or extracting them from one's mind. Such symptoms are often accompanied by a loss of "insight"; that is, a denial that these experiences might stem from an abnormal state of mind.

Negative symptoms refer to losses of normal function, including poverty of speech, reduced emotional expression, and, above all, a loss of motivation. They are distinct from depression, in which affect is very negative (i.e., the person feels very low and cries very easily, etc.), in that here affect is apparently reduced or absent. Disorganized symptoms are also known as "thought disorder" and refer to abnormal structure in a person's speech or writing (as thoughts cannot be directly assessed). These may be relatively mild, in the form of altered or new words (neologisms) or rather circumstantial answers to straightforward questions; more substantial, for example sudden tangents or breaks in one's train of thought, or statements that are connected by bizarre or irrelevant associations; or severe, in which it is difficult to discern any meaningful content from an utterance.

Alongside positive, negative, and disorganized symptoms, perhaps the commonest symptom of schizophrenia is of a generalized cognitive impairment: a loss of IQ of around 10–20 points (Meier et al. 2014). This decrement in cognitive function is hard to detect in a clinical interview, and so it does not form part of the diagnostic criteria (which were designed to maximize inter-rater reliability), but it seems fundamental to schizophrenia itself and poses a major public health problem, as returning to meaningful employment is often the biggest challenge for those diagnosed with the condition. Worse still, while antipsychotic drugs are reasonably effective for positive and disorganized symptoms, neither the cognitive impairment nor the negative symptoms have any effective medical therapy at present (although psychological interventions for both have been devised).

It should be stressed that the unitary diagnosis of "schizophrenia" is unlikely to stand the test of time, although it seems equally unlikely to be replaced in the near future. Psychiatry is gradually moving away from categorical diagnostic systems and toward more dimensional approaches, as it becomes clear that other psychotic disorders such as bipolar affective disorder and schizoaffective disorder share not just some symptoms but also some genetic risk variance (and presumably neurobiological mechanisms and psychosocial risk factors) with schizophrenia itself (Cross-Disorder Group of the Psychiatric Genomics Consortium 2013). Population surveys have also revealed that many psychotic symptom dimensions (e.g., positive, negative, cognitive and mood symptoms) are also continuous with the general population (Linscott and van Os 2010).

What part can computational psychiatry play in the future of schizophrenia research? It should make a major contribution to understanding how the different clusters of psychotic symptoms come about, by linking the biological, psychological, and social risk factors for the disorder to the brain's function as a model of its physical and social environment. Such understanding would benefit our categorization, diagnosis, and design of therapies for psychotic disorders.

6.2 Past and Current Computational Approaches

In describing the computational approaches to schizophrenia below, the negative, positive (and disorganized), and cognitive clusters will be considered in turn, as the models used to describe each are often quite different.

6.2.1 Negative Symptoms

Negative symptoms can be grouped into two domains: those involving the loss of emotional expression (in affect and in speech) and those involving the loss of motivation for behavior; crucially, the latter predict functional outcome and quality of life. The fundamental question they pose can be stated as: "Why do these subjects not pursue policies that would result in outcomes most people would find rewarding?"

One can easily see the relevance of reinforcement learning (RL) models (described in section 2.3 and chapter 5) to answering this question. Much more detailed accounts of RL in schizophrenia include Strauss, Waltz, and Gold (2014) and Deserno et al. (2013)—what follows is a précis of this highly recommended work.

There are numerous potential RL-based explanations of why those with negative symptoms might not act to obtain rewards:

i) They underestimate the value of rewards. Interestingly, although "anhedonia" (i.e., the loss of experience of pleasure) is listed as a negative symptom, subjects with schizophrenia actually show normal subjective and hedonic responses to rewards, so an explanation of negative symptoms is unlikely to be this straightforward (Strauss and Gold 2012).

ii) They learn more from negative feedback than positive feedback. If striatal dopamine release is disordered in schizophrenia, then one might expect greater difficulty in encoding positive reward-prediction errors (RPEs)—via increased phasic dopamine release—than negative RPEs, via pauses in dopamine neuron firing. The consequence of this would be an asymmetry in RL, in which relevant stimuli tend not to be associated with rewards but can still be associated with punishments or loss of reward, perhaps causing a loss of motivation for most actions over time. Such an asymmetry has indeed been demonstrated in subjects with high negative symptoms (Gold et al. 2012).

iii) They have difficulty building more accurate but complex models of the values of given actions. There are different ways of learning which action to take in a given situation: a simple way is using an actor–critic model to learn which actions are better or worse than average, while a more complex way is to use Q-learning to learn the expected values of specific action-stimulus pairs (see Box 10.1 in chapter 10 for a comparison of these methods). The latter is computationally more costly, but can differentiate between stimuli that are rewarding and those that merely avoid loss. Gold et al. (2012) showed that subjects with high negative symptoms learned optimal actions like the simpler actor–critic model—which may indicate pathology in orbitofrontal cortex, where representation of expected values is thought to occur—whereas controls and subjects with schizophrenia but without negative symptoms were fit best by a Q-learning model.

iv) They have difficulty comparing the values of different stimuli or the costs and benefits of a given action. Subjects with schizophrenia describe inconsistent preferences when judging between two stimuli even outside a cognitively demanding learning-based task, implying that their representation of expected values and its use in making decisions is corrupted in the disorder (Strauss et al. 2011). Similarly, subjects with high negative symptoms are less likely to select high-cost, high-reward actions (Gold et al. 2013), although whether this is due to problems in the valuation of reward or effort or the comparison of the two is unknown.

Of note, model-based fMRI studies of subjects with schizophrenia have also shown blunted ventral striatal activations to reward anticipation and RPEs, which in some cases correlate with the degree of negative symptoms (e.g., Juckel et al. 2006; meta-analyzed by Radua et al. 2015).

Motivational problems in schizophrenia show some similarities to anhedonia in major depression, in that in both disorders, basic reward experience and learning mechanisms seem largely preserved (e.g., hedonic responses to primary rewards and actor–critic reward learning), whereas inferences about—and hence affective responses to—more complex rewards are impaired.

6.2.2 Positive Symptoms

Given that delusions seem *a priori* to relate to abnormal learning, and the strong association between presynaptic striatal dopamine availability (measured using positron-emission tomography, or PET) and positive symptoms (Howes and Kapur 2009), one might be optimistic that delusions could also be explained in terms of aberrant RL mechanisms. The first attempt to link dopamine "hyperactivity," behavioral neuroscience and positive symptoms, however, was based not on RL but on the related field of motivational salience.

In the aberrant salience hypothesis, Kapur (2003) drew on Berridge and Robinson (1998)'s observations that some striatal dopamine innervation is crucial, not for learning the values of stimuli, but for motivating responses to stimuli *whose values have already been learned,* a property they termed "incentive salience." Kapur proposed that in early psychosis there is an increased release of dopamine, including at inappropriate times (i.e., to stimuli with no expected value). This would generate a state of "aberrant [incentive] salience" in the subject, in which various percepts, ideas, or memories have great (but unwarranted) importance. As a consequence, delusions could arise as (rational) attempts by the subject to explain these bizarre experiences. Hallucinations could also be a direct consequence of percepts (e.g., inner speech) or memories being imbued with too much salience.

A salience-attribution paradigm was devised to test Kapur's theory, and correlations between aberrant salience measures (speeding of reaction times to and/or incorrect beliefs about nonrewarding stimulus dimensions) and positive symptoms have been found. However, the most consistent finding in subjects with schizophrenia (and those with delusions in particular) is that of increased explicit aberrant salience (i.e., altered belief updating, measured via rating scales), although implicit aberrant salience (i.e., altered motivational signaling, measured via reaction times) has also been found (Roiser et al. 2009; Roiser et al. 2013; Smieskova et al. 2015; Abboud et al. 2016; Katthagen et al. 2018).

From a computational perspective, modeling aberrant salience is not straightforward, because the term "salience" is now used to describe many different things: not just motivation signals (or, in more computational terms, average reward rate), but also unsigned RPEs (some dopamine neurons respond equally to rewarding and aversive prediction errors), as well as either surprising or informative (Barto, Mirolli, and Baldassarre 2013) sensory states (unrelated to reward, but to which some dopamine neurons also respond). Interestingly, more evidence is emerging that dopamine neurons respond to changes in beliefs independent of any reward-prediction error (Corlett et al. 2007; Schwartenbeck, FitzGerald, and Dolan 2016; Nour et al. 2018), and indeed their role may be causal in this regard (Sharpe et al. 2017).

Maia and Frank (2017) produced a computationally simpler but still comprehensive account of how schizophrenia symptoms could arise from abnormal dopaminergic RPE signaling alone. They propose that negative symptoms could result from attenuated dopamine RPEs, while positive symptoms could result from increased "spontaneous" dopamine RPEs. Crucially, they observe that value and incentive salience depend mostly on dopaminergic signals in the limbic (ventral) striatum. However, in schizophrenia it is the associative striatum—where combined representations of states and actions may be learned—that is more consistently found to have increased dopamine synthesis and release (Howes and Kapur 2009). They therefore propose that delusions, hallucinations, and otherwise bizarre and disordered thoughts could come about through abnormal gating of random percepts, thoughts, or actions through the "Go" pathway in associative striatum.

This account is admirable for its clarity and for its explanation of abnormal cognition alongside abnormal value learning, which the aberrant salience hypothesis struggles to account for. Additional hypotheses may be required to account for some other findings in schizophrenia, however. This includes, in particular, the considerable genetic and neuropathological evidence for N-methyl-D-aspartate receptor (NMDAR) hypofunction in the disorder, as well as various empirical findings that seem to relate more to NMDAR dysfunction than to dopaminergic abnormalities. One such finding (also see below) is that in schizophrenia that is resistant to (antidopaminergic) treatment, PET imaging has not found evidence of increased striatal dopamine synthesis, but magnetic resonance spectroscopy (MRS) has found evidence of cortical glutamatergic abnormalities (Demjaha et al. 2014). Nevertheless, there are complex interactions between NMDARs and the dopamine system (Stephan, Friston, and Frith 2009) that careful empirical work is required to explore.

Hierarchical Bayesian predictive coding accounts of schizophrenia share Maia and Frank (2017)'s notion that prediction-error signaling is aberrant in schizophrenia, but propose that it is not just RPE signaling in the striatum that is affected, but prediction-error signaling throughout the cortex (Sterzer et al. 2018; Adams et al. 2013). This account is based on the idea that the brain uses (or approximates) Bayesian inference on its sensory inputs to infer their hidden causes in the environment (see section 2.4). To do so, it must use a hierarchical generative model of its sensations that encodes the sufficient statistics of the distributions over their causes—that is, both their means and their precisions (inverse variances). The most popular scheme for performing inference in such a model is known as "predictive coding"—in which higher levels pass predictions of activity down to lower levels, which return only errors to the higher levels, which correct their predictions, and so on—although other message-passing schemes can be used (see below and section 2.4.6).

The key pathology in the predictive coding account of schizophrenia is proposed to be the encoding of precision of the signals related to incoming information (the likelihood) and prior beliefs (in the cortex and elsewhere). Given that precision is used to weight one distribution over another in Bayesian inference, its neural substrate is likely to be synaptic gain (the factor by which an input to a neuron is multiplied to generate its output), which could likewise alter the influence (but not the content) of neural messages. Many neurobiological risk factors for schizophrenia affect synaptic gain, including neuromodulators such as dopamine and NMDARs, especially those on inhibitory interneurons, which affect the oscillatory properties of networks and hence their ease of communication with other brain areas.

In schizophrenia it seems that there is a hierarchical imbalance in synaptic gain, as primary sensory areas have been shown to be "hyperconnected" (i.e., show increased correlation with other brain areas compared with controls), whereas higher regions (e.g., prefrontal and medial temporal cortex) are "hypoconnected" (Anticevic et al. 2014). If this corresponds to a similar imbalance in the encoding of precision in a hierarchical model, then its effect would be to reduce the effect of priors on inference and cause larger belief updates in response to unexpected sensory evidence.

A loss of precision of prior beliefs could account for numerous phenomena in schizophrenia, including a resistance to visual illusions (which exploit prior beliefs to create their effects), impairments in smooth oculomotor pursuit of visual targets, abnormal electrophysiological responses to both predictable and oddball stimuli (e.g., the mismatch negativity) and a loss of attenuation of self-generated sensations (reviewed in Adams et al. 2013). Likewise, perceiving relatively inconsequential events as being imbued with significance (i.e., according too much precision to lower-level prediction errors) and updating one's beliefs as a result fits comfortably with this framework. Indeed, it may be that these kinds of higher-level updates, encouraged by the loss of precision encoding in those areas, are the source (or the consequence) of the apparently spontaneous dopamine transients in the striatum.

It is unlikely that there is a uniform loss of precision of prior beliefs in schizophrenia, however: two recent studies have shown that some prior beliefs (about visual stimuli) have a *greater* influence over sensory data in subjects with schizophrenia or schizotypal traits compared with controls (Teufel et al. 2015; Schmack et al. 2013), although this is not always the case (Valton et al. 2019). In the auditory domain, there is evidence that prior beliefs about sounds learned during a task are more strongly weighted in hallucinators, with or without psychosis (Powers, Mathys, and Corlett 2017), and that this increased weighting may relate to striatal dopamine (Cassidy et al. 2018).

How these apparently opposite imbalances between prior beliefs and sensory evidence might co-exist in schizophrenia is an open question: there are numerous possible explanations that can only be resolved by empirical studies. For example, loss of precision in the middle (e.g., cognitive) levels of a hierarchy might allow both sensory evidence and higher-level (e.g., affective) beliefs to dominate that level, causing sensory hypersensitivity and delusional ideas, respectively. Alternatively, it may be that there is a loss of ability to optimally adjust synaptic gain according to context, rather than a persistent over- or underestimation in any given area.

An alternative message-passing scheme that could perform Bayesian inference (on discrete, not continuous, states—unlike predictive coding) is belief propagation, in which ascending and descending messages are not prediction errors and predictions but likelihoods and prior expectations, respectively. Jardri et al. (2017) propose that a loss of inhibitory interneuron function in schizophrenia could allow ascending or descending messages to be passed back down or up the hierarchy, thus leading to "overcounting" of either sensory evidence or prior beliefs. They called their model the circular inference model, in reference to the loopy amplifications caused by the impaired inhibitory interneurons in the hierarchy (see also section 2.4.6). They demonstrate evidence for both overcounting of sensory evidence and prior beliefs using a task in which subjects with schizophrenia had to update some preliminary knowledge in the light of new data, and, interestingly, find that on the group level, these subjects showed more evidence for ascending loops (i.e., overcounting sensory evidence), but individual subjects showed evidence for both ascending and descending loops, which correlated with positive and negative symptom severity, respectively (both correlated with disorganization).

The overcounting (or increased precision) of sensory evidence may contribute to a well-described phenomenon in probabilistic belief updating in schizophrenia: the "jumping to conclusions" bias, which is also associated with the presence of delusions (Dudley et al. 2016). This bias is usually assessed with the urn or beads task (Garety, Hemsley, and Wessely 1991), in which subjects are shown two jars containing red and green beads in ratios of 80:20 and 20:80. The jars are hidden, and a sequence of beads is drawn (with replacement) from one jar. Participants need to guess which jar the beads are drawn from. Depending on the version of the task, participants either have to stop the sequence when they are sure of the jar's identity (the "draws to decision" version) or rate the probability of the jar after seeing each bead (the "probability estimates" version).

The best-replicated finding in this literature (Dudley et al. 2016) is that many more subjects with schizophrenia than controls decide on the jar in the "draws to decision" task after seeing only one or two beads (the "jumping to conclusions" bias). There are many other computational parameters, aside from sensory overcounting or precision, which could account for this effect, however: a lower decision threshold, an inability to inhibit a prepotent response, more stochastic decision making (i.e., higher decision "temperature"), a lower perceived cost of making a wrong decision, or a higher perceived cost of sampling. Unfortunately, most "draws to decision" paradigms have not controlled or manipulated these parameters, so it is not possible to distinguish conclusively between them.

Moutoussis et al. (2011) explored whether the last three parameters listed above—that is, decision temperature τ, cost of wrong decision C_W, or cost of sampling C_S—could explain the jumping-to-conclusions bias in subjects with schizophrenia and with or without active psychosis. The authors found that acutely psychotic subjects had much higher τ but no differences in C_W and C_S. In a subsequent study, first-episode psychosis subjects were found to have a higher C_S and only a borderline increase in τ (Ermakova et al. 2019). Note that a higher τ may mean that decisions are truly more stochastic, or it may mean that the source of variability in decision making has not been captured by the model.

One weakness of this model is that its τ, C_W, and C_S parameters don't allow for individual differences in belief updating: it assumes that all subjects update their beliefs in a Bayes-optimal fashion. However, there is evidence that subjects with schizophrenia update their beliefs differently from controls (neither of whom are Bayes-optimal). A scrupulous and well-controlled study of the beads task recently showed that while the main effect of schizophrenia diagnosis was more liberal (i.e., larger) belief updates, delusions were correlated with more conservative (i.e., smaller) belief updates—contrary to most interpretations of the "jumping to conclusions" bias (Baker et al. 2019).

In a similar vein, Averbeck et al. (2011) asked subjects with schizophrenia and controls to perform a sequence-learning task with probabilistic feedback. This allowed them to estimate how much subjects learned from positive and negative feedback. The subjects with schizophrenia learned *less* from positive feedback than controls, mirroring their reward-learning deficits described in the preceding section. Moreover, the less they learned, the *more* likely they were to show the jumping-to-conclusions bias. This apparently paradoxical finding is explored in greater detail in the next sections.

Although a significant amount of work has been done on belief-updating and value-learning in schizophrenia, there has been relatively little exploration of how language could be spontaneously created (as in auditory verbal hallucinations) or become disorganized, both in terms of its form (e.g., derailment—one subject changing into another without an obvious connection) or its content (e.g., attributing events to bizarre agents, such as famous people). In some pioneering studies, Hoffman and McGlashan (2006) showed that excessive pruning of connections and hypodopaminergia (i.e., disinhibition) in the hidden layer of a sentence-recognition network could reproduce speech-detection performance in human hallucinators, and that this excessive pruning could also lead to hallucinations (although these hallucinations were only of a single word appended to an existing sentence).

Hoffman et al. (2011) trained a more complex model comprised of multiple connected modules, each containing recurrent networks, to learn 28 narratives of varying emotional intensity and about different agents. They showed that of many possible perturbations, only enhancing prediction-error learning (i.e., increasing back-propagation learning rates) during memory-encoding matched errors made by subjects with schizophrenia in memories for narratives. These included exchanging the identities of agents (especially of similar social status) between autobiographical and other stories and derailments from one story to another, particularly between those of similar type or emotional valence.

6.2.3 Cognitive Symptoms

One implication of Hoffman's work is that abnormalities of working memory (WM) and memory-encoding processes may not just manifest in those processes, but also contribute to positive symptoms. In a landmark study, Collins et al. (2014) demonstrated that WM deficits could also contribute to apparent RL impairments in schizophrenia. Their subjects had to learn stimulus–response associations for reward, and the stimuli were presented in sets of size two to six. Under these conditions, smaller sets could possibly be learned through WM processes, but larger sets—exceeding WM capacity—would be more reliant on incremental (i.e., RL) mechanisms. Fitting an RL model with a WM component to individuals' data, they found that the subjects with schizophrenia had lower WM capacity and greater WM decay rate, but their RL and decision-stochasticity parameters were no different to those of controls. This demonstrates that unless WM is explicitly modeled, inferences about RL parameters in schizophrenia must be treated with caution. How WM relates to symptoms is unclear, though, as none of the model parameters or their principal components correlated with positive or negative symptoms.

In neurobiological terms, this implies that pathology in prefrontal cortex (PFC) and hippocampus might make a greater contribution than the striatum to abnormal inference and learning in schizophrenia. But what kind of pathology? A highly influential spiking network model of pyramidal cell and interneuron function in PFC during a spatial WM task contains excitatory pyramidal cells with bidirectional connections to a single inhibitory interneuron and recurrent excitatory connections to themselves (Rolls et al. 2008, see also chapter 3). Increased activity of one pyramidal cell is therefore a) self-sustaining, through the excitatory-excitatory (E-E) connection, and b) laterally inhibiting, through the excitatory-inhibitory (E-I) connection and subsequent inhibition of its neighboring pyramidal cells. These dynamics can be pictured as energy landscapes containing "basins" of attraction, the stability of which is determined by their depth and the level of "noise" in the network (Rolls et al. 2008). NMDAR hypofunction on pyramidal cells would reduce E-E strength and also self-sustaining activity. On the other hand, NMDAR hypofunction on interneurons would reduce E-I strength and increase the spread of excitation through the network. A model in which E-I strength is reduced more than E-E (i.e., an increased E/I ratio) captures the behavior of subjects with schizophrenia best: it increases "false alarms" to near (but not far) distractors during a spatial WM task (due to lateral spread of excitation) but not the rate of "misses" (see also chapter 3).

Other models of PFC function have also incorporated the recently demonstrated cortical dopamine hypofunction in schizophrenia (Slifstein et al. 2015). Dopamine hypofunction reduces activity in both pyramidal cells (via D_1 receptors) and interneurons (via unique excitatory D_2 receptors) in adult rats (O'Donnell 2012). Modeling studies suggest that this should exacerbate any NMDAR hypofunction and make PFC networks even more vulnerable to distraction (Durstewitz and Seamans 2008). An early connectionist model of dopamine's effects on gating inputs (e.g., sensory cues) into PFC proposed that greater variability of dopamine firing makes cues' effects on PFC less reliable (Braver, Barch, and Cohen 1999). There is clearly much still to be learned about cortical-dopaminergic interactions.

In the previous section, we encountered the puzzling finding that in subjects with schizophrenia, the jumping-to-conclusions bias correlates with a *reduced* tendency to learn from positive feedback (Averbeck et al. 2011). In addition, in the "probability estimates" versions of the beads task, numerous groups have demonstrated a "disconfirmatory bias" in schizophrenia; that is, a tendency to update more than controls on receipt of evidence *against* one's current hypothesis (Garety, Hemsley, and Wessely 1991; Peters and Garety 2006; Fear and Healy 1997; Young and Bentall 1997). However, when observing patients' behavior in this task, it appears that they update more to both a "disconfirmatory" bead *and* to the following bead (e.g., R-R-R-G-R; Langdon, Ward, and Coltheart 2010; Peters and Garety 2006). Yet like Averbeck and colleagues, others have observed *decreased* updating in patients to more consistent sequences both in this task (Baker et al. 2019) and in stimulus–reward-learning tasks, especially in patients with more negative symptoms (Gold et al. 2012). Likewise, healthy volunteers given ketamine (an NMDAR antagonist used to model psychosis in humans) show a decrement in updating to consistent stimulus associations (Vinckier et al. 2016).

To summarize, it appears that, compared with controls, subjects with schizophrenia may show greater belief updating in more uncertain contexts, but (sometimes) lower belief updating in less uncertain contexts, rather than a straightforward "disconfirmatory bias." These effects make sense in the light of attractor models of cortical function, in that NMDAR hypofunction on both pyramidal cells and inhibitory interneurons (to a greater extent) could both reduce recurrent excitation but also increase the E/I ratio. An increase in E/I ratio has been shown to cause more rapid updating and impulsive decision making in a perceptual task model (Lam et al. 2017). On the other hand, a reduction in recurrent excitation could reduce attractor stability (Rolls et al. 2008) and hence make it hard to reach maximum confidence in any one decision. This attractor hypothesis motivated the recent study described below.

6.3 Case Study Example: Attractor-like Dynamics in Belief Updating in Schizophrenia

Adams et al. (2018) tested Bayesian belief-updating models on "probability estimates" beads task data obtained from both healthy volunteers, subjects with schizophrenia, and psychiatric controls. Data set 1 was published previously (Peters and Garety 2006) and comprised 23 patients with delusions (18 diagnosed with schizophrenia), 22 patients with nonpsychotic mood disorders, and 36 nonclinical controls. 53 of those participants were also tested again once the clinical groups were no longer acutely unwell. Data set 2 was newly acquired and comprised 56 subjects with a diagnosis of schizophrenia and 111 controls. Subjects in data set 1 performed the "probability estimates" beads task with two urns with ratios of 85:15 and 15:85 green and red beads, respectively (figure 6.1, upper panel). They had to view a single sequence of 10 beads.

Figure 6.1

The "probability estimates" version of the beads task and the winning model.

Upper panel: This schematic illustrates the concept behind the beads task. A subject is shown two jars, each filled with opposite proportions of red and blue beads (e.g., 80:20 and 20:80 ratios), and the jars are then concealed from view. A sequence of beads is drawn, and the subject is asked to rate the probability that the beads are coming from one jar or another.

Middle panel: A schematic representation of the generative model in model 5 and model 6, the winning model. The black arrows denote the probabilistic network on trial k; the gray arrows denote the network at other points in time. The perceptual model lies above the dotted arrows, and the response model below them. The shaded circles are known quantities, and the parameters and states in unshaded circles are estimated. The dotted line represents the result of an inferential process (the response model builds on a perceptual model inference); the solid lines are generative processes. μ_2 denotes the estimated tendency toward the blue or red jar, and ω is a static source of variance at this level (greater variance means belief updates are larger). The bead seen by the subject, $u^{(k)}$, is generated by the estimated jar on trial k, $\mu_1^{(k)}$. The response model maps from $\hat{\mu}_1^{(k+1)}$—the predicted jar on the next trial, a sigmoid function s of $\mu_2^{(k)}$—to $y^{(k)}$, and the subject's indicated estimate of the probability the jar is blue. Variation in this mapping is modeled as the precision β of a beta distribution.

Lower panel: This figure illustrates the effects of κ_1 (used in models 5 and 6) on inference. It shows simulated perceptual model predictions; the second level μ_2 and simulated responses y have been omitted for clarity. The simulations use four different values of belief instability κ_1, which alters the sigmoid transformation: $\hat{\mu}_1^{(k+1)} = s\left(\kappa_1 \cdot \mu_2^{(k)}\right)$. When $\kappa_1 > \exp(0)$, updating is greater to unexpected evidence and lower to consistent evidence; when $\kappa_1 < \exp(0)$, the reverse is true. The red and brown lines $\left(\kappa_1 > \exp(0)\right)$ illustrate the effects of increasingly unstable attractor networks; that is, switching between states (jars) becomes more likely (see also figure 6.2, upper panel). The black line $\left(\kappa_1 = \exp(-1)\right)$ illustrates slower updating around $\hat{\mu}_1 = 0.5$, as was found in controls.

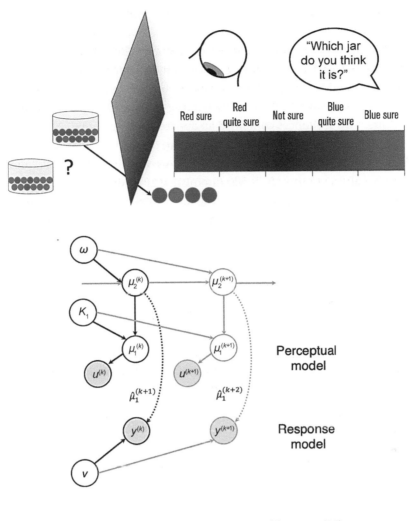

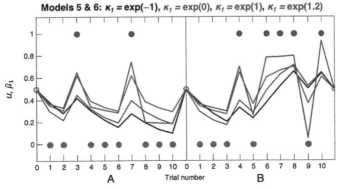

After each bead, they had to mark an analogue scale (from 1 to 100) denoting the probability that the urn was the 85% red one. Subjects in data set 2 performed the same task with two urns with ratios of 80:20 and 20:80 red and blue beads, respectively (figure 6.2, lower panel). Each subject viewed four separate sequences of 10 beads (an A and a B sequence, and A and B again, but with the bead colors inverted). After each bead, they had to mark a Likert scale (from 1 to 7) denoting the probability that the urn was the 80% blue one. Two sequences contained an apparent change of jar.

The behavioral differences between groups are detailed in Adams et al. (2018). In brief, subjects with schizophrenia showed increases in "disconfirmatory" updating in both data sets, although this effect was diminished at follow-up in data set 1.

The Bayesian belief-updating model was the hierarchical Gaussian filter, or HGF (Mathys et al. 2011; see section 2.4.6). The HGF contains numerous parameters that can vary between subjects, thus explaining individual differences in inferences while preserving the Bayes-optimality of inferences, given these parameters. The HGF has been used to demonstrate numerous interesting parameter differences between controls and groups with psychiatric diagnoses, such as ADHD (Hauser et al. 2014), autism (Lawson, Mathys, and Rees 2017), and schizophrenia (Powers, Mathys, and Corlett 2017). The models employed here are described in detail in Adams et al. (2018). In brief, the model's inputs are the bead shown $u^{(k)}$ and the subject's response $y^{(k)}$ on trials $k = 1 - 10$. From these inputs and its prior beliefs, the model infers the subject's beliefs about the jar $\mu_1^{(k)}$ (a logistic sigmoid function of the "tendency" of the jar $\mu_2^{(k)}$) on each trial, along with the model parameters (β, ω, φ or κ_1 and $\sigma_2^{(0)}$—see below, table 6.1, and figure 6.1). The response model generates the subject's response $y^{(k)}$ (i.e., where on the sliding scale they place the arrow on trial k), which is determined by $\mu_1^{(k)}$ and the precision of their response β (similar to inverse temperature; i.e., $1 / \tau$), which affects how much $y^{(k)}$ can deviate from $\mu_1^{(k)}$—that is, the (inverse) stochasticity of their responding, given their beliefs.

Using the HGF and the two data sets, the following questions were addressed. Can differences in belief updating in schizophrenia compared with controls be explained by i) group differences in general learning rate ω; ii) differences in response stochasticity β, or by additional parameters encoding; iii) the variance of beliefs about the jars at the start of the sequence $\sigma_2^{(0)}$; iv) a propensity φ to overweight disconfirmatory evidence specifically; or v) a parameter κ_1 that simulates unstable attractor states, making it easier to shift from believing in one jar to the other (figure 6.1, lower panel)?

Furthermore, are these findings consistent between different groups of schizophrenia, or within schizophrenia tested at different illness phases, and are they unique to schizophrenia or also present in other nonpsychotic mood disorders?

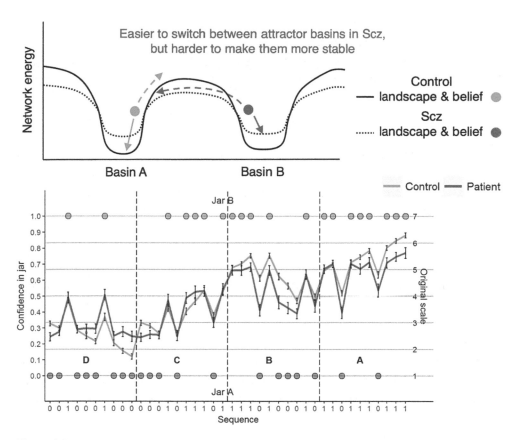

Figure 6.2

Attractors and belief updating, and data set 2 group-averaged beliefs.

Upper panel: This schematic illustrates the energy of a network with two attractors or fixed points—e.g., beliefs about blue and red jars—over a range of firing rates. The continuous line depicts a normal network whose "basins" of attraction are relatively deep. The dotted line depicts the effect of NMDAR (or cortical dopamine 1 receptor) hypofunction on the attractor dynamics. The dots depict initial belief states, and the full and dashed arrows depict the effects of confirmatory and disconfirmatory evidence, respectively. A shallower basin of attraction means its corresponding belief state is harder to stabilize but easier to change. See also similar schematics elsewhere (Durstewitz and Seamans 2008; Rolls et al. 2008).

Lower panel: This panel shows the mean (± standard error) confidence ratings in the blue jar averaged across each group in data set 2. These consist of four 10-bead sequences concatenated together (they were presented to the subjects separately during testing). The group with schizophrenia makes larger updates to unexpected beads but smaller updates to more consistent evidence at the end of sequences A and D.

Table 6.1

Six models tested on two beads-task data sets

Model	Free parameters (prior mean, var)	Description
1		Learning rate and response stochasticity only
2	$\sigma_2^{(0)}$ (exp(-5.1), 0.5)	Initial variance estimated
3	φ (0.1, 2)	Disconfirmatory bias
4	$\sigma_2^{(0)}$ (exp(-5.1), 0.5), φ (0.1, 2)	Disconfirmatory bias and initial variance estimated
5	κ_1 (0,1)	Attractor instability
6	$\sigma_2^{(0)}$ (exp(-5.1), 0.5), κ_1 (0,1)	Attractor instability and initial variance estimated

NB: all models also contained ω (–2, 16) and β (exp(4.85), 1). The brackets contain the prior mean and variance for each parameter used during model fitting.

Six models were tested, each containing a learning rate ω and response precision (similar to inverse temperature) β, and either φ or κ_1, or neither (each with or without σ_2); see table 6.1. Full details of the models and statistical and behavioral results are given elsewhere (Peters and Garety 2006; Adams et al. 2018). Bayesian model selection for data set 1 at both baseline and follow-up and data set 2 produced identical results: model 6 won in each case. In studies of schizophrenia, it is often the case that many patients are fit best by a different model to controls, usually a much simpler one (e.g., Moutoussis et al. 2011; Schlagenhauf et al. 2014). Performing model selection within each group separately, however, still found that model 6 best accounted for the data in all groups (figure 6.3).

In data set 1 at baseline, there were large group differences in the attractor instability κ_1 and response stochasticity β, but not in the initial variance $\sigma_2^{(0)}$ or the learning rate ω (figure 6.4, upper row): κ_1 was significantly larger in the nonclinical controls and the psychotic group than in the clinical control group, and β was smaller in these groups.

In data set 1 at follow-up (figure 6.4, middle row), the attractor instability κ_1 remained larger and response stochasticity β smaller in the psychotic group than the nonclinical control group, but now the clinical and nonclinical control groups were no longer significantly different. Similarly, in data set 2, κ_1 was significantly higher and β was lower in schizophrenia than in controls. There were no significant group differences in ω or $\sigma_2^{(0)}$ (figure 6.4, lower row). The model fits for two example subjects are shown in figure 6.5.

Neither κ_1 or β in data set 1 at baseline were predicted by any particular subgroup of (positive, negative, or affective) symptoms. In data set 2, there was only a weak relationship between β and negative symptoms.

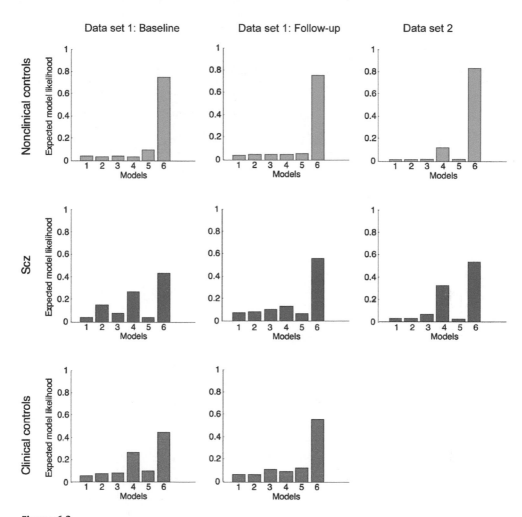

Figure 6.3
Expected model likelihoods for each group in each data set. This figure depicts the model likelihoods for the six models in each group in each data set. The model likelihood is the probability of that model being the best for any randomly selected subject (Stephan et al. 2009). Model 6 wins in all groups in both data sets.

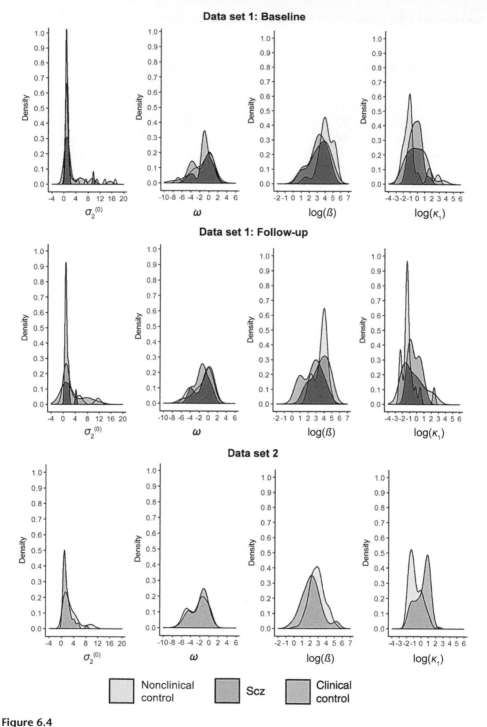

Figure 6.4
Probability density plots for the four model 6 parameters in each data set. The upper and middle rows show the parameter estimates for data set 1 at baseline ($n = 81$) and follow-up ($n = 53$), respectively, and the bottom row data set 2 ($n = 167$). There were significant group differences only in attractor instability κ_1 and β in each data set (see text).

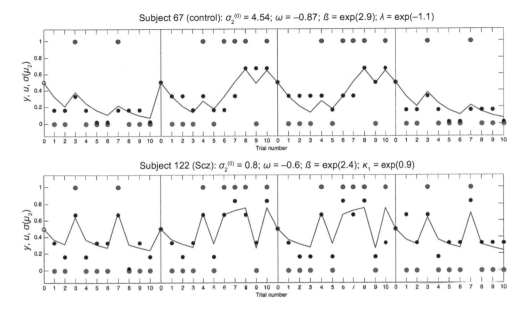

Figure 6.5

Model fits for two example subjects. These plots illustrate the beads seen by subjects (u, in blue and red), the ratings of the probability the jar is blue made by the subjects (y, in black), and the model fit line ($\sigma(\mu_2)$, in purple), for four 10-trial beads tasks concatenated together. The bead colors in two sequences have been swapped around for model-estimation purposes. The upper plot is a control subject, the lower plot a subject with schizophrenia. The two subjects illustrate the effects of attractor instability κ_1—their values of κ_1 (approximately $\exp(-1)$ and $\exp(1)$, respectively) are the modal values of κ_1 in each group (see figure 6.4, bottom row). The subject with schizophrenia makes much larger adjustments to changes in evidence (crossing the p(jar = blue) = 0.5 line repeatedly), explained by a higher κ_1. Note also that this patient's responses are also more stochastic, explained by a lower β. These parameter differences may both be the result of attractor network instability in prefrontal cortex.

We tested for correlations between the model 6 parameters: κ_1 and β were negatively correlated both at baseline and at follow-up in data set 1 and in data set 2. Note that if parameters are highly correlated, then it can be impossible to estimate them reliably; 200 data sets were therefore simulated using the HGF and the modal parameter values for the control and schizophrenia groups in data set 2, and then the parameters from these simulated data sets were reestimated in order to check we could estimate them reliably (parameter recovery; see section 2.5). With the exception of $\sigma_2^{(0)}$ in the simulated schizophrenia data set, the estimated parameter values closely matched their original values.

In summary, this study showed that in computational models of two independent data sets, all subjects—including subjects with schizophrenia—are best fit by a model simulating the effects of attractor-state dynamics on belief updating (model 6) rather than a model biased toward disconfirmatory updating alone (model 4). Medium-to-large differences were found between subjects with schizophrenia and controls in both data sets in both the attractor-instability parameter (κ_1 was greater in schizophrenia; i.e., more unstable) and the stochasticity of responding (β was smaller, i.e., noisier, in schizophrenia), and κ_1 correlated with β in both data sets. Furthermore, v correlated with κ_1 but not with ω or $\sigma_2^{(0)}$ in all three experiments, supporting the idea that β is measuring a stochasticity that is related to the attractor instability κ_1 by an underlying neurobiological process, rather than an effect that just isn't described by the model.

These findings are important because they connect numerous reasoning biases previously found in schizophrenia—for example, a disconfirmatory bias, increased initial certainty (Peters and Garety 2006), and decreased final certainty (Baker et al. 2019)—with model parameters that describe how nonlinear belief updating in cortex could be caused by unstable and noisy attractor states. (In this context, "nonlinear" refers to updating that isn't uniformly increased or decreased relative to controls; e.g., updating more to surprising evidence but less to unsurprising evidence).

Indeed, two recent studies of similar tasks in populations with schizophrenia have also demonstrated evidence of similar belief updating. Jardri et al. (2017) showed that the patients with schizophrenia on average "overcount" the likelihood in a single belief update. Jardri et al. attribute this effect to disinhibited cortical message-passing, but it could equally be attributed to attractor network instability. Stuke et al. (2017) showed in a very similar task that all subjects showed evidence of nonlinear updating, but the group with schizophrenia updated more than controls to "irrelevant information" (i.e., disconfirmatory evidence).

NMDAR hypofunction could contribute to an increased tendency to switch between beliefs and increased stochasticity in responding in several ways (Rolls et al. 2008, see also chapter 3): 1) by reducing inhibitory interneuron activity, such that other attractor states are less suppressed when one is active; 2) by reducing pyramidal cell activity, such that attractor states are harder to sustain; and 3) by reducing the NMDAR time constant, making states more vulnerable to random fluctuations in neural activity.

Another important aspect of data set 1 is the finding that κ_1 and β were also significantly different between the mood disorder clinical group and nonclinical control groups when the former were unwell, but not at follow-up, whereas the differences between the schizophrenia and nonclinical controls remained. This is interesting in light of past work indicating that neuromodulatory activity can have similar impacts on prefrontal network dynamics to NMDARs (Durstewitz and Seamans 2008). One might speculate that both the group with schizophrenia and clinical controls are affected by neuromodulatory changes when unwell, but only the former has an underlying NMDAR hypofunction that is still present once the acute disorder has resolved.

One might question why, given these relationships between parameters and cognition, there weren't strong relationships between κ_1 or β and positive or negative symptom domains (negative symptoms were weakly predictive of β in data set 2 only). One reason may be that the symptom analyses—conducted only on patients—were underpowered, but it is also possible that other pathological factors contribute to symptoms, beyond those measured here (e.g., striatal dopamine availability and positive symptoms). Of note, another study demonstrating clear WM parameter differences between subjects with schizophrenia and controls also failed to detect any relationship between those parameters and symptom domains (Collins et al. 2014).

An important future challenge will be to link belief-updating parameters to those of spiking network models in order to understand how NMDAR function in reference to both pyramidal cells and inhibitory interneurons as well as neural "noise" contributes to attractor instability, response stochasticity, and inference in general (Lam et al. 2017; Soltani and Wang 2010). Beyond that, a true understanding of the disorder will probably emerge once we gain a better understanding in computational terms of how the thalamus, striatum, and cortex all interact with each other, and with dopamine, in performing inference.

6.4 Chapter Summary

In this chapter, we have covered the positive, negative, and cognitive symptoms of schizophrenia and attempts to model them in computational terms. Negative symptoms—broadly, the failure to act to obtain reward—have been modeled using RL models with some success. Positive symptoms—delusions and hallucinations—are less straightforward to understand. Attempts to model them have concentrated either on abnormal dopamine signaling in striatum or abnormal synaptic gain at both ends of the cortical hierarchy. Abnormal dopamine signaling would contribute to delusional thoughts (through aberrant salience, aberrant RPEs, or aberrant gating of thoughts). Abnormal synaptic gain would lead to an imbalance (or alternatively a loss of adaptability) in the encoding of precision in the brain's model of the world, such that prior beliefs are underweighted, and sensory evidence is overweighed. Such models have not yet given a full account of positive symptoms, however. There is a sizable literature on psychological biases (e.g., jumping to conclusions) in schizophrenia, and these are beginning to be understood in modeling terms. Relevant to this may also be the modeling of cognitive symptoms—for example, concentration and working memory problems—using spiking network models with attractor dynamics. In such models, as described in chapter 3, NMDAR hypofunction, perhaps resulting in an increased E/I ratio (due to disinhibition), can make attractors unstable and easily affected by random fluctuations in neural firing. These changes can explain spatial working memory performance in subjects with schizophrenia, as well as apparent biases in probabilistic inference. Ultimately, to understand schizophrenia, we will need a deeper understanding of how the thalamus, striatum, and cortex all interact with each other, and with dopamine, in performing inference.

6.5 Further Study

Valton et al (2017) offers a comprehensive review of computational modeling in schizophrenia.

Strauss, Waltz, and Gold (2014) provide an excellent summary of RL models of negative symptoms.

Maia and Frank (2017) offer the most detailed and developed account of dopamine's potential contributions to positive and negative symptoms.

Adams, Huys, and Roiser (2015) contains a simplified version of the hierarchical predictive coding account of schizophrenia; for more equations and models, see Adams et al. (2013).

Rolls et al. (2008) is an excellent review of spiking and neural network models and how they relate to a dynamical system view of schizophrenia, containing unstable attractor states, and so on. For more on this theme, see also chapter 3 of this volume.

Collins et al. (2014) is a first-rate behavioral modeling paper, demonstrating the importance of including WM function in RL models, as performance in schizophrenia is explained by pathology in only the former.

7 Depressive Disorders from a Computational Perspective

Samuel Rupprechter, Vincent Valton, and Peggy Seriès
University of Edinburgh

7.1 Introduction

Depression and anxiety disorders are the two most common psychiatric disorders around the world (Alonso et al. 2004; Ayuso-Mateos et al. 2001; Üstün et al. 2004; Vos et al. 2012) and display a high level of comorbidity: patients suffering from one of these illnesses are often affected by the other one as well (Kessler et al. 2003). In the United States, Kessler et al. (2003) estimated the lifetime prevalence of major depressive disorder (MDD) at over 16%. Similar figures have been reported for Europe at 13% (Alonso et al. 2004).

Diagnosis for MDD is commonly based on the Diagnostics and Statistical Manual of mental disorders, or *DSM-V* (American Psychiatric Association 2013). The manual lists two core symptoms of MDD: depressed mood and loss of interest or pleasure (anhedonia), of which at least one has to be present for diagnosis. Other symptoms include a significant change in weight, insomnia, hypersomnia, psychomotor agitation or retardation, fatigue or loss of energy, feelings of worthlessness or guilt, a diminished ability to think or concentrate, and recurrent thoughts of death or suicide. Overall, five or more symptoms have to be present for at least two weeks, cause significant impairments in important areas of daily life, and should not be better explained by other psychiatric disorders. The International Classification of Diseases, or ICD-10 (World Health Organization 1992) has similar criteria for diagnosis of (single) depressive episodes and recurrent depressive disorder.

Strikingly, according to the *DSM* definition, it is possible for two people to receive the same diagnosis of MDD without sharing a single symptom. One MDD patient may experience depressed mood, weight gain, constant tiredness and fatigue, and regularly think about ending their life. Another MDD patient may experience anhedonia, lose a lot of weight, and go through psychomotor and concentration difficulties while being unable to sleep properly. The existence of these nonoverlapping profiles partly stems from the fact that categories and symptoms of depression originated from clinical consensus and do not necessarily have a basis in biology (Fried et al. 2014). As a consequence, research often focuses on individual symptoms—for example, anhedonia (Pizzagalli 2014; see also our case study)—in addition to categorical group differences. In the clinical and drug trial literature, the Hamilton Depression Rating (HRSD-17) and Montgomery-Åsberg Depression Rating are by far the most important rating scales. In research environments, the Beck Depression Inventory (BDI; Beck et al. 1961) is a popular choice to measure overall depressive severity, and a subscore can be extracted from items of the questionnaire to quantify anhedonic symptom severity.

7.2 Cognitive Neuroscience of Depression

Patients often show deficits on a broad range of tasks probing executive function and memory (Snyder 2013; Rock et al. 2014), and impairments often remain (to some degree) after remission (Rock et al. 2014).

An early influential theory, inspired by a wealth of animal studies, is that of learned helplessness (Seligman 1972; Maier and Seligman 1976; Abramson, Seligman, and Teasdale 1978). The theory suggests that continued exposure to aversive (stressful) environments over which animals do not have any control leads to behavioral deficits similar to those observed in depression. In such a framework, the patients' distress is believed to stem from their perception of a lack of control over the environment and ensuing rewards or penalties. This, in turn, could explain patients' distress and lack of motivation to initiate actions. Stress has been proposed as a mechanism for memory impairments in depression (Dillon and Pizzagalli 2018), and Pizzagalli (2014) hypothesized that dysfunctional interactions of stress with the brain reward system can lead to anhedonia.

An alternative influential theory about depression concentrated on the prevalence of negative biases involved in the development and maintenance of depression (Beck 2008), which led to the emergence of cognitive behavioral therapy (CBT). This line of research hypothesized that negative schemas about the self, the world, and the future would form due to adverse childhood experiences. According to this framework, negative schemas could lead patients to downplay the magnitude of positive events, or attribute negative valence to objectively neutral events. Patients would effectively perceive the world through "dark tainted" glasses.

It has been suggested that negative biases play a *causal* role in the development and maintenance of depression (Roiser, Elliott, and Sahakian 2012) and that antidepressant medications target these negative biases rather than targeting mood directly (Harmer, Goodwin, and Cowen 2009).

Recently, much cognitive research has focused on decreased sensitivity to reward in depression. There are at least two important reasons for this focus. First, reward processing appears to align with a lack of interest or pleasure (anhedonia), a core symptom of depression and one to which we will come back again in the case study of this chapter. Second, reward processes are better understood than mood processes, both at the neurobiological and at the behavioral level. Indeed, cognitive neuroscience has started to dissociate and delineate different subdomains of reward processing, which can be studied independently in relation to anhedonia (Treadway and Zald 2013). For example, "incentive salience" ("desire" or "want") can be distinguished from "motivation" and "hedonic response" (enjoyment), and we may want to independently study the association of each of these subdomains with depression. For instance, your driving attention and focus on a piece of chocolate (a potentially rewarding stimulus) is different from how much you enjoy that piece while you are eating it. These two subdomains may also be independent from your willingness to expend effort to obtain that piece of chocolate.

Cléry-Melin et al. (2011) tested depressed patients and healthy controls on a task in which they could exert physical effort (through grip force on a handle) to attain monetary rewards of varying magnitudes. They found that depressed participants did not exert more physical effort to obtain higher rewards (as opposed to lower rewards). However, they *believed* they had exerted more effort for higher rewards, as evidenced by their higher effort ratings. Controls, on the other hand, objectively exerted more effort for greater rewards, but reported subjectively reduced effort ratings for higher rewards compared to lower rewards. In another study (Treadway et al. 2012), participants were able to obtain varying amounts of money if they managed to make a large number of button presses within a short time window. Depressed patients exerted less effort (made fewer button presses) than controls in order to obtain reward. Together these studies suggest that depression, and anhedonia in particular, may be related to impairments in the motivation and willingness to exert effort for rewards. This may also explain why behavioral activation therapies have been reported to work well for depressed patients[1]: these practices specifically target decreased motivation (Treadway et al. 2012).

Overall, there is large overlap between different theories of depression. Most cognitive theories place a large emphasis on biases influencing emotional processing (Gotlib and Joormann 2010), but some differ in their explanation of the development of these biases; for example, whether they develop in response to early stressful life experiences

(Beck 2008, Pizzagalli 2014) or stem from biased perceptual and reinforcement processes (Roiser, Elliott, and Sahakian 2012).

Several neurotransmitters, most commonly serotonin and dopamine, are implicated in reward and punishment processing in depression (Eshel and Roiser 2010). Dopamine is heavily implicated in reinforcement learning processes (Schultz 2002) and has consistently been associated with depression in humans and animals (Pizzagalli 2014). Serotonin has long been implicated in the processing of aversive stimuli, and learned helplessness and depression may be related to a failure of stopping such aversive processes (Deakin 2013). Antidepressant medications commonly work by altering serotonin levels (Eshel and Roiser 2010). Neuroimaging studies have revealed abnormal activation and connectivity of many cortical and subcortical brain regions in depression (Pizzagalli 2014, Chen et al. 2015). Reporting of blunted striatal response to reward in MDD has been particularly consistent (Pizzagalli 2014, Arrondo et al. 2015). The orbitofrontal cortex (OFC) and ventromedial prefrontal cortex are implicated in the representation of internal values (Chase et al. 2015). Depression is associated with abnormal activation in these regions (Pizzagalli 2014, Cléry-Melin, Jollant, and Gorwood 2018), possibly related to abnormal use of reward values during decision making (Rupprechter et al. 2018). Large meta-analyses have concluded that MDD is associated with reduced hippocampal volume (Schmaal et al. 2017) and alterations in cortical thickness, especially in OFC (Schmaal et al. 2017).

7.3 Past and Current Computational Approaches

A variety of different computational approaches, ranging from connectionist and neural networks to drift-diffusion models, reinforcement learning, and Bayesian decision theory, have been used to study the behavior of MDD patients. We will, in turn, briefly describe findings from each of these approaches.

7.3.1 Connectionist Models

One early approach that has been used to model depression is a connectionist approach, which is inspired by the idea that complex functions can naturally arise from the interaction of simple units in a network (see section 2.1).

Siegle, Steinhauer, and Thase (2004) asked groups of depressed and healthy individuals to perform a Stroop color-naming task. In this task, color words are presented on each trial with different ink colors matching or not matching the word (e.g., the word "red" written in blue ink), and participants have to name the ink color while refraining from reading the word itself (figure 7.1). The task is typically used to probe attentional

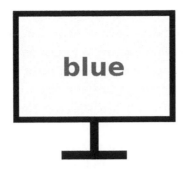

Figure 7.1
A sketch of the Stroop color-naming task, as used by Siegle et al. (2004). Participants had to respond by indicating the color of the ink of the word (here *red*), while ignoring the written word (here *blue*).

control. Pupil-dilation measurements were used as an indicator for cognitive load, because pupils reliably dilate under cognitively demanding conditions (Siegle et al. 2004). Previous studies had shown impairments within groups of depressed subjects, but the nature of these impairments varied, with patients sometimes showing slower responses and at other times increased error rates. Siegle et al. (2004) found similar performance patterns for the two groups, but differences in pupil dilation. Depressed individuals showed decreased pupil dilation, consistent with decreased cognitive control. A neural network was used to identify possible mechanisms that could have resulted in these group differences. The modeling suggested that decreased prefrontal cortex activity could lead to the observed cognitive control differences in this experiment. Such a disruption might also explain attentional deficits commonly observed in depression (Siegle et al. 2004).

Siegle and Hasselmo (2002) provided another example of how neural network models can be used to better understand deficits in depression during (negatively biased) emotional information processing. The task considered was one where emotional word stimuli were observed, which participants had to label as positive, negative, or neutral. Patients typically show biases in emotional information processing; for example, quicker responses to negative information (Siegle and Hasselmo 2002). A neural network model was used to simulate classification of emotional stimuli. It could reproduce the typically observed behavior of depressed patients: it was quicker to identify negative information than positive information and showed larger sustained activity when confronted with negative words. Different mechanisms could lead to these observed abnormalities in the network, including overlearning of negative information, which can be related to rumination—that is, the tendency to repetitively think about the causes, situational factors, and consequences of one's negative emotional experience. A network that had overlearned on negative information could be retrained using positive information (akin to a cognitive behavioral therapy), which resulted in the normalization of network activity in response to negative information. The longer the network had "ruminated," the longer it took for the "therapy" (i.e., retraining) to work, providing insights into the recovery from depression using CBT and its interactions with rumination. Siegle and Hasselmo (2002) therefore suggested that rumination can be predictive of treatment response and should be routinely assessed in depressed individuals.

7.3.2 Drift-Diffusion Models

Drift-diffusion models (DDMs; see section 2.2) have also been used to better understand the mechanisms underlying depressive illness. These models are especially useful when the modeling of reaction time and accuracy *in combination* is of primary interest.

For example, Pe, Vandekerckhove, and Kuppens (2013) modeled behavior on the emotional flanker task to analyze negative biases in depression. In this task, participants are shown a positively or negatively valenced word that they are asked to classify according to valence. The central stimulus is flanked by two additional words with positive, negative, or neutral valence (figure 7.2). The authors hypothesized that higher depressive symptomatology and rumination (as measured by self-report questionnaires)

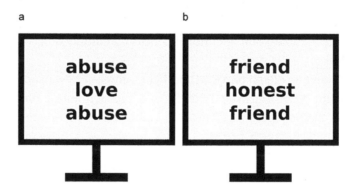

Figure 7.2
A sketch of two types of trials of the emotional flanker task, as used by Pe et al. (2013). Participants had to classify the word in the center according to its valence. (a) An incongruent trial, in which the target word *love* and the flanking word *abuse* have differing valence. (b) A congruent trial, in which the valence of the flanking word is the same as the valence of the target. (Note that Dutch, four-letter-long, monosyllabic words were used by Pe et al. 2013).

are related to negative attentional biases (i.e., a bias toward negative target words). Classical analyses showed that the higher the rumination score, the stronger the facilitation effect (computed from accuracy scores) of negative distracters on negative targets, and the weaker the facilitation effect of positive distracters on positive targets. After controlling for depression, only the former effect remained. A DDM analysis, on the other hand, revealed more effects involving the drift rate, which corresponds to the rate at which information is being processed. The drift rate was negatively correlated with rumination scores on trials where a negative target word was flanked by positive words and was positively correlated with rumination scores on trials where negative words flanked a negative or positive word. After controlling for depression scores, rumination still predicted attentional bias for negative information, but depression scores were no longer predictive after controlling for rumination. The computational modeling therefore revealed that rumination was associated with an enhanced processing of words flanked by negative words and decreased processing in the presence of positive flankers.

In addition to negative biases, depression is also associated with impairments in executive function (Snyder 2013). Dillon et al. (2015) used a combination of three drift-diffusion processes to account for behavior on a different (nonemotional) version of the flanker task. In this version, stimuli and distracters were three arrows pointing left or right. The central and flanking arrows could either be congruent (pointing in the same direction) or incongruent. Depressed and healthy participants had to indicate the direction of the arrow in the middle. The authors' goal was again to address inconsistent findings of previous studies, which had sometimes found enhanced executive functioning in depression during tasks that demand careful thought. Depression can lead to increased analytical information processing (c.f. rumination), which results in worse performance during tasks requiring fast decisions but can also lead to increased accuracy when a careful approach is necessitated and when reflexive responses need to be inhibited. Dillon et al. (2015) found that depressed participants were more accurate but slower than controls on incongruent trials. They decomposed behavior on the flanker task into three different mechanisms that might be affected by depression, and which were modeled by separate drift-diffusion processes: (1) a reflexive mechanism biased to respond according to the flankers; (2) a response-inhibition mechanism able to suppress the reflexive response; and (3) executive control responsible for correct responses in the presence of incongruent flankers. The analysis of model parameters showed that the drift rate for the executive control mechanism was lower in depression, which on its own would lead to slower, but also less accurate, responses. However, this executive control deficit was offset by an additional decreased drift rate in the reflexive mechanism. This could explain impaired executive function but highly accurate responses in MDD (Dillon et al. 2015).

One more example comes from Vallesi et al. (2015), who used DDMs to better understand deficits in the regulation of speed–accuracy trade-offs in depression. At the beginning of each trial, a cue signaled whether participants should focus on speed or accuracy. It was found that MDD patients, unlike controls, adjusted their decision threshold based on the instructions for the *previous* trial, with speed instructions decreasing the decision boundary (independently of the cue for the current trial). That is, patients had difficulties overcoming instructions from the previous trial and flexibly switching between fast and accurate decision making. In addition, drift rates within the patient group were generally lower than in the control group, indicating a slowing down of cognitive processing, which is commonly found in MDD patients.

7.3.3 Reinforcement Learning Models

In reinforcement learning models, behavior is captured on a trial-by-trial basis. An agent makes a decision based on some internal valuation of the objects in the environment, observes an outcome, and then uses this outcome to update the internal values (see section 2.3 and chapter 5). There exists substantial behavioral and neural evidence, often supported by computational modeling, for impaired reinforcement learning during depression (see Chen et al. 2015 for a review).

Chase et al. (2010) fitted a Q-learning model to the behavior of MDD patients and healthy controls on a probabilistic selection task. On each trial, one of three possible stimulus pairs was displayed, and participants had to choose one of the stimuli, each of which were followed by positive or negative feedback according to different probabilities. They did not find evidence for their initial hypothesis that patients would preferentially learn from negative outcomes due to a tendency in depression to focus on negative events. Participants' anhedonia scores, however, negatively correlated with positive and negative learning rate as well as the exploration–exploitation (softmax) parameter. The study therefore provided evidence that depression, and specifically anhedonia, is related to altered reinforcement learning.

Huys et al. (2013) performed a meta-analysis on the signal-detection task (Pizzagalli, Jahn, and O'Shea 2005). In contrast to the previous study, they concluded that anhedonia is principally associated with blunted sensitivity to reward as opposed to an impaired ability to learn from experienced rewards. The task and their approach will be covered in detail in the case study section of this chapter.

Temporal-difference (TD) prediction-error learning signals have been linked to the firing of dopamine neurons in the brain (Montague et al. 1996; Schultz 1998; Schultz

2002; O'Doherty et al. 2004), and there exists substantial evidence that these neurons play an important part in the experience of pleasure and reward (Dunlop and Nemeroff 2007). Using fMRI and a Pavlovian reward-learning task, Kumar et al. (2008) investigated whether TD learning signals are reduced in MDD patients. The authors indeed found blunted reward-prediction error signals in the patient group, and additionally a correlation between such blunting and illness severity ratings. This provides a link between an impaired physiological TD learning mechanism and reduced reward-learning behavior as observed in anhedonia.

The previous study (Kumar et al. 2008) investigated Pavlovian learning, during which participants passively observed stimulus-outcome associations. An early study to look at instrumental learning through active decision making in depression was performed by Gradin et al. (2011). Stimuli were associated with different reward probabilities, which slowly changed. Prediction errors and expected values of a Q-learning model were regressed against fMRI brain activity. Compared to healthy controls, depressed patients did not display behavioral differences. However, physiologically they showed reduced expected reward signals as well as blunted prediction-error encoding in dopamine-rich areas of the brain. This blunting correlated with anhedonia scores. This shows that model-based fMRI can reveal differences in reward learning, even in the absence of behavioral effects.

7.3.4 Bayesian Decision Theory

At a more abstract level, Bayesian decision theory (BDT) has been used to explain common symptoms of depression such as anhedonia, helplessness, and pessimism (Huys, Vogelstein, and Dayan 2009; Huys and Dayan 2009; Trimmer et al. 2015; Huys, Daw, and Dayan 2015a). Bayesian decision theory allows for formulating optimal behavior during a task and then analyzing how suboptimal behavior can arise (see section 2.4).

Huys, Vogelstein, and Dayan (2009) fitted a Bayesian reinforcement learning model to the behavior of depressed and healthy participants in two reward-learning tasks. Importantly, their formulation of the model included two parameters, describing sensitivity to reward and a prior belief about control (i.e., helplessness). Higher values of the control parameter corresponded to stronger beliefs about the predictability of outcomes following an action. Individuals who believe they have a lot of control over their environment would predict that previously rewarded actions will likely be rewarded again, while someone with a low control prior would expect weaker associations between action and reward. Huys, Vogelstein, and Dayan (2009) showed how a linear classifier could be used to distinguish between healthy and depressed participants after they had played a slot machine game, based purely on the two values of individuals' parameters.

This suggests that model parameters obtained by fitting a behavioral task, such as a probabilistic learning task, could be used to classify MDD to a high accuracy. The classification of diseases is an important goal of computational psychiatry (Stephan and Mathys 2014).

A comprehensive evaluation framework formulated through BDT was introduced by Huys et al. (2015a), in which they discuss how depressive symptoms can arise from impairments in utility evaluation and prior beliefs about (the control over) outcomes. They argued that it is primarily model-based reinforcement learning, rather than model-free learning, which is abnormal in depression.

A theoretical description of how optimal decision making can lead to (seemingly) depressed behavior and inaction similar to learned helplessness in a probabilistic environment can also be found in Trimmer et al. (2015). They concluded that to understand a patient's current depressed behavior, the history of the individual should be considered by describing it much further back in the past than what is the current norm. Imagine, for example, that Bob gets fired from his job due to "corporate restructuring" in an economic crisis. Further, no other company seems interested in hiring while the economy is in this downswing, which is unlikely to change for the foreseeable future. Best efforts and repeated attempts to get a new job fail, and adverse events in the environment increase (e.g., he loses friends or family or becomes homeless). Bob starts to learn that his actions do not seem to influence his environment. Negative outcomes appear unavoidable, and over time his willingness to try to escape his situation decreases. Distressed and desperate, Bob starts to show symptoms reminiscent of depression. He has "learned to be helpless."

7.4 Case Study: How Does Reward Learning Relate to Anhedonia?

The case study in this chapter is a meta-analysis published by Huys et al. (2013) of a behavioral task that has consistently revealed reward-learning impairments in depressed and anhedonic individuals and other closely related groups.

Anhedonia is a core symptom of depression. Different behavioral tasks have been used to show that reward feedback *objectively* has less impact on participants who *subjectively* report anhedonia (Huys et al. 2013). However, there are different ways through which such a relationship could be realized. The goal of the meta-analysis was to find out whether anhedonia was principally associated with the initial *rewarding experience* of stimuli, or the subsequent *learning* from these rewards. The two mechanisms are important to disentangle, as they would likely correspond to distinct etiologies and different strategies for therapies (Huys et al. 2013).

7.4.1 Signal-Detection Task

The signal-detection task (see figure 7.3) consists of many (often 300) trials. In each trial, one of two possible stimulus pictures (cartoon faces) is shown, and the participant is prompted to indicate which picture was observed. This can be quite difficult, because the stimuli look very similar—-they only differ slightly in the length of their mouth—-and are only displayed for a fraction of a second. If participants correctly identify a stimulus, they sometimes receive a reward (e.g., in the form of points) and sometimes receive no feedback. Participants are told to maximize their reward.

The most important aspect of the task is the *asymmetrical* reward structure. Unbeknownst to participants, one of the stimuli (called the "rich" stimulus) is followed by reward approximately three times as often as the alternative "lean" stimulus. If participants are not certain about the stimulus, they can incorporate knowledge about their reward history into their decision and choose the rich stimulus so as to maximize their chances to accumulate rewards. Healthy individuals have been consistently shown to develop a response bias toward the rich option (Huys et al. 2013).

Using this task, Pizzagalli et al. (2005) found a reduced ability in healthy participants with high depression (BDI) scores to adjust their behavior based on their reward

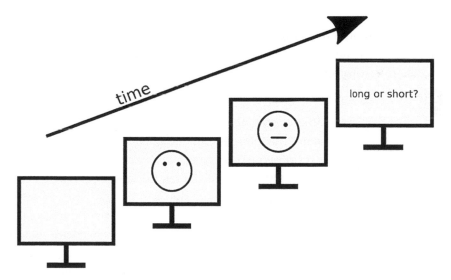

Figure 7.3
A sketch of the signal-detection task (Huys et al. 2013). On each trial, participants observe one of two possible cartoon faces, which only differ slightly in the lengths of their mouths. They have to indicate which face they observed. The reward structure is asymmetrical, with one of the stimuli being rewarded more frequently than the alternative.

history, while low BDI participants developed a stronger response bias toward the rich stimulus. Similarly, worse performance has been observed in MDD patients (Pizzagalli et al. 2008c), stressed individuals (Bogdan and Pizzagalli 2006), euthymic (i.e., neutral mood) bipolar outpatients (Pizzagalli et al. 2008b), as well as volunteers receiving medication (Pizzagalli et al. 2008a) and even healthy participants with a history of MDD (Pechtel et al. 2013).

These studies used signal-detection theory and summary statistics from raw behavior to analyze the data. Huys et al. (2013) extended this by using trial-by-trial reinforcement learning modeling to better understand the evolution of the behavior through time and get to a finer granularity in the analysis of the behavior.

While anhedonia has been associated with a diminished ability to use rewards to guide decision making (such as in studies listed above), there exist varied possibilities for this impairment. Of primary interest in this case study was the distinction between the primary reward sensitivity, the immediately experienced consummatory pleasure following reward, and the *learning* from reward. Huys et al. (2013) included these two factors as parameters into a reinforcement learning model. Figure 7.4 shows how changes in either reward sensitivity (ρ) or learning rate (ε) could lead to the empirically observed changes in response bias.

7.4.2 A Basic Reinforcement Learning Model

As described in section 2.3, a standard Q-learning update rule incorporates learning rate ε in the following way:

$$Q_{t+1}(a_t, s_t) = Q_t(a_t, s_t) + \varepsilon \times \delta_t \tag{7.1}$$

where s_t is the displayed stimulus on trial t, a_t is the action on trial t (i.e., which button was pressed), $Q_t(a_t, s_t)$ denotes the internal value assigned to the stimulus action pair (a_t, s_t) at trial t, $r \in (0, 1)$ is the observed outcome, and $\delta_t = \rho r_t - Q_t(a_t, s_t)$ is the prediction error. Note that Huys et al. (2013) included a reward sensitivity parameter ρ that scales the true value of the reward. A lowering of the learning rate ε increases the time needed to learn about the stimulus-action pairs, while a lowering of the reward sensitivity ρ alters the asymptotic (average) values of Q that are associated with each pair.

In addition, Huys et al. (2013) included a term, $\gamma I(a_t, s_t)$, encoding participants' ability to follow the task instructions (i.e., press one key for the short-mouth stimulus, and the other key for the long-mouth stimulus), where:

$I(a_t, s_t) = 1$ if stimulus s_t required action a_t, and

$I(a_t, s_t) = 0$ if action a_t is the wrong response to stimulus s_t \hfill (7.2)

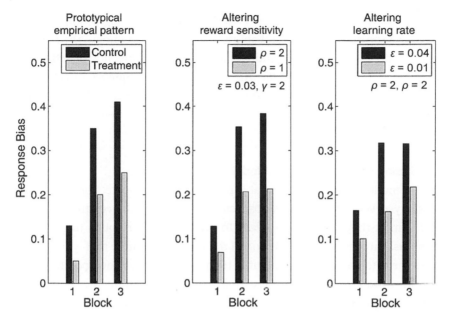

Figure 7.4
Modeling the signal-detection task. Response bias on simulated data (adapted from Huys et al. 2013). Three blocks of 100 trials were simulated, and the development of the response bias is shown across these blocks in each bar chart. On the left, a typical pattern of group differences is shown, with controls developing a strong response bias over the three blocks, and patients showing a reduced bias. The middle chart shows how a reduced reward sensitivity (ρ) could lead to these observed differences. The right chart shows how a reduced learning rate could also lead to similar differences.

Higher values for the parameter γ indicate a better ability to follow instructions and will result in generally higher accuracy. The two terms for I and Q were added together to form a "weight" for a particular stimulus-action pair (on trial t):

$$W_t(a_t, s_t) = \gamma I(a_t, s_t) + Q_t(a_t, s_t) \tag{7.3}$$

These weights are related to the probability of choosing action a when stimulus s was presented. From the above equation we can see that the probability of choosing an action depends not only on following the task instructions (I), but also on the internal value based on previous experience (Q). Huys et al. (2013) used the popular softmax decision function to map these weights to action probabilities:

$$p(a_t|s_t) = \frac{1}{1 + \exp\left(-\left(W_t(a_t, s_t) - W_t(\bar{a}_t, s_t)\right)\right)} \tag{7.4}$$

$W_t(\bar{a}_t, s_t)$ is the weight associated with choosing the wrong action for stimulus s at trial t. The softmax gives the probability that individuals choose the correct action given a certain stimulus. While individuals' parameters are not directly accessible, it is possible to infer them by *fitting* the model to their sequence of actions; that is, by finding parameters that maximize the probability the model would produce a similar sequence of actions when presented with the same sequence of stimuli (see section 2.5).[2]

7.4.3 Including Uncertainty in the Model

The above model ignores one central aspect of the signal-detection task: stimuli are only displayed very briefly, and so participants can never be certain about which of the two stimuli they actually observed. To account for perceptual uncertainty about the stimulus, Huys et al. (2013) expanded the model to assume that when participants compute the internal weights that guide their decision, they incorporate the possibility for both stimuli to have been presented. This leads to an updated equation for the weights, which now includes a term for stimulus s as well as a term for the alternative stimulus $\bar{s}$:

$$W_t(a_t, s_t) = \gamma I(a_t, s_t) + \zeta Q_t(a_t, s_t) + (1-\zeta)Q_t(a_t, \bar{s}_t) \tag{7.4}$$

Huys et al. (2013) use the parameter ζ to capture the average certainty (i.e., their belief) about which stimulus they actually observed and called this model "Belief."

7.4.4 Testing More Hypotheses

Reinforcement learning models can be used to describe specific hypotheses about the behavior of participants while performing the task. Model comparison (see also section 2.5) then allows one to find the model that "best fits" the data, by which is generally meant that the model is neither too simplistic nor too complex and can explain how the data was generated. Usually, model comparison is used to test different hypotheses, heuristics, or strategies that participants may employ to solve the task. One other such hypothesis about performance in the signal-detection task is that participants could feel as if they are being punished when they do not receive a reward on a given trial. In the models described above, the reward r was coded as 1 or 0 (presence or absence of reward). Huys et al. (2013) changed the model to test the possibility that participants would perceive a lack of reward as punishment by including a punishment sensitivity parameter $\bar{p}$. The prediction-error term therefore becomes

$$\delta_t = \rho r_t + \bar{p}(1-r_t) - Q_t(a_t, s_t) \tag{7.5}$$

Table 7.1
Summary of models

Model name	Prediction error	W update
Stimulus-action	$\delta_t = \rho r_t - Q_t(a_t, s_t)$	$W_t(a_t, s_t) = \gamma I(a_t, s_t) + Q_t(a_t, s_t)$
Belief	$\delta_t = \rho r_t - Q_t(a_t, s_t)$	$W_t(a_t, s_t) = \gamma I(a_t, s_t) + \zeta Q_t(a_t, s_t) + (1 - \zeta) Q_t(a_t, \bar{s}_t)$
Punishment	$\delta_t = \rho r_t + \bar{p}(1 - r_t)$ $\quad - Q_t(a_t, s_t)$	$W_t(a_t, s_t) = \gamma I(a_t, s_t) + \zeta Q_t(a_t, s_t) + (1 - \zeta) Q_t(a_t, \bar{s}_t)$
Action	$\delta_t = \rho r_t - Q_t(a_t, s_t)$	$W_t(a_t, s_t) = \gamma I(a_t, s_t) + 0.5 Q_t(a_t, s_t) + 0.5 Q_t(a_t, \bar{s}_t)$

The choice probability is always $p(a_t|s_t) = \sigma(W_t(a_t, s_t) - W_t(\bar{a}_t, s_t))$, and the Q update is always $Q_{t+1}(a_t, s_t) = Q_t(a_t, s_t) + \varepsilon \times \delta_t$.

A final possibility is that participants might completely ignore the stimuli and only focus on the values of actions. Huys et al. (2013) formalized an "Action" model by setting the ζ parameter of the Belief model (in equation 7.4) to 0.5, which results in the weights equation

$$W_t(a_t, s_t) = \gamma I(a_t, s_t) + \frac{1}{2} Q_t(a_t, s_t) + \frac{1}{2} Q_t(a_t, \bar{s}_t) \tag{7.6}$$

The ζ parameter captures the average "belief" about which stimulus they actually observed. By fixing the parameter at 0.5, participants are assumed to (on average) ignore the stimulus and only update the value of their actions. This means they would only learn about the values of a "left" or "right" button press.

Table 7.1 summarizes all four models.

7.4.5 Results

Huys et al. (2013) found that the Belief model best explained the data, and therefore focused further analysis on this single model (figure 7.5a). The authors also performed additional checks. For example, they confirmed that the model could explain more choices than a null model that assumed participants always chose options randomly. Huys et al. (2013) then attempted to relate the estimated model parameters to measures of depressive symptoms severity, and in particular to anhedonia. The authors used the anhedonic depression (AD) questionnaire. They performed a correlation analysis to investigate whether primary reward sensitivity (ρ) or learning (ε) was most associated with AD (figure 7.5b). They found a negative correlation between ρ and AD, but no significant correlation between ε and AD. This suggested that reward sensitivity rather than learning rate is primarily impaired in AD.

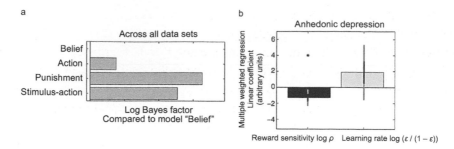

Figure 7.5
Results of the signal-detection task (adapted from Huys et al. 2013). (a) Results of the model comparison. Compared to the three alternative models, the "Belief" model was shown to be the most parsimonious explanation for the data. (b) Linear (correlation) coefficients between anhedonic depression and reward sensitivity (left; significant at $p < 0.05$) and learning rate (right; not significant) parameters. (See Huys et al. 2013 for details on this hierarchical regression analysis.)

There are limitations to these results. For example, Huys et al. (2013) found that reward sensitivity and learning rate were strongly negatively correlated. Additionally, the reward-sensitivity parameter could not be distinguished from a temperature parameter typically included in the softmax decision rule. This means that differences in the reward-sensitivity parameter might have masked differences in the exploration–exploitation behavior of participants. Another aspect of reward processing the study did not touch on is effort, which is a large part of everyday decision-making. Because in the signal-detection task participants always have to exert the same amount of effort (a button press) independent of the stimulus they chose, it was not possible to address this here.

7.5 Discussion

Depression is a devastating disease with a major societal impact and rising prevalence (Vos et al. 2012), making it an important area of study. Due to unclear boundaries between categorical definitions of psychiatric disorders, current research often focuses on individual personality traits, such as neuroticism, or depression symptoms, such as anhedonia, both of which have been identified as promising endophenotypes of depression (Pizzagalli 2014). However, it has been noted that anhedonia itself encompasses various subdomains (e.g., hedonic response to pleasurable stimuli, but also motivation to pursue such stimuli), and these also need to be teased apart (Treadway and Zald 2013).

Patients suffering from depression routinely display impairments in a range of different experimental paradigms (Snyder 2013; Rock et al. 2014; Chen et al. 2015; Rupprechter et al. 2018). Different computational tools and techniques (connectionist models, diffusion models, reinforcement learning techniques, Bayesian decision theory) have been used to describe this (abnormal) behavior and brain activity in depression to gain insight into cognitive and neural processes and to make predictions.

An important aim for computational psychiatry is the development of computational assays that can be used to separate patients into subgroups, generate treatment recommendations, and make predictions for the outcome of those treatments (Stephan, Baldeweg, and Friston 2006; Stephan and Mathys 2014; Chekroud et al. 2016). As Huys et al. (2016a) put it, "aspects of decision making that have predictive value may become useful for the guidance of treatment or for alternative (and complementary) classifications of psychiatric disorders and individual patients." Reinforcement learning has been described as especially promising in this regard (Hitchcock et al. 2017), and has indeed shown potential for classification of depression from purely behavioral data without the need for (subjective) questionnaires (Huys and Dayan 2009).

Commonly observed pessimistic cognitive biases in depression have been explained using prior beliefs within the framework of Bayesian decision theory (Huys et al. 2015a; Stankevicius et al. 2014). Simulations of neural network models have shown that biases could arise from a combination of different mechanisms, including overlearning of negative information and rumination (Siegle and Hasselmo 2002). Drift-diffusion models have been used to explain how aberrant behavior relates to executive control deficits (Dillon et al. 2015; Vallesi et al. 2015) and rumination (Pe et al. 2013).

Reinforcement learning models in which behavior is fitted on a trial-by-trial basis make it possible to measure group differences in behavior that are not obvious from raw data. Our case study (Huys et al. 2013) pooled data from various studies using the same experimental paradigm and fitted different reinforcement learning models according to hypotheses of the behavior of participants. The goal was to better understand anhedonia and how it is related to aberrant reward processing. Results indicated that the symptom is primarily associated with the initial experience of reward, rather than the reward-learning mechanism.

On the neuronal level, there is substantial evidence that dopamine neuron activity encodes reward-prediction errors (among other things; Schultz 1998; Iglesias et al. 2017). Work by Kumar et al. (2008) and Gradin et al. (2011) revealed that, in depression, prediction-error signals appear reduced in the striatum and other dopamine-rich regions of the brain, suggesting that symptoms of depression are associated with an abnormal encoding of reward-learning signals.

It is worth noting that in the meta-analysis of Huys et al. (2013), the authors found the two parameters of interest (reward sensitivity and learning rate) to be highly negatively correlated. Small changes in one of the parameters could therefore be compensated by changes in the other parameter, and Huys et al. (2013) had to perform additional analyses in order to increase their confidence in the fitted parameter values. The authors used the popular softmax function to model decision probabilities, but decided against adding a temperature (or exploration–exploitation) parameter, because it would have traded off against the important reward-sensitivity parameter. Changes in one of these parameters could have been compensated for by changes in the other parameter. The larger question here is how to reliably distinguish between parameters. At least some computational variables are thought to be encoded in the brain (Iglesias et al. 2017), for example dopamine neurons' activity is believed to encode prediction errors. However, to discover these biological correlates we need reliable estimates that are not confounded by other parameters. The signal-detection task was not initially designed with reinforcement learning modeling in mind, for example, and one could think about running a subtask to isolate exploration–exploitation behavior and estimate the temperature parameter independently. Replication of results, especially involving larger numbers of participants, will also be important before useful computational assays can be developed. Paulus, Huys, and Maia (2016) published a pipeline describing additional phases necessary for computational psychiatry to support the development for new drugs.

Current research has often focused on reward. While the omission of a reward might be felt as punishment by participants (as was assumed in Huys et al. 2013), Chen et al. (2015) point out that reward and punishment processing involve different neural bases. They hypothesize that depression might be characterized by a gain-loss asymmetry, so that patients experience decreased reward sensitivity but increased punishment sensitivity. As mentioned above, reward processing can also further be subdivided into different domains. The association between anhedonia and the motivation to exert effort could not be addressed in our case study. In natural settings, patients weigh the pros (reward outcome) against the cons (effort required) to make a decision (cost-benefit analysis). Therefore, when an individual displays an abnormally large effort sensitivity, perceiving efforts as more effortful than they objectively are, they may decide against engaging in a potentially rewarding activity. The effort cost might be perceived as outweighing the potential reward outcome. This is also related to what is observed in Parkinson's patients who display high levels of apathy (a symptom akin to anhedonia; Husain and Roiser 2018). In the future, scientists may want to design tasks that enable them to test hypotheses about different reward-learning domains such as effort sensitivity and reward sensitivity.

While much research points toward behavioral deficits of patients suffering from MDD, there is also evidence for improved performance in depression (Beevers et al. 2013). Replications and robust (computational) techniques will be needed to pinpoint exactly when impairments occur and how they relate to aberrant brain activity. Memory impairments are common in depression (Rock et al. 2014; Snyder 2013), but computationally they seem as of yet still largely unexplored. Notably, Dombrovski et al. (2010) included a memory parameter in their reinforcement learning model and found that depressed suicide attempters discounted previously observed rewards more than healthy controls. It has been proposed that many observed impairments in schizophrenia could potentially be explained by deficits in the memory of patients (Strauss et al. 2010; Collins et al. 2014). Future research might want to consider whether memory

Box 7.1

Open Questions in Computational Research Regarding Depressive Disorders

- Is there a more objective way to diagnose major depression, which does not rely on (subjective) interviews?
- Can we build automated assessment or screening tools using (computational modeling of) behavior during decision-making tasks?
- Should we focus on categorical definitions, individual symptoms, or networks of symptoms (Borsboom and Cramer 2013)? How are symptoms of depression related to other psychiatric disorders—especially anxiety?
- How far will brief experimental studies in the lab or clinical setting take us in the quest to better understand depression? How important is it to assess behavior within more ecologically valid environments (e.g., using mobile phones to collect data during day-to-day activities)?
- How can we combine machine-learning (data-driven) approaches with theory-driven computational modeling (Huys et al. 2016b) to make use of vast amounts of data?
- When is it sufficient to look at behavior, and at what point do we need to include the analysis of brain activity?
- How are abnormalities in brain function related to alterations in brain structure?
- What are the subdomains of reward and punishment processing, and how do these subdomains (e.g., "liking" and "wanting") relate to symptoms of depression?
- To what extent do memory impairments explain observed behavioral abnormalities in depression?
- Can we use the knowledge gained through the computational approach to depressive disorders to develop better pharmacological or psychological therapies or prevention strategies?

impairments could also be a (partial) explanation for many of the observed abnormalities in depression.

7.6 Chapter Summary

Behavioral impairments are prevalent in depression, and computational methods provide a useful tool to tease apart different (neural) mechanisms that might influence learning and decision making. Computational modeling of behavior in participants with depression has provided refinement and additional evidence for theories of MDD, which suggest that negative (perceptual) biases, deficient cognitive control, impaired reward learning, and beliefs about the controllability of the environment are all important aspects of the disease. Clever task design and replication involving larger samples, combined with robust computational techniques, are now needed to advance the field. It is important as well not to neglect the study of patients with moderate-to-severe mood disorders (rather than participants with low mood or mild forms of depression, who are often easier to study) and even of treatment-resistant patients. We want to move from findings that are able to distinguish between groups of patients and healthy control participants to results that show convincing individual differences along symptom dimensions. This will ultimately be necessary to make treatment recommendations and predictions of outcomes for individuals based on noninvasive measurements.

7.7 Further Study

Chen et al. (2015) review a large number of computational studies in depression, focusing on reinforcement learning approaches. Early model-based neuroimaging studies showing altered brain activity during Pavlovian and instrumental learning in depression can be found in Kumar et al. (2008) and Gradin et al. (2011). Huys et al. (2015a) provide a compelling decision-theoretic analysis of depression and its symptoms. A recent study by Pulcu and Browning (2017) suggests that affective biases (i.e., the tendency to differentially prioritize the processing of negative events relative to positive events, which is commonly observed in depression) may be related to individuals attributing higher information content to negative events than positive events. Recently, the availability of large amounts of data has enabled machine learning approaches to be used for treatment outcome predictions (Chekroud et al. 2016).

8   Anxiety Disorders from a Computational Perspective

Erdem Pulcu and Michael Browning
Department of Psychiatry, University of Oxford

8.1 Introduction

Anxiety disorders are among the most common psychiatric diagnoses, with the lifetime prevalence of any of the disorders estimated to be as high as 33% (Alonso, Lépine, and ESEMeD/MHEDEA 2000 Scientific Committee 2007). A range of specific diagnoses is included under the umbrella term of anxiety disorders (table 8.1). Many of these specific diagnoses are based around the context in which symptoms of anxiety are evoked. For example, social anxiety disorder describes a condition in which anxiety is evoked by social situations, whereas agoraphobia describes a condition in which anxiety is evoked by being in situations from which it is difficult to escape (or where help is not available). There has been some debate about the precise set of diagnoses which should be included as anxiety disorders, with the recent version of the *Diagnostic and Statistical Manual* (*DSM-V*) opting to move obsessive-compulsive disorder and post-traumatic stress disorder out of the anxiety category and into their own categories (see table 8.1 for summary of anxiety-related diagnoses in recent diagnostic manuals). Generally, a diagnosis of one of the anxiety disorders requires that significant symptoms of the disorder are present, often for at least six months, that the symptoms cause significant difficulties in everyday life, and that they cannot be better accounted for by other psychiatric or medical conditions or by the effects of drugs or alcohol.

A second approach to subdividing the anxiety disorders, other than the context in which symptoms are evoked, is whether symptoms of fear or worry are predominant in the presentation of the disorder. Fear describes a set of responses, including physiological, behavioral, and subjective, to a well-defined threat and is characteristically seen in the specific phobias, such as phobias of animals like spiders, or situations such as darkness. In contrast, worry describes a set of responses to less well-defined, often potential future threats and is characteristically seen in generalized anxiety disorder. It is generally easier to elicit fear responses in a laboratory setting or in animal models

Table 8.1

Brief descriptions of anxiety disorder diagnoses, including separate diagnoses classified as anxiety disorders in the DSM-IV

Disorder	Brief description
Obsessive-compulsive disorder*	Patients experience unpleasant, intrusive thoughts ("obsessions") and/or the need to perform associated actions ("compulsions")
PTSD*	Patients experience anxious symptoms following a threatening experience (e.g., being in a car crash, being attacked)
Specific phobia	Patients experience anxiety when faced with specific objects, places, animals, etc. (e.g., spider phobia)
Social anxiety disorder	Patients experience anxiety particularly when in social situations or when having to perform (e.g., give a talk)
Panic disorder	Patients experience recurrent "panic attacks," which include both catastrophic thoughts (e.g., feeling like they are going to die) and physical symptoms such as chest pain or shortness of breath. Often associated with agoraphobia
Agoraphobia	Patients experience anxiety particularly when in situations from which it would be difficult to escape (e.g., on airplanes) or where help may not be available (e.g., outside the home)
Generalized anxiety disorder	Patients worry about a range of activities and/or events. This is commonly associated with depression

*These disorders were moved to different categories in *DSM-V*. PTSD, post-traumatic stress disorder.

than it is to induce worry. As a result of this, much of the etiological work relevant to anxiety, including that reviewed below, has focused on the systems responsible for the production of fear responses rather than those implicated in worry.

Lastly, as with many psychiatric conditions, it is worth noting that symptoms of anxiety in the population appear to occur on a continuum, with little evidence of qualitative shifts in symptoms between "clinical" and "nonclinical" groups. Because of this, studies that examine "trait anxiety," the tendency to experience symptoms of anxiety in everyday life, can be informative when considering etiological processes in the anxiety disorders.

In this chapter, we provide a brief overview of the relevant conceptual background and results of recent studies that have taken a computational approach to study anxiety (for review, see also Raymond, Steele, and Seriès 2017; Grupe 2017; and Bishop and Gagne 2018) before describing one study (Browning et al. 2015) in more detail. We end by briefly summarizing the state of the literature and suggesting how it may most effectively be developed.

8.2 Past and Current Computational Approaches

The observation that underpins much of the mechanistic work investigating anxiety disorders is that individuals can learn to fear stimuli or situations they previously did not fear and, equally, can learn that previously feared stimuli or situations are in fact safe. This was memorably demonstrated a century ago in the experiments carried out by John Watson and Rosalie Rayner on the nine-month-old child known as "Little Albert." In these studies, Albert was allowed to play with a white laboratory rat, to which he showed no fear. Following this, whenever he touched the rat, the experimenters made a sudden loud noise by banging a hammer against a steel bar, which startled Albert. Subsequently, when the rat was shown to Albert, he would react with fear, even though no loud sounds were made. In other words, Albert had associated a neutral stimulus (the rat; in conditioning parlance, called the conditioned stimulus, or CS+) with an aversive stimulus (the loud sound, called the unconditioned stimulus, or US) and had thus learned to show a fear response (crying, the conditioned response, or CR) to the rat. Notwithstanding developments in the ethical oversight of experimental studies that have curtailed psychologists' freedom to traumatize infants, the same general experimental procedure has formed the basis of a large body of fear-conditioning studies in humans and animals. The methodology of the studies has been developed by including control stimuli (CS–) that are not paired with aversive outcomes and by examining extinction (i.e., the reduction of a previously learned fear association that occurs when the CS+ is presented in the absence of a US), which allows these studies to test some simple hypotheses about the etiology of anxiety disorders:

a. Do patients with anxiety disorders demonstrate an enhanced learning of fear association to the CS+?

b. Do patients with anxiety disorders demonstrate a reduced extinction of fear associations?

c. Do patients with anxiety disorders demonstrate a greater generalization of the fear CR (i.e., do patients respond to safe stimuli, CS–, as if they were associated with the aversive outcome)?

A recent meta-analysis of fear-conditioning studies in anxious participants (Duits et al. 2015) did not find evidence for enhanced fear learning to the CS+ (although see the earlier meta-analysis reported by Lissek et al. 2005 for slightly different conclusions), but did find evidence for reduced extinction of the CS+ and for increased generalization from the CS+ to the CS–.

The relative ease with which fear-conditioning paradigms can be deployed in animal models has stimulated a well-developed mechanistic literature on the amygdala-based neural systems that support fear learning (Duvarci and Pare 2014; Johansen et al. 2011) and a parallel clinical neuroimaging literature in anxious patients (LeDoux and Pine 2016; Craske et al. 2017). The overarching picture from the latter describes a tendency for anxious individuals to show increased limbic (including amygdala) and reduced frontal activity in response to aversive stimuli (Indovina et al. 2011). While this work has led to mechanistic models that describe specific roles for distinct neural systems in the anxiety disorders (LeDoux and Pine 2016), to date computational approaches have not been employed in this work. As a result, we focus in the rest of this chapter on studies that examine the behavior of anxious individuals and how computational techniques have been used to investigate this.

Conditioning studies such as those described above are well suited to computational descriptions, with much of the early models of reinforcement learning being used to capture learning behavior in animal conditioning studies (Rescorla and Wagner 1972). However, computational approaches have rarely been applied to behavioral or physiological measures in human fear-conditioning studies relevant to anxiety. One reason for this may be that traditional human fear-conditioning tends to employ "strong situations" (Lissek, Pine, and Grillon 2006) in which a CS+ (e.g., a shape on a screen) is paired deterministically with a unconditioned stimulus such as a shock. When faced with this sort of radically simple study design, human participants can generally learn the association between the CS+ and the aversive outcome in one or two trials. In this sort of simple learning situation, behavioral or physiological responses over only a handful of trials are generally collected. Such responses can be adequately captured using simple summary statistics, and computational analysis tends not to add much. However, concern regarding the ability of strong situations to capture the aspects of fear learning most relevant to anxiety has prompted recent studies to explore how anxiety is related to learning in more ambiguous situations. Such situations represent areas in which computational descriptions start to be more useful.

One approach to introducing ambiguity into fear-conditioning studies has been to utilize strong fear-conditioning procedures, with CS+/CS– stimuli strongly associated with the presence/absence of aversive outcomes, but then test participants' response to stimuli that are ambiguous with regard to their identity as CS+ or CS–. For example, Lissek and colleagues (Lissek et al. 2010) used a large ring stimulus as a CS+ and a small ring as an unambiguous CS– in patients with panic disorder and controls. Following this, participants were presented with stimuli of intermediate size, while startle response was measured using electromyography (EMG). In keeping with similar work in a variety of clinically anxious populations from the same laboratory, patients with panic disorder showed a greater degree of generalization of the CR than controls; that is, they reacted to a greater proportion of the ambiguous stimuli as if they were a CS+ than controls. This work suggests that anxiety may be associated with a difficulty in precisely representing states of the world, in accurately assigning credit for aversive outcomes or with a reduced belief in one's ability to avoid future aversive outcomes (Zorowitz, Momennejad, and Daw 2019). While finding the optimal approach to generalization and credit assignment is a core question tackled by the machine-learning literature (Alpaydin 2009), to date fear-conditioning studies in humans that examine generalization (see Dymond et al. 2015 for a recent review) have again tended to rely on summary statistics rather than computational approaches.

A second way in which ambiguity may be introduced to conditioning studies is by reducing the strength of the association between conditioned and unconditioned stimuli (i.e., by reducing the probability with which an aversive outcome follows a cue) and/or by employing designs in which the strength of this association changes over time (i.e., by changing which cue is most predictive of an outcome; Yu and Dayan 2005). These designs begin to capture some of the complexity missing from simple conditioning studies and highlight the real-world challenges faced by an individual trying to learn what may harm them in the environment. While the specific challenges introduced by this ambiguity are described in more detail in the case study example below, their effect is straightforward—they vastly increase how difficult it is to learn about the causes of aversive outcomes and therefore to select the optimal behaviors that avoid such outcomes. A number of lines of evidence suggest that humans employ various heuristics—simplified decision rules—in order to render this problem more tractable (Tversky and Kahneman 1992; Kahneman and Tversky 1979). The degree to which use of these heuristics is associated with anxiety has been examined in a number of studies using computational techniques.

Two of the most consistently reported heuristics are risk aversion—the tendency to select certain over probabilistic outcomes even when the expected value (i.e., the probability multiplied by the magnitude) of the certain outcome is lower; and loss aversion—the tendency to be more influenced when making a decision by potential losses than potential gains. Avoidance of perceived threatening situations is believed to be a causal process in the anxiety disorders (Barlow 2004), suggesting that both of these heuristics may be exaggerated in anxiety disorders and that reducing them may be an important component of treatment. In order to assess this possibility, Charpentier and colleagues (Charpentier et al. 2017) compared the behavior of a group of clinically anxious patients with nonanxious controls using a gambling task in which both risk and loss aversion could be independently estimated as parameters of a prospect theory (Tversky and Kahneman 1992) inspired decision rule. The authors reported significantly increased risk but not loss aversion in the anxious group, suggesting that the core process associated with anxiety is an aversion of risk rather than a general overweighting of negative outcomes, although the same group also report an increased loss learning rate in response to aversive stimuli (Aylward et al. 2019).

A complementary view of behavioral heuristics during learning and decision making suggests that humans (and animals) combine both a flexible instrumental learning system, which learns the best action to take in response to specific stimuli, with a stereotyped Pavlovian system that responds in an evolutionarily prespecified manner to stimuli (Dickinson and Balleine 2002). The Pavlovian system leads to fast, rigid responses to stimuli, such as generally withholding responses to punishments while facilitating responses to rewards. Mkrtchian and colleagues (Mkrtchian et al. 2017) probed these systems in patients with anxious or mood disorder and controls, using a task in which, on some trials, participants had to respond in line with Pavlovian biases, and other trials in which they had to generate opposing responses (e.g., withhold a response to gain a reward or respond to avoid a punishment). This design allowed the authors to separately estimate the impact of the instrumental and Pavlovian systems on participant behavior using a reinforcement learning model that included parameters that estimated the influence of both systems. The patient group was found to be more strongly influenced by the Pavlovian bias to withhold responses to a punishment, with other model parameters unchanged. The authors suggested that this reliance on Pavlovian inhibition provided mechanistic insight into the behavioral avoidance that is characteristic of anxiety disorders; that is, the avoidance arises because anxious individuals are more influenced by the automatic tendency to withhold responses in the face of punishment.

The final way in which computational approaches have been used in studies of anxiety is as a tool to further decompose cognitive processes that are associated with the disorders. Beyond the learning-based work described above, cognitive accounts of anxiety suggest that habitual threat-related biases—that is, the tendency to prioritize threat-related information at the expense of nonthreatening information—are causally linked to the disorders (Mathews and MacLeod 2005). For example, experimental studies suggest that a greater tendency to direct attention toward threat-related information is causally associated with anxiety (MacLeod et al. 2002). Three separate studies have used drift-diffusion models to decompose reaction-time data from tasks investigating such negative biases in anxiety. As described in section 2.2, drift-diffusion models attempt to capture the process by which decisions (generally perceptual decisions) are made (Ratcliff et al. 2016), breaking this process into an initial non–decision-making stage and a later stage in which evidence is noisily accumulated over time until a decision boundary is crossed. Firstly, White and colleagues (White et al. 2010a) reported that high anxious subjects demonstrated a higher drift rate for threatening, relative to neutral, stimuli, with a later result providing similar evidence using a slightly different metric (White et al. 2016). Aylward and colleagues (Aylward et al. 2017) report similar findings using positive outcomes, with higher anxiety being associated with a lower drift rate for positive stimuli. Together these results are consistent with two possible interpretations: a) that anxious participants view the threatening stimuli as more threatening (and positive stimuli as less positive); or b) that anxious individuals use a lower threshold to classify a stimulus as threatening and a higher threshold to classify positive stimuli. By reparameterizing the traditional measures of negative bias reported for anxious participants, these studies hint at "where" in the process of evidence accumulation biases may be created.

In summary, the centrality of learning and decision-making to the mechanistic literature on anxiety and its disorders makes them well placed to benefit from the insights provided by computational approaches. However, to date relatively few studies of anxiety have employed computational techniques. In the following section, we describe in more detail the results from a study that investigated how anxious individuals deal with the uncertainty caused by learning about an association that changes over time.

8.3 Case Study Example: Anxious Individuals Have Difficulty in Learning about the Uncertainty Associated with Negative Outcomes (from Browning et al. 2015)

8.3.1 Theoretical Background and Expected and Unexpected Uncertainty
As described in the previous section, learning in the real world is more challenging than that captured by traditional conditioning studies (see Pulcu and Browning 2019 for a general discussion of uncertainty estimation). Below we present an example to illustrate the different sources of uncertainty that complicate learning and then describe how this uncertainty can be dealt with.

Imagine trying to learn what mood your cat is in based purely on observing whether it does or does not scratch you when you stroke it (figure 8.1). When the cat is in a good mood, it will only scratch you when it is play-fighting, say on 10% of the times you stroke it (figure 8.1, green areas), whereas when it is in a bad mood it will scratch you on 80% of the times you stroke it (figure 8.1, red areas). The cat's mood is therefore useful to know—because it will help you predict how likely you are to be scratched in the future. However, given that you can't directly observe the cat's mood, you need to

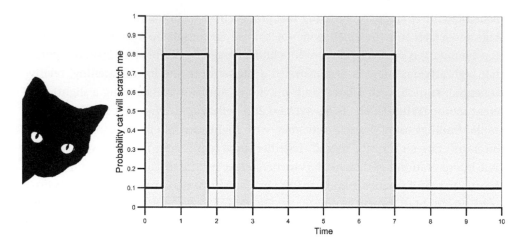

Figure 8.1

Ambiguity in fear learning (Pulcu and Browning 2019). Your cat scratches you 10% of the times you stroke it when it is in a good mood (green areas), and 80% of the time you stroke it when it is in a bad mood (red areas). You can't observe the cat's mood; all you can observe is whether it has scratched you when you previously stroked it. In order to learn what the cat's mood is and therefore how likely it is to scratch you the next time you stroke it, you need to account for two sources of uncertainty: 1) even if you know exactly what the cat's mood is, you can't be certain what its behavior will be (e.g., even when it is in a good mood it will scratch you 10% of the times you stroked it); and 2) the cat's mood changes over time.

infer it based on previous events (whether it scratches you when you stroke it). The first challenge in this task is that being scratched (or not) by the cat is an ambiguous measure of the cat's mood—if you are scratched, it may be because the cat is in a bad mood (and is therefore more likely to scratch you) or it may be because it is play-fighting. Similarly, if you are not scratched, it may be because the cat is in a good mood or that you were just lucky and this time, for whatever reason, it chose not to scratch you even though it was in a bad mood. One way to get a better estimate of the cat's mood is to study its behavior over a longer time period; if you have stroked it 10 times and it has only scratched you once, then it is probably in a good mood (although you still can't be certain of this). However, a further challenge limits how useful collecting data over a longer time period is, since the cat's mood is characterized by some degree of volatility—that is, it will change over time, so even if the cat was in a good mood the last time you stroked it, it may be in a bad mood now, which means you can't rely on the cat's previous behavior, particularly in the distant past, as being representative of its current mood.

In order to learn as accurately as possible what the cat's mood is and therefore how likely it is that you will be scratched, you need to deal with the uncertainty generated by the two challenges described above; first, the cat's behavior is probabilistic rather than deterministic, so even if you know precisely what its mood is, you will not be able to predict with certainty whether it will scratch you when you stroke it. This form of uncertainty is sometimes called "expected uncertainty" (Yu and Dayan 2005), since, after sufficient experience, it can be precisely determined (e.g., you can know that the probability of the cat scratching you is exactly 10% when it is in a good mood, even though you can't say with certainty what will happen on each occasion you stroke it). Expected uncertainty erodes how informative each individual event is when you are learning. For example, imagine your cat's behavior had low expected uncertainty, so that it never scratched you when it was in a good mood but always scratched you when it was in a bad mood. In this case you can instantly tell what mood the cat is in after you have stroked it once. On the other hand, if the cat's behavior has high expected uncertainty, so that it scratches you 40% of the time when it is in a good mood and 60% of the time when it is in a bad mood, it becomes much more challenging to estimate its mood. In other words, the higher the expected uncertainty, the less informative each particular event (i.e., stroking the cat and observing whether it scratches you) is. A second form of uncertainty is produced by changes in the underlying association that you are learning and is sometimes called "unexpected uncertainty" (Yu and Dayan 2005). This occurs when the cat's mood changes from good to bad or vice versa, so that the probability that it will scratch you changes. The effect of unexpected uncertainty is to reduce how informative previous events are during learning. For example, imagine your cat's mood never changes, and the probability that it will scratch you is always 30%. In this case, the unexpected uncertainty is low, and the most accurate way to precisely estimate how likely it is to scratch you (and therefore its mood) is to estimate over many trials the average rate at which it scratches you. In contrast, when learning about a cat whose mood changes frequently—that is, whose behavior has high unexpected uncertainty— you can't rely on distant events, since it is likely that they occurred when the cat was in a different mood than currently, and you have to rely more on recent events. In other words, previous events become increasingly less informative the higher the unexpected uncertainty. In the next section, we introduce a simple learning model to illustrate how one should adapt to these sources of uncertainty during learning.

8.3.2 Learning as a Rational Combination of New and Old Information

The Rescorla-Wagner learning rule (Rescorla and Wagner 1972) provides a simple description of how one might learn what the cat's mood is:

$$r_{(t+1)} = r_{(t)} + \alpha \left(s_{(t)} - r_{(t)} \right) \tag{8.1}$$

In this equation, $r_{(t)}$ is the model's estimate of the probability the cat will scratch you at time t, which we will use as a metric of its mood (i.e., when r is 1, the cat's mood is as bad as it can be, and when it is 0, the cat's mood is as good as it can be). We initialize this so $r_1 = 0.5$ and then update the model's belief every time the cat is stroked using the outcome information $s_{(t)}$, which equals 1 if the cat scratches and 0 otherwise. A single parameter is included, the learning rate α, which lies between 0 and 1. Generally the learning rate is treated as a free parameter or is arbitrarily set at some value. However, in order to learn as efficiently as possible, the learning rate used should adapt to the two sources of uncertainty described above (or, at least, to the learner's estimates of these uncertainties).

Note that in the above equation, $s_{(t)}$, the outcome, represents the new information presented to the model each time the cat is stroked, and $r_{(t)}$ is the model's current belief about the mood of the cat, which has been influenced by all the previous times it has been stroked. If we rearrange the above equation to separate these two variables, we get:

$$r_{(t+1)} = (1 - \alpha) r_{(t)} + \alpha \left(s_{(t)} \right) \tag{8.2}$$

This demonstrates that the Rescorla-Wagner model's belief after each event is simply a weighted mean of the information provided by the recent event $\left(s_{(t)} \right)$ and the model's previous belief $\left(r_{(t)} \right)$, with the learning rate acting as the weight. When the learning rate is 1, all the weight is placed on the new information and the model discards its previous belief, whereas when the learning rate is 0, the model places all the weight on its previous belief and ignores the new information.

In the previous section, we described how expected and unexpected uncertainty influence how informative events are—a high expected uncertainty reduces how informative new events are, while a high unexpected uncertainty reduces how informative previous events are. Efficient learning requires beliefs to be more influenced by informative than noninformative events, indicating how expected and unexpected uncertainty should influence learning rate. High expected uncertainty (i.e., a noisy relationship between cue and outcome) reduces how informative current events are, indicating that a lower learning rate should be used to reflect the fact that previous events are relatively more informative. On the other hand, high unexpected uncertainty (volatility) reduces how informative previous events are, indicating that a higher learning rate should be used. The relationship between unexpected uncertainty and learning rate is illustrated in figure 8.2, in which it can be seen that a model with a high learning rate is better at learning about a volatile cat, whereas a low learning rate is better for a stable cat.

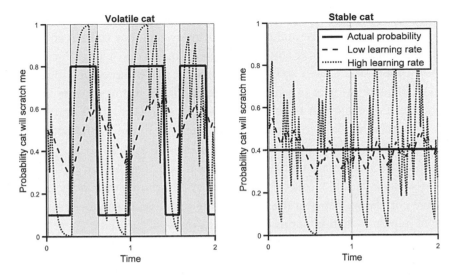

Figure 8.2

The optimal learning rate to use depends on the volatility of the association being learned (Pulcu and Browning 2019). Two Rescorla-Wagner models try to learn how likely two cats are to scratch them. The first cat (left panel) is volatile, with periods of better mood (scratch probability 10%) and worse mood (scratch probability 80%). The second cat (right panel) is stable, with one mood (scratch probability 40%). One model uses a low learning rate (dashed line), the other a high learning rate (dotted line); the solid black line is the underlying truth the models are trying to learn. For the volatile cat (left panel), the model with the high learning rate captures the cat's behavior more accurately than the low learning rate model. This is because the high learning rate model puts more weight on new events than previous events, and the volatility of the cat's behavior reduces how informative previous events are. For the stable cat (right panel), the low learning rate model more accurately captures its behavior, because previous events are more informative.

8.3.3 Effect of Volatility on Human Learning

As explained above, learning about a volatile process is more efficiently achieved with a higher learning rate. A number of studies (Behrens et al. 2007, 2008; Nassar et al. 2012) have examined whether humans adapt their learning as described above; that is, whether humans estimate the volatility of the process they are learning about and tune their learning rate to increase learning efficiency. In all of these studies, participants were required to learn about the association between a cue and a reward during periods in which the association between the two was either volatile or stable. The consistent findings of the studies are that participants adapted the learning rate they used precisely as described above, employing a higher learning rate in volatile rather than stable contexts. Interest has also focused on physiological markers of this volatility estimation process. An early synthesis of animal work (Yu and Dayan 2005) suggested that phasic activity of the central norepinephrine system may contain an estimate of volatility or unexpected uncertainty. This proposition is consistent with current theories (Aston-Jones and Cohen 2005) on the broader role of norepinephrine, which is argued to increase the gain of sensory representations and thus increase their impact on behavior (i.e., analogous to an increased learning rate, which, as described above, is an appropriate response to volatility). Phasic activity of the central norepinephrine system is correlated with pupil dilation in primates (Joshi et al. 2016), suggesting that it may be possible to estimate activity of this system using pupillometry. Nassar and colleagues (Nassar et al. 2012) collected pupillometry data during their study and reported a positive correlation between the learning rate participants employed and the magnitude of pupillary dilation during the outcome phase of their task. These findings are in line with the proposal by Yu and Dayan (2005) and suggest that estimates of central norepinephrine may provide a physiological marker of the neural process that adapts learning rate to estimated volatility.

8.3.4 Summary of Browning et al. (2015) Study

The background presented above suggests that humans adapt their learning to statistical aspects of their environment—such as the stability or volatility of the association they are learning. This observation raises the possibility that anxiety may be associated with difficulties in implementing this adaptation, rather than (or as well as) gross differences in learning about or extinguishing fear associations.

In order to test this possibility, Browning and colleagues (Browning et al. 2015) recruited a group of nonclinical participants who had been prescreened to ensure a range of trait anxiety scores. Participants completed an aversive learning task (figure 8.3) in which two shapes were probabilistically associated with receiving an electric shock while pupillometry data was collected. The crucial manipulation of the task is that it was formed of two blocks (figure 8.3b)—one volatile and one stable.

The learning rate for each participant and each block was estimated by fitting a computational model to participant choice in that block. The model consisted of three stages, with a single free parameter in each stage. First, a simple Rescorla-Wagner rule was used to learn the probability that the shock was associated with "shape A":

$$r_{shapeA(i+1)} = r_{shapeA(i)} + \alpha \varepsilon_{shapeA(i)} \tag{8.3}$$

In this stage, $r_{shapeA(i)}$ is the model's belief on trial i that the shock would be associated with shape A (note that the belief for shape B is simply 1—that for shape A), $\varepsilon_{shapeA(i)}$ is the prediction error and the free parameter α is the learning rate. The second

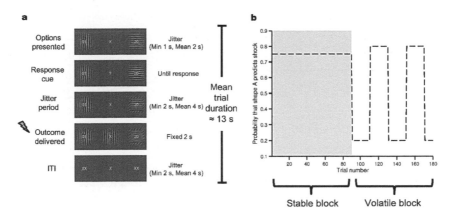

Figure 8.3
Task used in Browning et al. (2015) study. (a) Example trial from the task. Participants were presented with two shapes, each with a number in the center. They chose one shape; if the chosen shape was associated with the electric shock for that trial, they then received the shock after a short delay. The magnitude of the delivered shock was reported by the number in the center of each shape (shock intensity had been calibrated for each participant before the task). Participants therefore had to learn which shape was most likely to be associated with the shock and combine this information with the displayed intensities of the shock for each shape when deciding which shape to choose. (b) Structure of the task. The y axis reports the probability that the shock was associated with "shape a" (the probability that the shock was associated with the other shape is 1 minus these values). The task consisted of 180 trials divided into two blocks. In one block, the shock was stably associated with one shape on 75% of trials. In the other block, the association reversed every 20 trials, from 20% to 80% and back again. Block order (stable, volatile) was counterbalanced across participants.

stage calculated the value g_{shape} of each shape by combining this learned probability, $r_{shapeA(i+1)}$, with the shock magnitude, $I_{shapeA(i+1)}$:

$$g_{shapeA(i+1)} = F\left(r_{shapeA(i+1)}, \gamma\right) * I_{shapeA(i+1)}$$
$$F(r, \gamma) = \max\left[\min\left[\left(\gamma(r-0.5)+0.5\right), 1\right], 0\right]$$

(8.4)

In this stage, $F(r, \gamma)$ transforms the learned probability using the free parameter γ. The effect of this parameter is to either increase or decrease the relative weight of the probability versus the magnitude when calculating the value ($g_{shapeA(i+1)}$) of each shape [i.e., this allows for the possibility that participants did not use the exact product of probability and magnitude when making decisions, but rather could be more influenced by outcome probability ($\gamma > 1$) or magnitude ($\gamma < 1$)]. Finally, the two values are combined using a softmax equation:

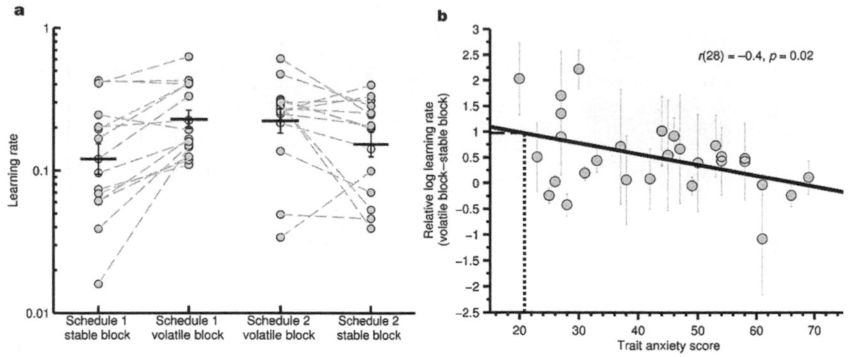

Figure 8.4
Estimated learning rates from the Browning et al. (2015) study. (a) Individual learning rates from the stable and volatile blocks for all participants. As expected, learning rates were significantly higher in the volatile than in the stable blocks. (b) Relationship between trait anxiety (*x* axis) and the degree to which an individual adjusted their learning rate between the volatile and stable blocks (*y* axis). A significant negative correlation was seen: the more anxious a participant, the less they adjusted their learning rate between blocks. The dashed line shows the behavior of a normative Bayesian learner (Behrens et al. 2007) that performs the task optimally; the dotted line illustrates that the behavior of the learner is similar to those participants with low levels of anxiety. The behavior of participants with low anxiety is more like this learner than participants with high anxiety. Anxiety was not associated with differences in any of the other model parameters.

$$P_{(\text{choice=shape}A)} = \frac{1}{1+\exp^{\left(-\beta\left(g_{\text{shape}B}-g_{\text{shape}A}\right)\right)}} \tag{8.5}$$

This stage has a single free parameter, β, the inverse temperature that controls the degree to which the values influence choice. The results derived from fitting this model are displayed in figure 8.4. The critical result is displayed in panel B, which shows the relationship between trait anxiety and the degree to which participants altered their learning rate between the volatile and stable blocks. As can be seen, participants with lower anxiety adjusted their learning rate to a greater extent than participants with high anxiety. In other words, anxiety was not associated with a grossly increased or decreased learning rate during this task; rather, anxious participants were less sensitive to the volatility of the task and adjusted their learning rate less.

The second question addressed in the study was the degree to which the physiological measure of central norepinephrine function, pupil dilation, was related to the behavioral measure of learning rate and to trait anxiety (figure 8.5). This was assessed using a two-stage analysis of the pupil data, similar to that employed in fMRI studies.

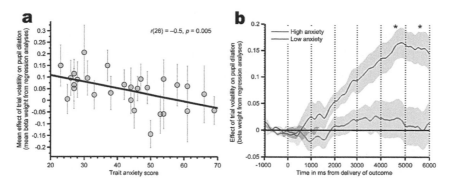

Figure 8.5

Relationship between pupil dilation and trait anxiety. The degree to which pupil dilation during the outcome of a trial was influenced by trial volatility was estimated using regression analyses performed separately for each participant; the larger the beta weights from these analyses, the more that participant's pupil dilated during volatile relative to stable trials. Panels (a) and (b) illustrate the same results. Panel (a) demonstrates that the mean effect of volatility on a participant's pupil dilation across the entire 6-second outcome period was negatively correlated with trait anxiety. Panel (b) uses a median split on participant anxiety to illustrate the mean (shaded area is SEM) time course of the volatility effect in participants with high and low trait anxiety. These results demonstrate that the pupils of participants with high anxiety show less differentiation between volatile and stable trials than those of low-anxiety participants. Asterisks (*) indicate significant difference between the groups after Bonferroni correction for number of time bins.

At the first level, regression analyses were performed for each subject that estimated the degree to which a range of explanatory variables, including estimated volatility, influenced pupil dilation on a trial-by-trial basis. Separate regression analyses were performed for each time point of pupillary data over six seconds after outcomes were presented. These analyses produced time series of beta weights, which estimate the degree to which pupil dilation in an individual participant was influenced by a particular explanatory variable. A second level of analysis then combined these time series across all participants to test whether the explanatory variables influenced pupil dilation across the population of participants. These analyses demonstrated that a greater differential pupil dilation between volatile and stable blocks was positively associated with a greater behaviorally estimated learning rate difference between blocks (results not shown), which is consistent with Yu and Dayan's proposal for the role of norepinephrine (Yu and Dayan 2005). Critically, the analysis also revealed that the pupils of participants with higher anxiety differentiated between volatile and stable blocks less than those of low-anxiety participants.

Overall, this study provided initial evidence that computational approaches may be usefully used to unpick the abnormal fear learning associated with anxiety. Specifically, it suggested that anxiety may be associated with difficulties in estimating the unexpected uncertainty of an environment or in using these estimates to guide learning.

8.4 Discussion

As reviewed in this chapter, anxiety disorders are a prime target for investigations that utilize computational approaches, largely because there is clear evidence for a role for abnormal learning and decision making in their etiology. To date, relatively few studies using computational approaches in anxiety have been published. Although preliminary, the computational work that has been completed has begun to describe differential use of decision-making and learning heuristics in anxious individuals (Charpentier et al. 2017; Mkrtchian et al. 2017), reduced sensitivity to statistical aspects of the environment (Browning et al. 2015), and biased evidence-accumulation processes during threat perception (White et al. 2016; White et al. 2010a; Aylward et al. 2017).

A common theme across these studies is that computational approaches have been used to identify and describe cognitive processes linked to anxiety that are not readily apparent using traditional analytic strategies. For example, the study by Mkrtchian and colleagues sought to separately estimate the impact of an automatic Pavlovian and a more flexible instrumental learning system on decision-making in anxiety, which would be difficult to achieve without some formal estimation of the effects of the two systems. The motivation for identifying and characterizing such cognitive processes is that they may improve our etiological understanding of anxiety, which, it is hoped, will ultimately facilitate better patient care by improving our ability to stratify diagnoses and/or by guiding the development of novel treatments.

A related observation about the published computational studies is that they have all used case-control designs to investigate and delineate cognitive differences between anxious and nonanxious groups. This is clearly a reasonable first step in identifying processes that are perturbed in anxiety; however, these designs rarely provide tangible clinical benefit, as they don't provide strong evidence for a causal relationship between the processes and symptoms of anxiety or provide the sort of information that might usefully guide treatment. We believe that progress in realizing the clinical benefit of computational studies will require a broader range of study designs to be implemented in the future and suggest two specific examples. First, having identified computationally defined processes associated with anxiety, it will be important to test whether measurement of these processes may be useful in clinical situations. For example, do they predict prognosis or treatment response, suggesting that they may be used to guide treatment decisions? Longitudinal studies in depression have begun to find associations between computationally defined processes and treatment response, suggesting that this approach is feasible (Huys et al. 2016a) and may be usefully deployed in anxiety disorders. The second example concerns the development of novel treatments. Relationships between a cognitive process and anxiety, such as those described in this chapter, are particularly interesting when the relationship is causal. Causality is most clearly established using experimental designs in which the computational process is manipulated and the effects of this on symptoms are then measured. Conceivably, computationally defined processes that are causally related to symptoms may provide a new class of treatment targets for anxiety, so it will be important to establish which of the identified processes are indeed causally related to symptoms rather than simply being associated with them. Manipulation of computational processes may be achieved using targeted cognitive interventions, such as those used in the cognitive bias modification literature (Browning et al. 2012). However, an advantage of computational approaches generally is that they have been successful in linking cognitive processes to the underlying neural and neurochemical systems that produce them. This raises the possibility of also using pharmacological interventions to manipulate the computational processes, such as using norepinepheric agents to alter learning rate (Jepma et al. 2016). Currently, the most commonly used pharmacological treatments for anxiety are benzodiazepines, which enhance central GABA transmission, and serotonin-reuptake inhibitors, which increase synaptic serotonin. While the molecular effects of these agents have been well characterized, their impact on cognitive processes is less clear. Computational approaches may also be used to extend our understanding of these drugs' mechanism of action, possibly by examining their impact on the computational outcomes described in this chapter.

A final observation is that, if a clinical impact is to be achieved, it will be essential to ensure that published computational results are as robust and reliable as possible. Reliability is demonstrated by the replication of results, and robustness requires the collection of large clinical data sets. Both of these goals will be facilitated by closer collaboration between disparate research teams in the computational field. Such collaborations are becoming increasingly feasible with developments in online communication technology as well as stimulus presentation and analysis software that facilitates the sharing of tasks and code as well as general communication between centers. The nascent field of computational psychiatry is well placed to take advantage of these developments (Browning et al. 2019).

To conclude, computational approaches in anxiety are in their infancy, and they have shown early promise in being able to identify and describe novel cognitive processes related to anxiety. Translation of this promise into clinical benefit will require the adoption of robust study methodology and a willingness to employ a broader range of study design.

8.5 Chapter Summary

A large amount of previous work has demonstrated that anxiety and its disorders are associated with abnormal learning about aversive outcomes. Computational approaches can be particularly useful when investigating both learning and decision making although relatively few studies to date have employed these techniques in anxious populations. The studies that have been published suggest that anxious individuals utilize different decision-making and learning heuristics, show reduced sensitivity to statistical aspects of the environment, and biased evidence accumulation during threat perception. While computational work in anxiety is in its infancy, it shows promise in being able to identify novel cognitive processes that are relevant to the disorders and are not apparent using standard analytic approaches. Future work needs to employ robust methodology and a broader range of study design if this promise is to be realized.

8.6 Further Study

Craske and colleagues (Craske et al. 2017) provide a recent and broad (although not computational) review of diagnostic, mechanistic, and treatment-related issues in the anxiety disorders, including a section on the neural, genetic, and cognitive associations of the disorders. This paper would be of interest to those who want a broad introduction to issues in anxiety research. A more focused review on the neurobiology of subjective versus behavioral fear is provided by LeDoux and Pine (LeDoux and Pine 2016). The example study in this chapter measured the changes in learning rate induced by volatility by fitting a simple learning model to a stable and a volatile block of trials. However, computational approaches can also be used to describe the underlying calculations necessary to estimate volatility. A number of previous papers have described different approaches to this problem. While these papers don't specifically focus on anxiety disorders, they provide a useful computational background on how the volatility effect described in this chapter may be conceptualized. First, a seminal study by Pearce and Hall (Pearce and Hall 1980) describe how the Rescorla-Wagner model may be modified such that it adapts to how surprising stimuli are (one way of estimating volatility is as the frequency with which surprising outcomes are observed). Second, a neuroimaging paper by Li and colleagues (Li et al. 2011) suggested that a smoothed version of a Pearce–Hall signal was present in the human amygdala. Behrens and colleagues (Behrens et al. 2007) describe a fully Bayesian approach to this problem. For other reviews of computational studies regarding anxiety, the reader can also consult Raymond, Steele, and Seriès (2017) and Sharp and Eldar (2019).

9 Addiction from a Computational Perspective

A. David Redish
University of Minnesota

9.1 Introduction: What Is Addiction?

Everyone knows what addiction is. We all know people whose lives have been ruined by drugs, and we all have behaviors that we wish we could stop, but don't. However, the definition of addiction remains elusive. Early definitions related to a "lack of will" and suggested addiction was a moral failing. However, this theory did not lead to reliable treatments and left many incapable of ending their addictions. Later definitions defined addiction as a disease and suggested that behavioral and chemical treatments could alleviate it. In particular, these disease-related theories suggested that many drug addictions arose from biological responses to chemical imbalances that could be treated pharmacologically. Some of these pharmacological treatments, such as methadone treatment for heroin addictions (Meyer and Mirin 1979) and the nicotine patch for smoking (Hanson et al. 2003), have been very successful, but other addictions (stimulants, alcohol) have been much more difficult to treat pharmacologically. Furthermore, pharmacological definitions do not include the possibility of nonchemical addictions, such as gambling, which is now seen as an addiction-like problem.

Current definitions of addiction are based on conceptualizations of addiction as a problem with decision-making systems (Heyman 2009; Redish 2013), often evidenced as continued use despite stated preferences (Goldstein 2001; Ainslie 2001) and as continued use despite high cost (Robinson and Berridge 2003; Koob and Le Moal 2006). The most recent models identify addiction as arising from vulnerabilities leading to failure modes in decision-making algorithms (Redish, Jensen, and Johnson 2008).

One of the most common popular descriptions of addiction lies in the addict's continued use despite making explicit statements of a desire to stop. Current theories of decision making reject the hypothesis of the unitary decision-maker—each individual is actually a multiplicity of decision-making systems (algorithms, processes) competing for behavioral control (O'Keefe and Nadel 1978; Daw et al. 2005; Rangel, Camerer, and Montague 2008; Redish et al. 2008; Kahneman 2011; van der Meer, Kurth-Nelson, and Redish 2012; Redish 2013). While this theory provides an explanation for this conflict (Kurzban 2010), computational models of addiction have not emphasized this conflict because it is hard to study in nonlinguistic animals (i.e., nonhumans), while human rights limitations make it difficult to do controlled studies of addiction in humans. Nevertheless, the study of decision-making systems and their interaction is well established in both human and nonhuman animals and has been used computationally to guide treatment.

One of the classic descriptions of addiction is based on the observation that addicts will continue to use even in the face of high costs. This can be quantified through the economic concept of elasticity as a measure of how much one's willingness to buy something changes by its cost (Bickel, DeGrandpre, and Higgins 1993; Hursh 2005). Things that diminish slowly by cost are inelastic. Researchers have suggested that drugs are fundamentally inelastic: as costs increase, the number of rewards paid for decrease less than they should. Of course, there are many things that are inelastic that are not considered addictive—oxygen, for example (where the withdrawal symptoms are particularly traumatic), but also some behaviors continued even in the face of high costs are celebrated, such as Kerri Strug's 1996 Olympic vault performed on a sprained ankle, or Osip Mandelstam continuing to write poetry even after Stalin had thrown him in the gulag for it.

A key to the question of addiction is to separate the science of why an agent continues its behavior from the decision to treat and change that behavior. This conceptualization parallels Jerome Wakefield's conceptualization of psychiatry as depending on harmful dysfunction (Wakefield 1992). "Dysfunction" reflects a system not working as it was intended to. For example, mu-opioid activation signals pleasure in mammalian brains (Berridge and Robinson 2003). These receptors were certainly not evolved to respond to heroin, but they do. "Harmful" reflects a society's choice of what to change. For example, American society is currently transitioning from treating marijuana as so dangerous as to be illegal with severe penalties to something that can better be handled under legal regulation. Things can be harmful without being dysfunctional, such as tribal wars, which are extremely harmful, but likely reflect the natural evolution of human behavior (Turchin 2003; Diamond 2006), and dysfunctional without being harmful, such as synesthesia (Cytowic 1998).

Computational models of addiction are aimed at understanding the science of why an agent continues its behavior and the science of how one could change that behavior if one so desired. Importantly, the decision of whether to change that behavior has not been computationally assessed. Such a decision would depend on sociological models, which are not the focus of this chapter. Instead, this chapter will focus on computational approaches to addictive behavior and its modification.

9.2 Past Approaches

Past computational approaches to addiction can be divided into three broad categories: economic models, in which drugs are seen as economic objects that have feedback properties that make them overvalued; homeostatic models, in which drugs change intrinsic biological properties and shift allostatic set-points, which subsequently require drugs to reach that set-point; and reinforcement learning models, in which drugs hijack learning algorithms to produce aberrant learning. Current views on addiction suggest that these three hypotheses are all failure modes of decision-making systems, and that there are many endophenotypes of drug addiction.

9.2.1 Economic Models

Although popular descriptions of drug use (e.g., *Reefer Madness* [Gasnier 1936], *Long Day's Journey into Night* [O'Neill 1956], *The Lost Weekend* [Wilder and Brackett 1945], *Sid and Nancy* [Cox 1986]) have suggested that drugs are overwhelming and addicts would go to any cost to achieve drug-taking, experimental studies have long suggested that drugs are economic objects and that drug use decreases with increasing costs (Bickel et al. 1993; Liu et al. 1999; Grossman and Chaloupka 1998; Hursh 2005). The first economic model of drug use is Becker and Murphy's (1988) "Rational Addiction" model, which is an economic utility model in which subjects are assumed to select the most cost-effective choice with the highest value. Drugs are assumed to have a positive feedback, so that the more one takes those drugs, the more valuable they become. Becker and Murphy show that under these assumptions, a hypothetical user could be shown to become addicted when the positive feedback overwhelms the negative consequences of the drug use.

These models led to quantitative analyses of drug use, asking direct questions of the economic demand curves of drug use. Demand curves are quantitative measures of elasticity. This can be measured either through effort (how many lever presses will a nonhuman animal push for reward?) or through monetary costs (how many grams of drug will you buy?). In a typical demand curve (figure 9.1), there is an inelastic portion, where increases in cost have little effect on number of rewards bought, and an elastic portion, where the number of rewards bought falls off very quickly. These are separated by an inflection point (*pMax*). Addicts can be defined as people for whom

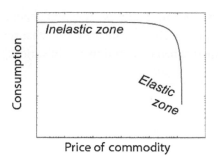

Figure 9.1
The shape of a typical demand curve. As the price of the commodity increases, the number of samples consumed decreases. There is typically an inelastic zone, where large ratio changes have little effect, and an elastic zone, where large ratio changes have a larger effect. Note that both axes are logarithmic. Compare this, for example, to real demand curves as seen in Bruner and Johnson (2013), where subjects were asked how much cocaine they would buy at a hypothetical given price.

this inflection point has shifted far to the right, but nevertheless, their demand curves do have this typical, canonical shape.

A key insight from this economic perspective on drug use is that drugs provide fast rewards and slow consequences. All animals (human and nonhuman) discount future rewards, valuing rewards more if they are delivered in a shorter time frame (Ainslie 1992; Madden and Bickel 2010). Economically, this makes sense, since immediate rewards can be invested, and consequences can prevent the use of later rewards. Importantly, as described in section 5.2, all animals (human and nonhuman) show nonexponential discounting curves (figure 9.2), which means that preferences can cross—thus, it is possible both to prefer to smoke the cigarette in your hand and to prefer to not smoke in the future. (Of course, when the future becomes now, one will want to smoke the cigarette now again.) Addicts show particularly fast discounting functions, which can exacerbate this problem (Bickel and Marsch 2001). There is some evidence that successful treatment modifies these discounting rates in subjects with particularly fast discounting functions (Bickel et al. 2014) and that these discounting rates are predictive of relapse (Sheffer et al. 2014). It is possible to modify discounting rates, guiding the subject's attention to delayed rewards by providing episodic cues about the delayed rewards to make those delayed rewards more concrete (Peters and Büchel 2010). Recent evidence has suggested that these changes can reduce drug use (Stein et al. 2018; Snider et al. 2018). However, whether these changes are due to changes in discounting rates per se or to changes in interacting multiple decision systems remains an open question.

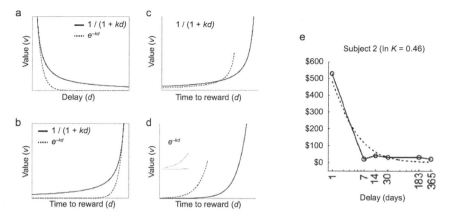

Figure 9.2
Delay discounting. (a) Delay discounting entails a loss of value as a function of delay to an event. Two discounting functions are typically used, hyperbolic [$V = r/(1 + kd)$], and exponential [e^{-kd}], where d is the delay to the event and k is a parameterization factor. (b) Logically, this can be understood in terms of value of an expected event as one approaches the event in time. (c) Hyperbolic discounting functions can create a preference reversal where one prefers one option (the larger, later, solid line) to another (the smaller, sooner, dashed line) that reverses as one approaches the options in time. (d) Exponential discounting, however, does not reverse, even when both options are far away (see inset), showing an expansion of the far-left edge of the graph. (e) A real discounting curve from an individual, reprinted from Kurth-Nelson and Redish (2009).

While the basic economic story that drugs are economic objects that are discounted quickly is clearly correct, drug use is context-sensitive in ways that make these simple economic descriptions incomplete (Bernheim and Rangel 2004). We will return to the question of these economics later, when we come to the interacting multiple systems models below.

9.2.2 Homeostatic Models
All drugs that are reliably self-administered, either by humans or other animals, are pharmacologically similar in some way to endogenous chemicals used in neural processing (Koob and Le Moal 2006). For example, active opioids such as morphine, heroin, or oxycodone activate the mu-opiate receptor; cocaine blocks dopamine reuptake in the synapse, which increases dopamine in the synapse; amphetamine encourages release of dopaminergic vesicles; and nicotine activates acetylcholine receptors. Biological systems in general and neural systems in particular are very sensitive to levels of these endogenous chemicals and have extensive negative feedback processes (such as

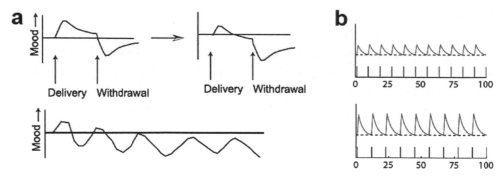

Figure 9.3
Homeostatic/allostatic processes. (a) Drug delivery produces a positive reaction state, which then adapts and collapses to a negative state when the drug is removed. Over time, the user is hypothesized to adapt to the positive state, producing a shift in the allostatic set-point toward the negative state. Redrawn after Koob (2013). (b) Tsibulsky and Norman (1999) and Keramati et al. (2017) modeled self-administration as an attempt to maintain the total level of drug at a given set-point. As the drug was processed internally and reduced beyond the set-point, the animal was hypothesized to seek the drug through lever-pressing. This model explains the different rates of lever-pressing as a function of the drug dose. Redrawn after Tsibulsky and Norman (1999) and Keramati et al. (2017).

trafficking of receptors in and out of the synaptic membrane) that keep the sensitivity balanced. In situations where receptors are flooded, they will normalize their levels, requiring more activation to produce the same effects.

For example, many self-administration experiments (in which animals are trained to press a lever for drug reward) can be described quantitatively in terms of maintenance of pharmacological levels of the drug (Tsibulsky and Norman 1999, Keramati et al. 2017). Negative feedback processes driving maintenance interact with the positive feedback processes of drug utility (as suggested by Becker and Murphy) to produce dramatic differences in valuation between drugs and nondrug rewards (with drugs being valued much higher than nondrugs, leading to overtaking of drug rewards.)

Three quantitative models based on issues of homeostatic balance are the Tsibulsky and Norman (1999), the Keramati et al. (2017), and the Dezfouli et al. (2009) models (figure 9.3). The Tsibulsky and Norman model explicitly hypothesizes that animals are attempting to maintain a specific level of cocaine, which explains quantitatively the observed shifts in response to changes in the dosages given with each lever press. Keramati et al. notes, however, that there are short-term dynamics when the changes actually occur that are not explicable by a simple set-point hypothesis, particularly in the transition that occurs with increased access to drug. They therefore add in a learning component based on the reinforcement learning models detailed below. The Dezfouli et al. model is based on a homeostatic expansion of the Redish (2004) model (see below), particularly looking at the effect of homeostatic set-points driving pharmacological effects of dopamine on learning. While the Redish model is based on the temporal-difference, reinforcement learning dopamine-as-delta model of Montague et al. 1996, and is thus a hijacked-learning model, the Dezfouli et al. model is based on the average reward dopamine hypothesis of Daw and Touretzky (2000), and becomes a homeostatic model.

9.2.3 Opponent Process Theory

One of the earliest models of drug use is the opponent process theory of Solomon and Corbit (1974; see Koob and Le Moal 2006 for extensive discussion of this model), in which drugs are assumed to produce a strong positive reward followed by a strong negative recovery. Homeostatic processes are assumed to normalize the excess drug to decrease the positive factors, and increase the negative factors, which leads to increased need for drugs to return the homeostatic process to baseline. These models have been supported by evidence that chronic drug use leads to enhancement of positive-valuation neuron activity in the nucleus accumbens (Kourrich et al. 2007; Volman et al. 2013) and evidence that the emotional crash after drug use is an important factor in driving self-administration (Rothwell, Gewirtz, and Thomas 2010).

While the Solomon and Corbit (1974) and the Koob and Le Moal (2006) models are not quantitative, Gutkin, Dehaene, and Changeux (2006) proposed an opponent process model in which there is habituation of response processes to a continuous delivery of nicotine—a phasic increase at the start and a phasic decrease at the end, and a decrease in the overall tonic dopamine levels. The normalization caused by the assumed decrease in dopamine levels leads to a decrease in ability to learn non–drug-related cues, which leads to an increase in attention to and learning of drug-related cues. Thus, Gutkin et al. show how an opponent process model can hijack learning process by disrupting the difference between learning on and off drug.

9.2.4 Reinforcement Models

The third family of computational models is based on the concept that learning depends on physical processes, and those physical processes can be modulated by external chemicals and other processes. In animal learning theory, the concept of reinforcement is separate from the concept of reward. Reinforcement is any mechanism that makes an agent more likely to return to an action. An external chemical that increases reinforcement would increase drug-seeking and drug-taking (di Chiara 1999, Redish 2004).

In the 1950s, it was discovered that electrical stimulation of specific neural sites was reinforcing, in that both human and nonhuman animals would activate the stimulation (Olds and Milner 1954), even to the extent of avoiding many other rewards. Interestingly, in humans (who could rate "pleasure" linguistically), these studies found that the most reinforcing stimulations were not always the most pleasant (Heath 1963).

An important breakthrough in the understanding of reinforcement came when Berridge and Robinson directly measured reinforcement and pleasure in nonhuman animals and discovered that they were separable. It was well-known that many drugs of abuse affected dopaminergic functioning and that the stimulation drove dopamine release, and it was thought that dopamine would drive pleasure signals. However, when Berridge and Robinson (2003) directly tested this hypothesis, it was discovered that this was wrong—dopamine and pleasure were dissociable. In their elegant studies, they measured facial expressions of pleasure and disgust in rats under manipulations of dopamine and opiate signals. Dopamine manipulations affected reinforcement but did not affect facial expressions of pleasure. In contrast, manipulations of opiate signals (e.g., mu-opiate and kappa-opiate agonists and antagonists) affected pleasure responses. This led them to hypothesize that drugs that affected dopamine increased the "incentive salience" or "value" of a reward, which drove seeking, independently of the pleasure experienced by that reward.

Around this time, a major breakthrough occurred in the understanding of dopamine function in animal learning—Wolfram Schultz and his team discovered that dopamine cells burst when provided a surprising reward but did not fire when the reward was predicted by a cue (Ljungberg, Apicella, and Schultz 1992). Read Montague and colleagues (1996) realized that this signal was the value-prediction error (VPE)[1] signal δ (delta) that underlay a theory of robotic learning called temporal-difference reinforcement learning (TDRL) that had become very successful in the field of computer science[2] (Sutton and Barto 1998; see also section 2.3).

As described in section 2.3, the TDRL algorithm defines value as the total reward one can expect to achieve given a policy of actions to be taken in given situations. TDRL maintains a representation of the currently believed value for each situation, and then calculates the difference between that remembered value and the observed value. This difference is the value-prediction error, or VPE. Positive VPE occurs anytime a value is better than expected and drives an increased willingness to take an action, while negative VPE occurs anytime a value is worse than expected and drives a decreased willingness to take an action. The concept of VPE is best understood through an example.

Imagine a soda machine. If you put your money in the soda machine and get two sodas out, then you will be more willing to put money in that soda machine next time. (You have positive VPE.) If you put your money in the soda machine and get nothing out, then you will be less willing to put money in that soda machine next time. (You have negative VPE.) And, most importantly, if you put the correct amount of money in the soda machine, get your expected soda out, then you understand how that machine works and you don't need to learn anything about it. (You have zero VPE.) Notice that you still get the pleasure (such as it is) of drinking the soda, but you don't need to change your willingness to put money in that machine. VPE is about learning the value of actions. Computer simulations had shown that VPE would allow an agent to learn to behave in simulated environments (Sutton and Barto 1998). These processes can be expressed in the following equations (see also section 2.3):

$$V(S_k) = \int_t^{\infty} \gamma^{\tau-t} E[R(\tau)] d\tau$$
$$\delta(t) = \gamma^d [R(S_l) + V(S_l)] - V(S_k)$$
$$V(S_k) \leftarrow V(S_k) + \eta\delta$$

(9.1)

Where $V(S_k)$ is the value of state S_k, γ^d is a discounting parameter,[3] reflecting expected value decreases over observed delay d; $R(S_l) + V(S_l)$ is the value achieved on entering state S_l; and $\delta(t)$ is the value-prediction error (the difference between the observed and expected value). By changing the value of state S_k toward the observed value (with learning rate η), $V(S_k)$ will approach the observed value. Theories hypothesized that dopamine signaled the value-prediction error $\delta(t)$.

Redish (2004) proposed that if drugs were providing a dopamine signal pharmacologically, then taking drugs would lead to positive VPE, even if the neural calculation of VPE should have been 0 (figure 9.4). Effectively, Redish's model predicted that the dopamine signal at reward contained two components, one from the calculation of $\delta(t)$, and the other from the pharmacological action of the drug. This meant that even with experience, there would always be a noncompensable VPE signal at the reward, which would increase the predicted value of the reward, driving that value to infinity. (Or with normalization, normalizing all other values to zero.)

$$\delta = \max\{\gamma^d [R(S_l) + V(S_l)] - V(S_k) + D(S_l), D(S_l)\}$$

(9.2)

where $D(S_l)$ reflects the effect of the pharmacological dopamine from the drug.

In his 2004 paper, Redish used computer simulations to show that this model would lead to developing inelasticity (as in the Becker and Murphy hypothesis) and made several untested predictions. The first prediction was that there would be a double

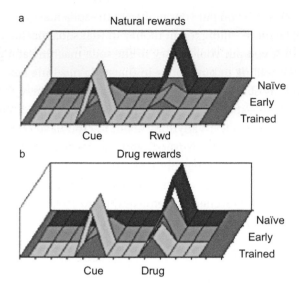

Figure 9.4
The delta signal—dopamine and delta. Diagram of delta (vertical axis) by time (horizontal axis) over three conditions: naïve (untrained), early (with limited training), and trained. (a) With normal rewards, the delta signal shifts from appearing at the unexpected reward to the unexpected cue-that-predicts-reward. (b) In the Redish (2004) model, there are two components in the delta signal, a reward-related component that shifts and a pharmacological component that remains at the reward time. Compare the classic data from Schultz (1998). When the expected reward is not delivered, dopamine cells pause their firing. Aragona et al. (2009) tested the double-bump hypothesis and found that the cue-related signal occurred in accumbens core, while the pharmacological component occurred in shell.

surge of dopamine in drug experiments. In the TDRL theory, $\delta(t)$ first appeared at the time of reward (as it was initially unexpected), and then it shifted to earlier cues that reliably predicted the reward (because the reward was now expected—thus $\delta = 0$, but the cues indicated an unexpected increase in value—thus $\delta > 0$). Similarly, Schultz and colleagues (see Schultz 2002) had found that dopamine shifted from the reward (when unexpected) to the cue (once the animal learned that the cue predicted the reward). In Redish's model, the extra pharmacological component would always appear, even as the dopamine signal appeared at the cue. Since then, this double surge of dopamine has been observed, but as with any theory, reality is more complex than the model, and each component of the double surge occurs separately, with the reward-related surge appearing in accumbens shell and the cue-related surge appearing in accumbens core (Aragona et al. 2009).

The two other key predictions of the Redish 2004 model were (1) that additional drug use would always lead to increased valuation of the drug and (2) that drugs would not show Kamin blocking. As detailed below, these predictions have since been tested and provide insight into the mechanisms of drug addiction.

In the Redish (2004) model, the excess dopamine provides additional value, no matter what. Marks et al. (2010) directly tested this hypothesis in an elegant experiment, where rats were trained to press two levers for a certain dose of cocaine (both levers being equal). One lever was then removed and the other provided smaller doses of cocaine. The Redish (2004) theory predicts that the second lever should gain value, while expectation or homeostatic theories like those discussed earlier would predict that the second lever should lose value (because animals would learn the second lever was providing smaller doses). The Marks et al. data was not consistent with the Redish excess-delta model. However, as noted above, a key factor in drug addiction is that not everyone who takes drugs loses control over their drug use and becomes an addict. Studies of drug use in both human and nonhuman animals suggest that most animals in self-administration experiments continue to show elasticity in drug-taking, stopping in response to high cost, but that a small proportion (interestingly similar to the proportion of humans who become addicted to drugs) become inelastic to drug-taking, being willing to pay excessive costs for their drugs (Anthony, Warner, and Kessler 1994; Hart 2013). One possibility is that the homeostatic models (like that of Tsibulsky and Norman 1999) are a good description of nonaddicted animals, which have a goal of maintaining a satiety level, but that addiction is different.

The Redish (2004) model also predicted that drugs would not show Kamin blocking. Kamin blocking is a phenomenon where animals don't learn that a second cue predicts reward if a first cue already predicts it (Kamin 1969). This phenomenon is well-described by value-prediction error (VPE)—once the animal learns that the first cue predicts the reward, there is no more VPE (because it's predicted!) and the animal does not learn about the second cue (Rescorla and Wagner 1972). Redish noted that because drugs provided dopamine, and dopamine was hypothesized to be that VPE delta signal, then when drugs were the "reward," there was always VPE. Thus, drug outcomes should not show Kamin blocking. The first tests of this, like the Marks et al. study, did not conform to the prediction—animals showed Kamin blocking, even with drug outcomes (Panlilio, Thorndike, and Schindler 2007). However, Jaffe et al. (2014) wondered whether this was related to the subset problem—that only some animals were actually overvaluing the drug. Jaffe et al. tested rats in Kamin blocking for food and nicotine. All rats showed normal Kamin blocking for food. Most rats showed normal Kamin blocking for nicotine. But the subset of rats that were high responders to nicotine did not show Kamin blocking to nicotine, even though they did to food, exactly as predicted by the Redish model.

9.3 Interacting Multisystem Theories

Studies of decision making in both human and nonhuman animals have, for a long time, found that there are multiple decision-making processes that can drive behavior (O'Keefe and Nadel 1978; Daw et al. 2005; Rangel et al. 2008; Redish et al. 2008; Kahneman 2011; van der Meer et al. 2012; see Redish 2013 for review). These processes are sometimes referred to as different algorithms because they process information differently. They are accessed at different times and in different situations; they depend on different neural systems. How an animal is trained and how a question is asked can change which system drives behavior. Damage to one neural structure or another can shift which system drives behavior.

The key to these different systems lies in how they process information. Decision making can be understood as a consequence of three different kinds of information—what has happened in similar situations in the past (memory), the current situation (perception), and the needs/desires/goals (teleology). How information about each of these aspects is stored can change the selected action—for example, what defines "similar situations" in the past? What parameters of the current situation matter? Are the goals explicitly represented or not? Each system answers these questions differently.

Almost all current decision-making taxonomies differentiate between planning (deliberative) systems and procedural (habit) systems. Planning systems include information about consequences—if I take this action, then I expect to receive that outcome, which can then be evaluated in the context of explicitly encoded needs. Planning systems are slow but flexible. Procedural systems cache those actions—in this situation, this is the best action to take, which is fast but inflexible. As described earlier (sections 2.3 and 5.2), many current computational models refer to planning systems as model-based (because they depend on a model of the consequences in the world), while procedural systems are model-free (which is an unfortunate term because procedural systems still depend on an ability to categorize the current situation, which depends on a model of the world; Redish et al. 2007; Gershman, Blei, and Niv 2010). Some taxonomies also include reflex systems, in which the past experience, the parameters of the current situation that matter, and the action to be taken are all hard-wired within a given organism and are learned genetically over generations. Most taxonomies also include a fourth decision system, variously termed Pavlovian, emotional, affective, or instinctual, in which a species-important action (e.g., salivating, running away, approaching food) is released as a consequence of a learned perception (context or cue).

The importance of these systems is threefold. (1) How a question is asked can change which system controls behavior; (2) damage to one system can drive behavior to be controlled by another (intact) system; and (3) there are multiple failure modes of each of these systems and their interaction. We will address each of these in turn.

9.3.1 How a Question Is Asked Can Change Which System Controls Behavior

One way to measure how much rats value a reward such as cocaine is to test them in a progressive ratio self-administration experiment (Hodos 1961). In this experiment, the first hit of cocaine costs one lever press, but the second costs two, the third costs four, the fourth eight, and so on. Eventually a rat has to press the lever a thousand times for its hit of cocaine. Measuring when the rat stops pressing the lever indicates the willingness-to-pay and the value of the cocaine to the rat. Not surprisingly, many experiments have found that rats will pay more for cocaine than for other rewards such as saccharine, indicating that cocaine was more valuable than saccharine. However, Serge Ahmed's laboratory found that if those same rats were offered a choice between two levers, one of which provided saccharine while the other provided cocaine, the rats would reliably choose the saccharine lever over the cocaine lever, indicating that saccharine was more valuable than cocaine (Lenoir et al. 2007, see Ahmed 2010). The most logical explanation for this contradiction is that the progressive ratio accesses one decision system (probably procedural) while the choice accesses another (probably deliberative), and that the two systems value cocaine differently. Interestingly, Perry, Westenbroek, and Becker (2013) found that a subset of rats will choose the cocaine, even in the two-option paradigm. These are the same subset of rats that overvalue cocaine in other contexts, such as being willing to cross a shock to get to the cocaine (Deroche-Gamonet 2004). Whether they are also the high responders or whether they no longer show Kamin blocking remains unknown.

9.3.2 Damage to One System Can Drive Behavior to Another

Imagine an animal pressing a lever for an outcome (say, cheese). If the animal is using a planning system to make its decisions, then it is effectively saying, "If I push this lever, I get cheese. Cheese is good. Let's press the lever!" If the animal is using the procedural system, then it is effectively saying, "Pressing the lever is a good thing. Let's press the lever!"—and cheese never enters into the calculation. What this means is that if we make cheese bad (by devaluing it, which we can do by pairing cheese with a nauseating agent like lithium chloride), then rats using planning systems won't press the lever anymore ("If I push this lever, I get cheese. Yuck!"), but rats using procedural systems will ("Pressing the lever is a good thing. Let's press the lever!"). (See, for example, Niv, Joel, and Dayan 2006 for a model of this dichotomy.) Many experiments have determined that with limited experience, animals are sensitive to devaluation (i.e., they are using a planning system), while with extended experience they are not (i.e., they are using a procedural system), and that lesions to various neural systems can shift this behavior (Killcross and Coutureau 2003; Schoenbaum, Roesch, and Stalnaker 2006). A number of studies have suggested that many drugs (cocaine, amphetamine, alcohol) drive behavior to procedural devaluation-insensitive systems, which has led some theoreticians to argue that drug addiction entails a switch from planning to habit modes (Everitt and Robbins 2005).

Building on the anatomical data known to drive the typical shift from planning to procedural decision systems, Piray et al. (2010) proposed a computational model in which drugs disrupted the planning-valuation systems and accelerated learning in the procedural-valuation systems. This model suggested that known changes in dopaminergic function in the nucleus accumbens as a consequence of chronic drug use could lead to overly fast learning of habit behaviors in the dorsal striatum and would produce a shift from planning to habit systems due to changes in valuation between the two systems.

9.3.3 There Are Multiple Failure Modes of Each of These Systems and Their Interaction

However, rats and humans will take drugs even when they plan. A drug addict who robs a convenience store to get money to buy drugs is not using a well-practiced procedural learning system. A teenager who starts smoking because he (incorrectly) thinks it will make him look cool and make him attractive to girls is making a mistake about outcomes and taking drugs because of an error in the planning system (the error is in his understanding of the structure of the world.)

Some researchers have argued that craving depends on the ability to plan, because craving is transitive (one always craves *something*), and thus it must be depend on expectations and a model-based process (Tiffany 1999; Redish and Johnson 2007). In fact, there are many ways that these different decision systems could drive drug-seeking and drug-taking (Redish et al. 2008). Some of those processes would depend on expectations (i.e., would be model-based, and depend on planning) and explicit representations of outcomes, and could involve craving, while other processes would not (i.e., would be model-free, depending, for example, on habit systems). (An important consequence of this is the observation that seems to get rediscovered every decade or so that craving and relapse are dissociable—you can crave without relapsing and you can relapse without craving.)

In 2008, Redish and colleagues surveyed the theories of addiction and found that all theories of addiction could be restated in terms of different failure modes of this multi-algorithm decision-making system. An agent that succumbed to overproduction of dopamine signals (Redish 2004) from drug delivery would overvalue drugs and would make economic mistakes to take those drugs. An agent that switched decision systems to habit faster under drugs (Everitt and Robbins 2005; Piray et al. 2010) would become inflexible in response to drug offerings and take drugs even while knowing better. An agent with incorrect expectations ("smoking makes you cool," "I won't get cancer") would make planning mistakes and take drugs in incorrect situations. An agent who discounted the future ("I don't care what happens tomorrow, I want my pleasure today") would be more likely to take drugs than an agent who included future consequences in its plans (Bickel and Marsch 2001). All of these are different examples of vulnerabilities within the decision-making algorithms. Redish et al. (2008) proposed that drug addiction was a symptom, not a disease—that there were many potential causes that could drive an agent to return to drug use, and that efficacious treatment would depend on which causes were active within any given individual.

9.4 Implications

9.4.1 Drug Use and Addiction Are Different Things

At this point, the evidence that a subset of subjects have runaway valuations in response to drugs is overwhelming (Anthony et al. 1994; Deroche-Gamonet 2004, Koob and Le Moal 2006; Hart 2013; Perry et al. 2013; Jaffe et al. 2014). This is true both of animal models of drug addiction and humans self-administering drugs. This suggests a very important point, which is that drug use and addiction are different things. If we, as a society, want to address the health and sociological harm that drugs cause, then we may want to tackle drug use rather than addiction, which would require sociological changes (Hart 2013). As noted above, these sociological models are beyond the scope of this chapter, which is addressing computational models of addiction.

9.4.2 Failure Modes

This chapter has discussed three families of models. The first family was *economic models*, which simply define addiction as inelasticity, particularly due to misvaluations. However, these models do not identify what would cause that misvaluation. The second family was *pharmacological models*, which define addiction as a shift in a pharmacological set-point that drives value in an attempt to return the pharmacological levels back to that set-point. The third family was *learning and memory models*, which suggest that addiction derives from vulnerabilities in the neural implementations of these algorithms, which drives errors in action-selection.

The multiple-failure-modes model suggests that all three families provide important insights into addiction. It suggests that there are multiple potential vulnerabilities that could drive drug use (which could lie in pharmacological changes in set-points or in many potential failure modes of these learning systems). The multiple vulnerabilities model suggests that addiction is a symptom, not a disease. Many failure modes can create addiction. Importantly, identifying which failure modes occur within any given individual would require specially designed probe tests; this model suggests that it would not be enough to merely identify extended drug use. In fact, these failure modes are likely to depend on specific interactions between the drug and the individual and the specific decision processes driving the drug-seeking/drug-taking behavior.

9.4.3 Behavioral Addictions

If addictions are due to failure modes within neural implementations of decision-making algorithms, then addiction does not require pharmacological effects (even if pharmacological effects can cause addictions), and it becomes possible to define behavioral problems as addictions. For example, problem gambling is now considered an addiction, and other behaviors (such as internet gaming, porn, or even shopping) are now being considered as possible addictions. As noted at the beginning of the chapter, the definition of addiction is difficult. Nevertheless, computational models of addiction have provided insight into problem gambling and behavioral change in general, whether we call those behaviors addictive or not.

Classic computational models of problem gambling have been based on the certainty and uncertainty of reward delivery, but these models have been unable to explain observed properties of gamblers, such as that gamblers tend to have had a large win in their past (Custer 1984; Wagenaar 1988), that they are notoriously superstitious about their gambling (Griffiths 1994), or that they often show hindsight bias (in which they "explain away losses"; Parke and Griffiths 2004), or the illusion of control (in which they believe they can control random effects; Langer 1975).

Redish and colleagues (2007) noted that most models of decision making were based on learning value functions over worlds in which the potential states were already defined. Furthermore, they noted that most animal learning experiments took place in cue-poor environments, where the question the animal faced was *"What is the consequence of this cue?"* However, most lives (both human and nonhuman) are lived in cue-rich environments, in which the repeated structure of the world is not given to the subject. Instead, subjects have to identify which cues are critical to the definition of the situation the subjects finds themselves in. Redish and colleagues (2007) noted that this becomes a categorization problem and had been well studied in computational models of perception. Attaching a perceptual categorization process based on competitive-learning models (Hertz et al. 1991) to a reinforcement learning algorithm, Redish and colleagues built a model in which the tonic levels of dopamine [i.e., longer-term averages of $\delta(t)$] controlled the stability of the situation-categorization process. This identified two important vulnerabilities in the system depending on over- and under-categorization, particularly in different responses to wins and losses. In their model, wins produced learning of value, while losses produced recategorizations of situations. Their simulated agents were particularly susceptible to near-misses and surprising wins, leading to models of hindsight bias and the illusion of control.

In general, these multi-system models suggest that addiction is a question of harmful dysfunction—dysfunction (vulnerabilities leading to active failure modes) within a system that causes sufficient harm to suggest we need to treat it. They permit both behavioral and pharmacological drivers of addiction.

9.4.4 Using the Multisystem Model to Treat Patients

The suggestion that different decision-making systems can drive behavior provides a very interesting treatment possibility, which is that one could potentially use one decision-system to correct for errors in another. Three computational analyses of this have been done—changing discounting rates with episodic future thinking (Peters and Büchel 2010; Snider et al. 2018; Stein et al. 2018), analyses of contingency management (Petry 2012; Regier and Redish 2015), and analyses of precommitment (Kurth-Nelson and Redish 2009).

Episodic future thinking is a process in which one imagines a future world (Atance and O'Neill 2001), which is the key to planning and model-based decision making, in which one simulates (imagines) an outcome, and then makes one's decision based on that imagined future world (Niv et al. 2006; Redish 2013, 2016). Models of planning suggest that discounting rates may depend in part on the ability to imagine those concrete futures. Part of the discounting may arise from the intangibility of that future (Rick and Loewenstein 2008; Trope and Liberman 2010; Kurth-Nelson, Bickel, and Redish 2012), which may explain why making future outcomes more concrete reduces discounting rates (Peters and Büchel 2010). Other models have suggested that these discounting rate decreases occur through changes in the balance between impulsive and more cognitive decision systems (McClure and Bickel 2014). Nevertheless, recent work has found that treatments in which subjects are provided concrete episodic future outcomes to guide episodic future thinking can decrease discounting rates (providing a more future-oriented attitude) and decrease drug use (Snider et al. 2018; Stein et al. 2018). Whether this effect comes from the changes in discounting rates per se or whether those changes are reflective of other processes (such as an increased ability to use planning and deliberative systems) is currently unknown.

Contingency management is a treatment to create behavioral change (such as stopping use of drugs) through the direct payment of rewards for achieving that behavioral change—effectively paying people to stop taking drugs (Petry 2012). Contingency management was originally conceived of economically: if drugs have some elasticity (which they do; see figure 9.1), then paying people not to take drugs increases the cost of taking drugs by creating lost opportunity costs. In psychology, this would be called an alternate reinforcer.

However, Regier and Redish (2015) noted that the rewards that produced success in contingency management did not match the inelasticity seen in either animal models of addiction nor in real world measures of inelasticity due to changes of drug costs in the street. Building on the idea that choosing to take a drug or not (a go/no-go task, asking one's willingness-to-pay) accesses different decision-making algorithms than choosing between two options (take the drug or get the alternate reward), Regier and Redish suggested that contingency management had effectively nudged the subject to use their deliberative decision-making systems. They then suggested that this could provide improvements to standard contingency-management methods, including testing for prefrontal-hippocampal integrity (critical to deliberative systems) and providing concrete alternatives with reminders (making it easier to imagine those potential futures). Whether these suggestions actually improve contingency management has not yet been tested.

The fact that addicts show fast discounting functions with preferences that change over time suggests two interesting related treatments: bundling and precommitment. Bundling is a process whereby multiple rewards are grouped together so as to calculate the value of the full set rather than each individually (Ainslie 2001). For example, an alcoholic may want to go to the bar to drink one beer, but recognizing that going to the bar will entail lots of drinking may reduce the value of going to the bar relative to staying home. This can shift the person's preferences from going to the bar to staying home.

A similar process is that of precommitment, where a subject who knows in advance that if given a later option, the subject will take the poor choice, prevents the

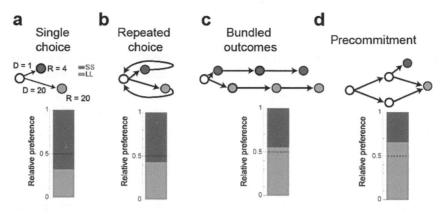

Figure 9.5

Changing state spaces. (a) Imagine a single choice between a smaller reward ($R = 4$) delivered sooner (after 1 second), compared to a larger reward ($R = 20$) delivered later (after 20 seconds). A typical agent might prefer the smaller-sooner over the larger-later reward. (b) If the agent realizes that this is going to be a repeated choice, then it is possible to drive the relative preference to 50/50 with a long look ahead, but it is impossible to change the actual preference. An agent that prefers the smaller-sooner option in (a) will still prefer it in (b). (c) Bundling creates new options such that there are consequences to one's decision. An agent can switch preferences by bundling. (d) Precommitment adds a new option to skip the choice. An agent making a decision at the earlier option can prefer the larger-later and learn to skip the choice in the right conditions. After models in Kurth-Nelson and Redish (2012).

opportunity in the first place. The classic example is that a person who knows they will drink too much at the bar decides not to go to the bar in the first place. Economically, precommitment depends on the hyperbolic discounting factors that lead to preference reversals (Ainslie 2001). Preference reversals imply that the earlier person wants one option (to not drink) while the later person wants a different one (to drink). Although many experiments have found that the average subject shows hyperbolic discounting (Madden and Bickel 2010), individuals can show large deviations from good hyperbolic fits. Computationally, an individual's willingness to precommit should depend on the specific shape of their discounting function (Kurth-Nelson and Redish 2010).

Furthermore, Kurth-Nelson and Redish (2010) proved that, neurophysiologically, precommitment depends on having a multifaceted value function—that is, the neural implementation of valuation has to be able to represent multiple values simultaneously. One obvious possibility is that the multiple decision-making systems each value options differently, and conflict between these options can be used to drive precommitment to prevent being offered the addictive option in the first place.

9.5 Chapter Summary

Because addiction is fundamentally a problem with decision making, computational models of decision making (whether economic, motivational [pharmacological], or neurosystem) have been important to our definitions and understanding of addiction. These theories have led to new treatments and new modifications that could improve those treatments.

9.6 Further Study

Koob and Le Moal (2006) provide a thorough description of the known neurobiology of addiction.

Bickel et al. (1993) is a seminal article showing that behavioral economics provides a conceptual framework that has utility for the study of drug dependence.

Redish (2004) was the first explicitly computational model of drug addiction and set the stage for considering addiction as computational dysfunction in decision systems.

Redish et al. (2008) provides evidence that addiction is a symptom rather than a fundamental disease and proposed that the concept of vulnerabilities in decision processes offers a unified framework for thinking about addiction.

10 Tourette Syndrome from a Computational Perspective

Vasco A. Conceição and Tiago V. Maia
Institute of Molecular Medicine, School of Medicine, University of Lisbon

10.1. Introduction

10.1.1 Disorder Definition and Clinical Manifestations

Tourette syndrome (TS) is a disorder characterized by tics—repetitive, stereotyped movements and oral-nasopharyngeal noises—that are usually preceded by aversive sensations called premonitory urges (American Psychiatric Association 2013; Leckman, Walker, and Cohen 1993; Robertson et al. 2017). Tics have sometimes been characterized as involuntary, but they may instead be voluntary (or "semi-voluntary") responses aimed at alleviating the preceding premonitory urges (Hashemiyoon, Kuhn, and Visser-Vandewalle 2017; Jankovic 2001). Tics may be motor or phonic; they are classified as simple if they involve only a small group of muscles or simple oral-nasopharyngeal noises such as sniffing or grunting, or as complex if they instead involve several muscle groups or more elaborate phonic phenomena such as the utterance of words or phrases (American Psychiatric Association 2013; Robertson et al. 2017). TS has an estimated prevalence of 0.3–1% (Robertson et al. 2017).

10.1.2 Pathophysiology

TS is strongly (Conceição et al. 2017; Neuner, Schneider, and Shah 2013; Worbe, Lehericy, and Hartmann 2015a) and likely causally (Caligiore et al. 2017; Pogorelov et al. 2015; Tremblay et al. 2015) mediated by disturbances in the motor cortico-basal ganglia-thalamo-cortical (CBGTC) loop, which seems to be strongly implicated in both simple and complex tics (Conceição et al. 2017; Pogorelov et al. 2015; Tremblay et al. 2015). The associative and limbic CBGTC loops are strongly implicated in attention-deficit/hyperactivity disorder (ADHD) and obsessive-compulsive disorder (OCD; Castellanos et al. 2006; Fineberg et al. 2018; Maia, Cooney, and Peterson 2008; Makris et al. 2009; Norman et al. 2016; Tremblay et al. 2015), which occur in approximately half or even more of patients with TS (Hashemiyoon, Kuhn, and Visser-Vandewalle 2017; Robertson et al. 2017). Studies in animals, in fact, suggest that the same disruption in CBGTC loops may produce tics, complex tics and inattention with hyperactivity-impulsivity, or obsessive-compulsive symptoms, depending on whether that disruption affects motor, associative, or limbic CBGTC loops, respectively (Grabli et al. 2004; Tremblay et al. 2015; Worbe et al. 2009).

The motor loop is implicated in the learning and execution of habits (Horga et al. 2015; Yin and Knowlton 2006). Habits correspond to stimulus–response associations that initially are learned on the basis of outcomes but then become independent from such outcomes, thereby implementing "cached" action values (Daw, Niv, and Dayan 2006; Delorme et al. 2016; Yin and Knowlton 2006). Learning stimulus–response associations bypasses the need to learn a model of the environment, so habit learning is often called "model-free" (Daw et al. 2011; Delorme et al. 2016). Such designation contrasts with that used for goal-directed learning, which relies on internal models of the world and is thereby often called "model-based" (Daw et al. 2011). The use of the term "model-free" can be somewhat confusing because many reinforcement learning (RL) models work in a model-free way (box 10.1). The term "model-free" refers to the absence of an explicit internal model of contingencies in the world, not to the absence of a computational model.

The implication of the motor loop in both habits and tics is consistent with the idea that "tics are exaggerated, maladaptive, and persistent motor habits" (Maia and Conceição 2017, 401). Habit learning and execution, moreover, are strongly modulated by dopamine, which likely explains the role of dopamine in TS (Maia and Conceição 2017, 2018; Nespoli et al. 2018), as we will discuss in detail below (section 10.3).

Cortical motor areas are organized hierarchically, with lower- and higher-order motor cortices being responsible for simpler and more complex movements, respectively (Kalaska and Rizzolatti 2013; Rizzolatti and Kalaska 2013; Rizzolatti and Strick 2013). This hierarchical organization likely explains why primary and higher-order motor cortices seem to be implicated in simple and complex tics, respectively (Worbe et al. 2010). Interestingly, and consistent with the implication of somatosensory regions in the premonitory urges that typically precede tics (Conceição et al. 2017; Cox, Seri, and Cavanna 2018), simple tics are associated with disturbances in somatosensory cortices that may be more restricted to primary somatosensory cortex (Sowell et al. 2008), whereas for complex tics, those disturbances extend farther into higher-order somatosensory cortices (Worbe et al. 2010).

As briefly mentioned above, some evidence suggests that the associative CBGTC loop may also be implicated in complex tics (Tremblay et al. 2015; Worbe et al. 2012,

Box 10.1

Commonly Used Reinforcement Learning Models

Two standard computational models from the machine learning literature—Q-learning (QL) and the actor–critic (Barto 1995; Sutton and Barto 1998; Watkins 1989)—have been used commonly and with considerable success to capture reinforcement learning (RL) in animals, healthy humans, and patients with Tourette syndrome (TS) and several other disorders (see, for example, Frank et al. 2007; Maia 2009; Roesch, Calu, and Schoenbaum 2007; Worbe et al. 2011). We briefly review those models here for two reasons: (1) understanding these models is necessary to understand the alterations in model parameters that have been described in TS (reviewed in section 10.2.1); (2) these models—specifically, the actor–critic—provide the backbone for a more elaborate model that we have used to provide an integrated, mechanistic account of multiple aspects of TS (as discussed in section 10.3).

Both QL and the actor–critic perform "model-free RL": a potentially misleading term, because these are computational models, but a reflection of the fact that these models do not explicitly learn a model of world contingencies. Instead, they use *prediction errors* (commonly represented by δ) to learn directly the equivalent of Thorndikian stimulus–response associations. In RL, it is common to speak of *states* rather than stimuli; states are more general because they include stimuli, situations, and contexts (which may be external and/or internal). In addition, although in psychology "responses" can be distinguished from "actions" (Dickinson 1985), in RL there is typically no such distinction, so responses—the accurate psychological term in the context of stimulus–response associations (Dickinson 1985)—are also called *actions*. Thus, in RL, learning stimulus–response associations corresponds to learning weights linking states and actions, $w_t(s,a)$ (where the subscript t indicates that these weights will vary over time with learning). QL and the actor–critic learn such weights in slightly different ways (described below). In both cases, however, those weights can be converted into action probabilities: $P_t(a_i|s_t)$, which gives the probability of selecting action a_i in the state s_t at time t. A common formula to convert the weights into probabilities is the softmax (Sutton and Barto 1998):

$$P_t(a_i|s_t) = \frac{e^{\beta w_t(s_t,a_i)}}{\sum_{a_j} e^{\beta w_t(s_t,a_j)}},$$

(10.1)

where β is the inverse temperature or gain ($\beta \geq 0$). This equation ensures that actions with greater weights tend to be selected more often, with the degree to which that happens being controlled by β, which therefore controls the degree of exploration (trying out random actions regardless of their weights) versus exploitation (always selecting the action or actions with the greatest learned weights; Daw 2011; Sutton and Barto 1998).

QL and the actor–critic both learn the weights $w_t(s,a)$ in a way that seeks to maximize the expected total sum of future reinforcements (although, as noted above, they do so slightly differently):

$$E\left[\sum_{\tau=t}^{\infty} \gamma^{\tau-t} r_\tau\right],$$

(10.2)

Box 10.1 (continued)

where t denotes the current time, and r_τ denotes the reinforcement at time τ. This expected total sum of future reinforcements is formally called a *value*. The sum has an infinite number of terms because, formally, values consider all future reinforcements. The discount factor, γ ($0 < \gamma < 1$), which discounts future reinforcements, is therefore usually necessary to ensure that the sum converges.

We turn next to the specific meaning of the weights and the mechanism that supports their learning in QL (next subsection) and the actor–critic (subsequent subsection) models.

a) The Standard QL Model

In QL, the weight $w_t(s,a)$ corresponds to an estimate at time t of the value of performing action a in state s—that is, the expected total sum of future reinforcements obtained by performing action a in state s. Such state-action values are commonly called Q values and represented as $Q_t(s,a)$ (Maia 2009; Sutton and Barto 1998; Watkins 1989). Q values are learned using prediction errors (δs) that consist of the difference between (1) the sum of the obtained reinforcement with the discounted estimated state-action value for the best action in the next state and (2) the state-action value estimated prior to action execution (Maia 2009; Watkins 1989):

$$Q_{t+1}(s_t,a_t) = Q_t(s_t,a_t) + \alpha\delta_t,$$
$$\delta_t = r_t + \gamma\max_{a_i} Q_t(s_{t+1},a_i) - Q_t(s_t,a_t),$$

(10.3)

where s_t and a_t are the state and the action executed at time t, respectively, α is a learning rate ($0 \leq \alpha \leq 1$), r_t is the reinforcement obtained at time t, γ is the future-discount factor, and the $\max_{a_i} Q_t(s_{t+1},a_i)$ term represents the estimated state-action value of performing the best action in the subsequent state (Maia 2009; Sutton and Barto 1998; Watkins 1989).

b) The Standard Actor–Critic Model

Instead of estimating state-action values, the actor–critic estimates the values of states, $V(s)$, which correspond to the expected sum of future reinforcements starting in state s (essentially marginalizing all actions that can be performed in that state). State values are stored and learned in the *critic* component of the actor–critic. As in QL, state values are also learned using prediction errors (δs) but correspond to the difference between (1) the sum of the obtained reinforcement with the discounted estimated value of the next state and (2) the prior value of the state (Barto 1995; Maia 2009; Sutton and Barto 1998):

$$V_{t+1}(s_t) = V_t(s_t) + \alpha_C\delta_t,$$
$$\delta_t = r_t + \gamma V_t(s_{t+1}) - V_t(s_t),$$

(10.4)

where α_C is the critic learning rate.

In the actor–critic, the weights $w_t(s,a)$ therefore do *not* directly correspond to state-action values. Instead, these weights, commonly called preferences, $p_t(s,a)$, and stored and

Box 10.1 (continued)

learned in the *actor* component, are learned using the prediction errors calculated in the critic component (Barto 1995; Maia 2009; Sutton and Barto 1998):

$$p_{t+1}(s_t, a_t) = p_t(s_t, a_t) + \alpha_A \delta_t, \tag{10.5}$$

where α_A is the actor learning rate. Contrary to state values, which in time should converge to the value of the state, the preferences are unbounded.

c) Simplifying Prediction-Error Calculation

In so-called *bandit tasks*, action execution under the current state (s_t) does not affect the transition to subsequent states ($s_{t+1}, s_{t+2}, ...$; Sutton and Barto 1998). In such cases, the equations for prediction-error calculation may be simplified into

$$\delta_t = r_t - Q_t(s_t, a_t) \tag{10.6}$$

in Q-learning models, or

$$\delta_t = r_t - V_t(s_t) \tag{10.7}$$

in actor–critic models.

For simplicity, in this chapter we generally adopt these simplified equations, except where otherwise noted.

d) Extending QL and Actor–Critic Models to Be More Realistic Biologically

Positive and negative prediction errors are signaled differently by dopaminergic neurons: positive prediction errors are signaled via burst-firing of dopamine neurons, and negative prediction errors are likely signaled via the duration of pauses in the firing of dopamine neurons (Maia 2009; Maia and Frank 2011). Specific dopaminergic disturbances may therefore affect the signaling of positive and negative prediction errors differently; thus, models intended to capture these effects need to distinguish between positive and negative prediction errors computationally. In addition, it is sometimes of interest to assess individual or between-group differences in the internal representation of reinforcements (e.g., a $1 reward may have a very different effect on different participants). These extensions may be captured by the following set of generalized equations:

$$Q_{t+1}(s_t, a_t) = Q_t(s_t, a_t) + \alpha(\delta_t)\delta_t,$$

$$\delta_t = f(r_t) - Q_t(s_t, a_t),$$

$$\alpha(\delta_t) = \begin{cases} \alpha^+, \text{ if } \delta_t \geq 0 \\ \alpha^-, \text{ otherwise} \end{cases}, \tag{10.8}$$

where α^+ and α^- are positive and negative learning rates, respectively, which capture learning following positive and negative prediction errors, respectively (Frank et al. 2007), and $f(r_t)$ denotes the internal value of the reinforcement obtained at time t. In tasks in which the only non-negligible reinforcement is a positive reward, r, $f(r_t)$ may be simplified to:

Box 10.1 (continued)

$$f(r_t) = \begin{cases} R^+, & \text{if } r_t = r \\ 0, & \text{otherwise} \end{cases}.$$ (10.9)

We mention this special case because the latter equation was used by two studies that assessed RL in TS (Palminteri et al. 2011; Worbe et al. 2011), and so we refer specifically to R^+ in section 10.2.1. Unpacking the actor learning rate into two prediction-error-dependent learning rates, or capturing the internal values of reinforcements, can be done similarly in actor–critic models.

Although using two learning rates to capture differential learning from positive versus negative prediction errors is a step in the right direction to make the models more realistic biologically, it is likely insufficient. Direct, or Go, and indirect, or NoGo, motor (and associative) CBGTC pathways respectively mediate motor (and cognitive) action facilitation and inhibition (figure 10.1; Collins and Frank 2014; Maia and Frank 2011, 2017). Both phasic increases and phasic decreases of dopamine (see box 10.2)—signaling positive and negative δs, respectively—may simultaneously affect the Go and NoGo motor (and associative) CBGTC pathways in opposite directions, and not necessarily with the same magnitudes. Thus, (at least) four learning rates—besides the critic learning rate(s) in the actor–critic, or analogous, frameworks—may be needed to appropriately model RL via the CBGTC loops (see section 10.3.2; Maia and Conceição 2017).

It would similarly be possible to unpack the critic learning rate into two prediction-error-dependent learning rates or, indeed, into four learning rates that depended on both the sign of the prediction error and the pathway affected (Go or NoGo). Such unpacking, however, could be slightly trickier to interpret because the critic is often associated with the ventral (limbic) striatum (Maia 2009; O'Doherty et al. 2004; Rothenhoefer et al. 2017), and the limbic indirect pathway presents considerable anatomical and neurochemical differences from motor and associative indirect pathways (Soares-Cunha et al. 2016). We therefore do not address α_C unpacking in this chapter.

Concerning action selection, there are alternatives to the softmax, some of which better orthogonalize the processes implicated in action selection (see, e.g., Guitart-Masip et al. 2012). Here, however, we focus exclusively on the softmax because it is widely used in the literature and because expanding it to use two inverse temperatures (or gains), rather than a single gain, has been used to model the differential effects of dopamine in the expression of the positive and negative values of actions learned through the Go and NoGo pathways, respectively (Collins and Frank 2014; Maia and Conceição 2017; Maia and Frank 2017). Striatal dopamine at the time of action selection promotes the expression of the learned positive values of actions while suppressing the expression of the learned negative values of actions by increasing the gain of the Go pathway (β_G) and suppressing the gain of the NoGo pathway (β_N), respectively (as comprehensively explained in section 10.3.2, figure 10.1; Collins and Frank 2014; Maia and Conceição 2017; Maia and Frank 2017). Irrespective of the chosen action-selection equation, several other processes (not addressed here) may also be considered during action selection (see, for example, Daw 2011; Guitart-Masip et al. 2012).

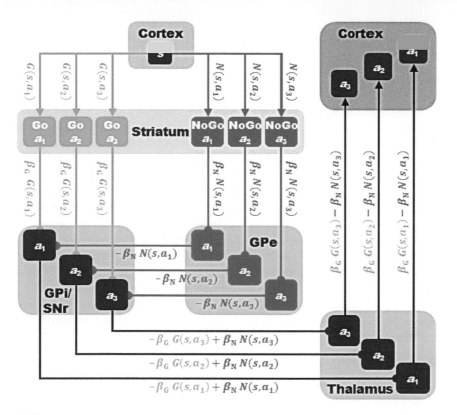

Figure 10.1

Computational roles of the direct (or Go) and indirect (or NoGo) motor pathways in action learning and selection. The situation or state, s, is a potentially rich, multidimensional representation encompassing representations of the external world (perception), interoception, motivational and emotional states, etc., potentially represented in a wide range of cortical (and some subcortical) regions—which likely explains why many regions project to the striatum (Choi, Yeo, and Buckner 2012; Postuma and Dagher 2006). The figure represents three possible actions (a_1, a_2, and a_3); their representation is kept separate in each anatomical region as required to have action specificity. The striatum contains two populations of neurons: D_1-expressing (Go) and D_2-expressing (NoGo) medium spiny neurons (MSNs), which are represented in green and red, respectively. Each of these populations contains a representation of the three actions. Go (G) and NoGo (N) values that represent the learned associations between state s and each of the actions are represented in corticostriatal synapses onto Go and NoGo MSNs, respectively. The gains of Go and NoGo MSNs (β_G and β_N respectively) are modulated by striatal dopamine levels. The activation, and therefore the output, of Go and NoGo MSNs is thus given by $\beta_G G(s,a_i)$ and $\beta_N N(s,a_i)$, respectively. Mathematically, inhibitory projections (GABAergic projections, represented by circles) flip the sign of the information (provided that there is intrinsic activity in the target structures, as is the case here). The anatomy of the basal ganglia seems therefore precisely suited to represent the difference between Go and NoGo activations, $\beta_G G(s,a_i) - \beta_N N(s,a_i)$, in the thalamus. The latter, in turn, helps to select actions in cortex in proportion to this difference. Internal variables, structures, and projections related to the direct and indirect pathways are coded in green and red, respectively. Glutamatergic (excitatory) projections are represented by arrowheads. GPe: external segment of the globus pallidus; GPi: internal segment of the globus pallidus; SNr: substantia nigra pars reticulata. Figure reprinted, with minor alterations, from *Biological Psychiatry*, 82(6), Maia, T. V., and Conceição, V. A., The roles of phasic and tonic dopamine in tic learning and expression, pp. 332–344, 2017, with permission from Elsevier.

Box 10.1 (continued)

Although we have highlighted how models with more parameters might be more realistic biologically, increasing the number of parameters in a model can create problems with model identifiability—especially when the parameters are far from being orthogonal, as in RL. Either extreme care must be exercised in task design to ensure that the parameters in models with a larger number of parameters are identifiable, or one must resort to simpler models. Still, the physiological basis for the use of (at least) four learning rates and (at least) two inverse temperatures (Maia and Conceição 2017) means that careful interpretation of the results from simpler models is needed, even when they seem to nicely capture physiological processes. For example, suppose that a given pathology or medication causes an impairment in long-term depression of the Go pathway (which should normally occur following negative prediction errors; Maia and Conceição 2017). In a model with only two learning rates, α^+ and α^-, such an effect would likely be captured by a reduced α^-; if, naively, one assumed that α^- was only associated with the NoGo pathway, this might be interpreted as suggestive of a NoGo-pathway-related abnormality, which would not be correct in this specific case.

e) Differences between QL and Actor–Critic Models

The differences between QL and actor–critic models, although seemingly subtle, have important implications. Indeed, QL and actor–critic models may, in some circumstances, lead systematically to prediction errors with distinct signs for the same action in the same state (because only actor–critic models consider the past outcomes of all actions in a given state, via state-values, when calculating prediction errors). Such a difference is extremely relevant when considering the role of dopamine in TS—and, indeed, in psychiatric disorders more generally—because, as noted previously, positive and negative prediction errors are coded differently by dopaminergic neurons.

One case that illustrates these differences is that of active-avoidance learning. In active-avoidance learning, animals have to learn to perform a response that avoids an aversive outcome that would otherwise occur. Under the actor–critic framework, the expectation of the aversive outcome elicits a negative value $[V(s) < 0]$. When the animal performs the avoidance response, the successful avoidance of the aversive outcome elicits a positive prediction error because the observed outcome is null but the predicted outcome was negative $[\delta = 0 - V(s) > 0$ because $V(s) < 0]$; it is this positive prediction error that reinforces the avoidance response (Maia 2010). In QL, however, the prediction error is 0: the state-action value is 0 [i.e., $Q(s, a) = 0$ when a is the avoidance response] because the avoidance response has itself never been associated with a negative outcome, so the prediction error is also 0 $[\delta = 0 - Q(s,a) = 0$ because $Q(s,a) = 0]$. This null prediction error is therefore unable to reinforce the response. Thus, for the response to be learned, the subject needs to execute a potentially infinite number of candidate actions—all possible actions other than the avoidance response—and to learn that the execution of all such actions leads to a negative outcome. Only after all other actions have negative Q values will the avoidance response, with its zero Q value, become preferred to the other actions (see the softmax equation at

Box 10.1 (continued)

the beginning of this box). Although in very constrained laboratory situations the set of candidate actions may be fairly constrained—especially in experiments with humans, who can be instructed about the possible actions (e.g., two possible buttons to press)—such a learning process clearly does not generalize to the real world.

This line of reasoning, together with the fact that nonoverlapping implementations of both the actor and the critic have been identified (Maia 2009; O'Doherty et al. 2004), seems to suggest that actor–critic models capture the actual biological implementation in animals and humans better than QL models do. However, the superiority of actor–critic over QL models is still debated, with some electrophysiological data in animals actually favoring the latter (Roesch, Calu, and Schoenbaum 2007).

Box 10.2

Tonic and Phasic Dopamine

In this chapter, we often mention *tonic* and *phasic* dopamine, as well as differences in the specific contributions of tonic and phasic striatal dopamine to action selection and learning. Here, we briefly explain the difference between tonic and phasic dopamine. This distinction arises because dopaminergic neurons may fire in two distinct manners: in a spontaneous, low-frequency, single-spike manner or in a high-frequency, burst manner (Grace and Bunney 1984b; 1984a).

Spontaneously active neurons fire at a baseline frequency of approximately 5 Hz (Grace and Bunney 1984b; Sulzer, Cragg, and Rice 2016; Wightman and Robinson 2002) due to the alternation between a slow, pacemaker-like depolarizing current and an ensuing after-hyperpolarization (Grace and Bunney 1984b). Such firing, together with the mechanisms underlying the synthesis, release, reuptake, and degradation of dopamine, defines the tonic dopamine levels, which are relatively stable and spatially homogeneous (Venton et al. 2003; Sulzer, Cragg, and Rice 2016). In the striatum, tonic dopamine levels range between 10–30 nM (Sulzer, Cragg, and Rice 2016).

Dopaminergic neurons that are tonically active can be driven to burst-fire, provided that there is incoming excitatory drive to those neurons (Grace and Bunney 1984b; Lodge and Grace 2011). Bursts correspond to a small number of action potentials (typically up to 10) at high frequencies, sometimes exceeding 30 Hz (Grace and Bunney 1984a; Wightman and Robinson 2002); thus, burst firing may cause abrupt, spatially heterogeneous, and massive increases in dopamine release (Grace and Bunney 1984a; Sulzer, Cragg, and Rice 2016; Venton et al. 2003). These large increases are called *phasic*; they are typically in the micromolar range and often—albeit not always (da Silva et al. 2018; Matsumoto and Hikosaka 2009; Wenzel et al. 2015)—signal positive prediction errors (Maia 2009; Schultz 2016). In addition to these phasic increases in dopamine, there are also phasic decreases. These occur when dopaminergic neurons temporarily pause firing, such as when a negative prediction error occurs (Maia 2009).

Worbe et al. 2009). The associative CBGTC loop is involved in goal-directed behaviors (Yin and Knowlton 2006), which may explain why complex tics often seem to have a more intentional character than simple tics do (American Psychiatric Association 2013).

10.1.3 Treatment

TS can be treated pharmacologically (Ganos, Martino, and Pringsheim 2017; Mogwitz et al. 2018; the ESSTS Guidelines Group et al. 2011a) or behaviorally (Fründt, Woods, and Ganos 2017; Robertson et al. 2017; the ESSTS Guidelines Group et al. 2011b). Consistent with the likely implication of dopaminergic hyperinnervation in TS (Buse et al. 2013; Hienert et al. 2018; Maia and Conceição 2018), patients with TS are typically prescribed antipsychotics (dopamine D_2 antagonists), because of their greater efficacy (Ganos, Martino, and Pringsheim 2017; the ESSTS Guidelines Group et al. 2011a), or α_2 agonists, which also reduce dopaminergic transmission (Maia and Conceição 2018), because of their more favorable side effects (Ganos, Martino, and Pringsheim 2017). Aripiprazole, an antipsychotic with a different mechanism of action (Casey and Canal 2017; Mailman and Murthy 2010), may be particularly efficacious for TS (Mogwitz et al. 2018). Indeed, in the striatum, aripiprazole may combine favorable actions both on postsynaptic D_2 receptors, where it may partially block the effects of endogenous dopamine, and on presynaptic D_2 receptors, where its effects may be more akin to those of an agonist, thereby reducing dopamine release (Maia and Conceição 2018).

Behaviorally, the treatments with most evidence for efficacy are habit reversal therapy (HRT) and exposure with response prevention (ExRP), both of which are recommended as first-line treatments for TS (Fründt, Woods, and Ganos 2017). HRT trains patients to suppress tics by executing tic-competing responses, via the use of antagonistic muscles, following the detection of premonitory urges and/or early movements that precede tic execution (McGuire et al. 2014; Rizzo et al. 2018; the ESSTS Guidelines Group et al. 2011b). In ExRP, patients are encouraged to suppress all tics while focusing on the premonitory urges, so as to promote premonitory-urge habituation; in addition, the patient is often exposed to situations (in vivo or imaginarily) that tend to elicit tics, while being encouraged to suppress the tics and focus on the premonitory urges (Fründt, Woods, and Ganos 2017; Rizzo et al. 2018; the ESSTS Guidelines Group et al. 2011b). Although clinically the protocols for HRT and ExRP are different, their mechanisms of action might be similar or even the same (van de Griendt et al. 2013). Indeed, premonitory-urge habituation is also a key component of HRT (McGuire et al. 2014), and both therapies involve suppressing tics (through a competing response in HRT and through the patient's own strategies in ExRP). Both HRT and ExRP may also be administered within broader behavioral interventions (Fründt, Woods, and Ganos 2017). HRT, for example, is a primary component of the comprehensive behavioral intervention for tics (CBIT; Fründt, Woods, and Ganos 2017; McGuire et al. 2014), which is also currently recommended as a first-line treatment for TS (Fründt, Woods, and Ganos 2017). Although HRT and ExRP have the advantage of avoiding medication's side effects, pharmacological treatment, or the combination of behavioral and pharmacological treatments, may be necessary for, at least, the most severely affected patients (Ganos et al. 2017).

Some patients are refractory to all pharmacological and behavioral treatments (Kious, Jimenez-Shahed, and Shprecher 2016). In such cases, for very severely affected patients, invasive treatments, such as deep-brain stimulation (Akbarian-Tefaghi, Zrinzo, and Foltynie 2016; Baldermann et al. 2016; Hashemiyoon, Kuhn, and Visser-Vandewalle 2017) or even psychosurgery (Hashemiyoon, Kuhn, and Visser-Vandewalle 2017), may be justified. The best targets for these treatments are still under investigation but generally involve nodes or fibers in the CBGTC loops (Akbarian-Tefaghi, Zrinzo, and Foltynie 2016; Baldermann et al. 2016; Hashemiyoon, Kuhn, and Visser-Vandewalle 2017). Even such invasive treatments, however, can sometimes be only moderately successful (Akbarian-Tefaghi, Zrinzo, and Foltynie 2016; Baldermann et al. 2016; Hashemiyoon, Kuhn, and Visser-Vandewalle 2017).

10.1.4 Contributions of Computational Psychiatry

Despite substantial progress, fundamental questions concerning the etiology, pathophysiology, and, more importantly, the adequate treatment of TS remain (Hashemiyoon, Kuhn, and Visser-Vandewalle 2017; Robertson et al. 2017; Thenganatt and Jankovic 2016). There is a pressing need both for a more detailed and integrative mechanistic understanding of TS (and its treatment) and for practical, clinically relevant predictive tools (whether based on an understanding of mechanism or not). These two needs align closely with the two main branches of computational psychiatry, which are theory- and data-driven computational psychiatry, respectively (Huys et al. 2016b; Maia 2015). Moreover, the potential of the combined fulfillment of these two needs relates to the potential of combining these two approaches to computational psychiatry (Huys et al. 2016b; Maia 2015).

As described in the remainder of this chapter, computational-psychiatry work in TS has already started to address these needs. While these efforts are still in their early days, with much work remaining to be done, theory-driven computational psychiatry has already yielded a mathematically rigorous theory of multiple aspects of TS (section 10.3); data-driven computational psychiatry has started to yield proof-of-concept classifiers for automated TS diagnosis (section 10.2.3); and the combination of these approaches has started to characterize computationally the neurocognitive disturbances that may underpin TS (section 10.2.1).

10.2 Past and Current Computational Approaches to Tourette Syndrome

Consistent with the implication in TS of disturbances in the dopaminergic system (reviewed below; see section 10.3) and in the motor loop (reviewed above; see section 10.1.2), multiple studies have reported alterations in RL and in habit learning in TS. Studies that have used data-driven approaches to automatically classify patients with TS, moreover, have offered additional evidence for the involvement of the motor loop in TS. In this section, we review the findings from these three lines of research: RL, habit learning, and automated classification in TS. Then, in the next section, we show how all those findings may be reconciled under the hypothesis that TS involves dopaminergic hyperinnervation.

10.2.1 Reinforcement Learning in Tourette Syndrome

Unmedicated patients with TS seem to have increased learning from rewards: they learned from rewards but not from punishments in a subliminal task (Palminteri et al. 2009), and they had increased internal reward values (R^+, box 10.1) relative to controls in a motor skill–learning task (Palminteri et al. 2011). Two studies failed to find significant differences between unmedicated patients and controls in learning from rewards (Salvador et al. 2017; Worbe et al. 2011), including specifically in R^+ (Worbe et al. 2011). Both of those studies, however, had a substantially greater proportion of males in the patient group than in the control group: the ratio of males to females in patients versus controls was 2.16 versus 1.17, respectively, in one study (Worbe et al. 2011), and 3.25 versus 1.22, respectively, in the other (Salvador et al. 2017)[1]. The increased proportion of females in the control group in these studies could have masked increased learning from rewards in patients, because females learn better from rewards than males do (Evans and Hampson 2015)—a finding that is consistent with higher striatal presynaptic dopamine synthesis capacity (Laakso et al. 2002) and possibly higher striatal dopaminergic innervation, as assessed by dopamine transporter binding (Wong et al. 2012), in females relative to males. Furthermore, the study that found no differences in R^+ between unmedicated patients and controls (Worbe et al. 2011) suffered from model identifiability issues (Maia and Conceição 2017) that we discuss briefly below (section 10.2.2). A third study did not find differences in learning from rewards between patients with TS, many of whom were unmedicated, and controls, other than differences due to ADHD comorbidity (Shephard, Jackson, and Groom 2016). That study, however, used a simple deterministic task, and accuracy throughout the task was very high for all participants; the task therefore likely engaged explicit, rule-based learning, which may be largely unaffected in unmedicated patients with TS (Maia and Conceição 2017).

Patients with TS on antipsychotics other than aripiprazole have consistently been reported to be impaired at learning from rewards: they learned from punishments but not from rewards in a subliminal task (Palminteri et al. 2009), and they had decreased R^+ relative to controls in two studies (Palminteri et al. 2011; Worbe 2011). These findings are most likely due to the medication, because antipsychotics also decrease learning from rewards in healthy humans, patients with other disorders, and animals (Maia and Conceição 2017; Maia and Frank 2017). Patients on aripiprazole, unlike those on other antipsychotics, seem to have preserved simple learning from rewards (Salvador et al. 2017; Worbe 2011). The mechanisms of action of aripiprazole are different from those of other antipsychotics (Casey and Canal 2017; Maia and Conceição 2018), as aripiprazole is characterized by "functional selectivity" (Mailman and Murthy 2010), which may explain this difference in effects. Aripiprazole does impair more complex forms of learning—namely, counterfactual learning—in a dose-dependent manner, but that may be due to detrimental effects on executive function (Salvador et al. 2017). Indeed, counterfactual learning involves learning from the outcomes of actions that one did not take but could have taken, which requires more complex inference and therefore executive function.

10.2.2 Habits in Tourette Syndrome

As noted above, the motor loop is associated with both habits and tics, which suggests that "tics are exaggerated, maladaptive, and persistent motor habits" (Maia and Conceição 2017, 401). Further support for that idea comes from a study that found that patients with TS overrely on habits relative to goal-directed behaviors (Delorme et al. 2016). The same study, moreover, found positive correlations between (1) overreliance on habits and tic severity, (2) overreliance on habits and structural connectivity between motor cortex and putamen, and (3) tic severity and structural connectivity between supplementary motor cortex and putamen (the latter two in unmedicated patients only), thereby demonstrating an association among habits, tics, and increased structural connectivity within the motor loop. Other studies have also shown positive correlations between structural connectivity within the motor loop and both (1) tics in patients with TS (with patients, moreover, having increased structural connectivity within the motor loop relative to controls; Worbe et al. 2015b) and (2) habit learning in healthy controls (de Wit et al. 2012).

Two older studies found that patients with TS performed worse than healthy controls in the weather prediction task (Kéri et al. 2002; Marsh et al. 2004), a probabilistic classification task that was designed with the goal of probing the gradual learning of stimulus–response associations (Knowlton, Squire, and Gluck 1994). Moreover, this impaired performance did not seem attributable to medication or comorbidities. Those articles interpreted the impaired performance as indicative of impaired habit learning; however, neither study included any of the tests that are now considered necessary to classify a behavior as a habit (Yin and Knowlton 2006), a particularly pertinent concern because performance in the weather prediction task may also rely on other cognitive processes (Price 2009). Neither study, moreover, disentangled learning from positive versus negative prediction errors (box 10.1); as we will discuss later (section 10.3.2), the reported impairments might therefore be a consequence of impaired learning from negative, but not positive, prediction errors in TS.

10.2.3 Data-Driven Automated Diagnosis in Tourette Syndrome

As noted in section 10.1.2, somatosensory and motor regions are strongly implicated in premonitory urges and tics, respectively (Conceição et al. 2017; Cox et al. 2018; Worbe et al. 2015a). Consistent with such involvement, studies that have applied data-driven computational-psychiatry approaches to build classifiers using data from magnetic resonance imaging (MRI) suggest that sensorimotor regions are key to distinguish patients with TS from healthy controls or from patients with other neuropsychiatric disorders, as described next.

Three studies used MRI data to automatically distinguish medication-naïve children with TS from healthy children. The three studies were conducted by the same research group using substantially overlapping samples and the same machine-learning approach: support vector machines with cross-validation. The studies differed in the specific MRI modalities used: resting-state functional MRI (rs-fMRI; Wen et al. 2018), diffusion MRI (Wen et al. 2017b), and both structural and diffusion MRI (Wen et al. 2017a). In one of the studies, children with TS had no comorbidities (Wen et al. 2018), and in the other two they had no comorbidities other than ADHD (Wen et al. 2017a; Wen et al. 2017b). All three studies achieved classification accuracies above 85%, and they all implicated sensorimotor regions, or their connectivity, as key discriminating features between children with TS and healthy children. They also implicated several other regions—for example, the inferior frontal gyrus, which is strongly implicated in inhibitory control (Aron, Robbins, and Poldrack 2014)—or their connectivity as discriminating features.

Two additional studies used rs-fMRI data to distinguish children with TS from healthy children but using samples in which a considerable percentage of the children with TS was medicated (Greene et al. 2016; Liao et al. 2017). Both studies also used support vector machines with cross-validation. One study used inter-hemispheric intrinsic functional connectivity and included only boys without comorbid ADHD or OCD; that study strongly implicated sensorimotor and limbic regions in successful discrimination, and it achieved a classification accuracy of over 90% (Liao et al. 2017). The other study, which did not exclude patients with comorbidities, strongly implicated connectivity within and between sensorimotor and/or cognitive-control regions in successful discrimination (Greene et al. 2016), but it had a much lower classification accuracy (~70%) than the other studies.

A final study used cortical and subcortical morphological variations to classify children or adults who were either healthy or diagnosed with one of several neuropsychiatric disorders, including TS (Bansal et al. 2012). The medication status of patients with TS was not reported. For each pair (or set) of groups to be compared, the discriminating features were preselected as those that differed with high significance between those specific groups. For children with TS versus healthy children, the chosen features involved the surface morphology of the right globus pallidus and hippocampus; for adults with TS versus healthy adults, they involved only the surface morphology of the right hippocampus. Classification accuracy was remarkably high when grouping features into two groups (e.g., adults with TS vs. healthy adults), but not into three groups (e.g., adults with TS vs. adults with schizophrenia vs. healthy adults). Although the study used both leave-one-out cross-validation and multiple independent split-half replication analyses, the preselection of features for each discrimination seems to have used the full sample of subjects to be discriminated—including, as far as we can tell, the subjects held out for test in the leave-one-out cross-validation and split-half analyses—which may have introduced overfitting.

In short, consistent with the main theme of this chapter, automated classification studies highlight the importance of sensorimotor regions for the classification of patients with TS, although they also point to other potentially relevant regions. In terms of clinical application, however—the aim of applied computational psychiatry (Huys et al. 2016b; Paulus et al. 2016)—this work has important limitations. Arguably, the most fundamental limitation of this work is that the nearly exclusive focus on classification of patients with TS versus healthy controls does not respond to a real clinical need; clinicians face many difficult tasks in which they could use the help of computational psychiatry—for example, prognosis, prediction of treatment outcome, or differential diagnosis (Huys et al. 2016b)—but distinguishing patients from controls usually is not a primary concern. Amongst all of the studies reviewed above, only one tried to tackle the more realistic problem of distinguishing between different disorders, and it even tried to tackle classification into more than two groups (Bansal et al. 2012). Unfortunately, as noted above, that study might have suffered from overfitting; moreover, even with the possible overfitting allowed by the feature-selection process, the study had very limited success in the classification into more than two groups, which highlights the difficulties inherent in that process. Ultimately, we hope that more researchers interested in automated classification turn their attention to problems with potential for real clinical impact (Huys et al. 2016b; Paulus et al. 2016).

10.3 Case Study: An Integrative, Theory-Driven Account of Tourette Syndrome

CBGTC (Neuner, Schneider, and Shah 2013; Worbe et al. 2015a) and dopaminergic (Buse et al. 2013) disturbances have long been implicated in TS. To the best of our knowledge, however, there was no cohesive, integrated account capable of explaining the multiple findings in TS obtained with various methods: molecular imaging, pharmacology, structural imaging, tic-related and resting-state functional imaging, and experimental behavioral data. Given that parsimony is a fundamental principle of science, we recently suggested a mechanistic, integrated theory of TS that provides a unified explanation for these multiple findings (Conceição et al. 2017; Maia and Conceição 2017, 2018). First, we conducted a systematic review of all positron emission tomography (PET) and single-photon emission computed tomography (SPECT) studies of the dopaminergic system in TS and considered related postmortem studies and the mechanisms of action of all medications with proven efficacy in TS; we showed that the hypothesis that TS involves dopaminergic hyperinnervation—that is, an increased number of dopaminergic terminals—provides a simple and unified explanation for all of those findings (Maia and Conceição 2018). Second, we used insights concerning the computational roles of phasic and tonic dopamine in action learning and selection (Collins and Frank 2014; Maia and Frank 2017) to formulate a computational description of how increases in phasic and tonic dopamine—themselves resultant from dopaminergic hyperinnervation—may promote tic learning and expression and also explain the findings from the studies that have assessed RL and habits in TS. This formulation also allowed us to explain detailed observations concerning the time course of action of antipsychotics in the treatment of TS that had previously been unappreciated (Maia and Conceição 2017). Third, we reviewed studies that used anatomical imaging, resting-state functional imaging, and tic-related functional imaging in TS, focusing on the relation between such data and the genesis and severity of tics and premonitory urges (Conceição et al. 2017); using that information, we expanded the theory that we had formulated (Maia and Conceição 2017) to explain the neural substrates of premonitory urges and the computational roles of such urges in tic learning and execution (Conceição et al. 2017). We review each of these three steps below (sections 10.3.1–10.3.3).

10.3.1 Dopaminergic Hyperinnervation as a Parsimonious Explanation for Neurochemical and Pharmacological Data in Tourette Syndrome

PET/SPECT studies of the dopaminergic system suggest that patients with TS have increases in dopamine transporter (DAT) binding, in amphetamine-induced dopamine release, and possibly also in vesicular monoamine transporter 2 (VMAT2) binding and F-DOPA accumulation (Maia and Conceição 2018). Dopaminergic hyperinnervation would be expected to cause all of these findings (figure 10.2; Maia and Conceição 2018). The full ensemble of findings of PET/SPECT studies of the dopaminergic system in TS presents important interpretational challenges, and typically there are about as many studies with null findings as studies with positive findings supporting the disturbances we mentioned above. Careful consideration of the studies with null findings, however, shows, first, a widespread and unmistakable lack of power—most studies used extremely small samples—and, second, in several studies, important age-, sex-, and/ or medication-related confounds (Maia and Conceição 2018). At the moment, therefore, the dopaminergic-hyperinnervation hypothesis seems to successfully reconcile all extant PET/SPECT findings (Maia and Conceição 2018). This hypothesis has recently received additional support from a meta-analysis that confirmed increased striatal DAT binding in TS (Hienert et al. 2018). Furthermore, the dopaminergic-hyperinnervation hypothesis explains why all medications with well-established efficacy for TS— antipsychotics, low-doses of certain dopamine agonists like pergolide (which act mostly on presynaptic D_2 receptors), ecopipam (a selective D_1 antagonist), VMAT2 inhibitors, and even α_2 / α_{2A} agonists—reduce dopaminergic transmission (Maia and Conceição 2018). Moreover, if indeed TS involves dopaminergic hyperinnervation, then it can be expected to involve increased tonic and increased phasic dopamine. As we will discuss in the next section, such increases explain a wide range of clinical and experimental findings in TS.

10.3.2 The Roles of Phasic and Tonic Dopamine in Tourette Syndrome

Extensive evidence implicates phasic and tonic dopamine (box 10.2) in action learning and selection (box 10.1; figure 10.1), and these effects have been elegantly captured

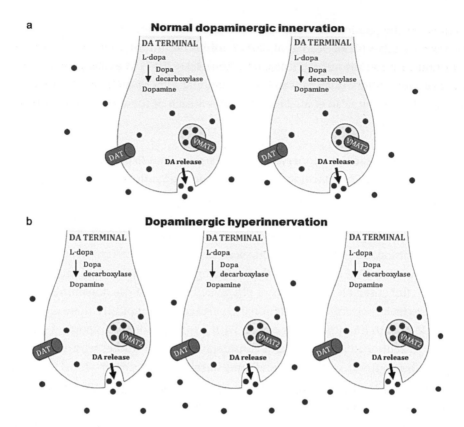

Figure 10.2
The dopaminergic-hyperinnervation hypothesis of Tourette syndrome (TS). (a) Normal dopa-minergic innervation. Multiple characteristics of dopamine terminals can be investigated using molecular imaging *in vivo*: the dopamine transporter (DAT), the vesicular monoamine transporter 2 (VMAT2), the activity of dopa decarboxylase (by measuring F-dopa uptake), and the extent of amphetamine-induced dopamine (DA) release. (b) The hypothesis that TS involves dopaminergic hyperinnervation—that is, an increased number of DA terminals—explains why all of these mark-ers (DAT and VMAT2 binding, F-dopa uptake, and amphetamine-induced DA release) seem to be increased in TS (section 10.3.1; Maia and Conceição 2018).

computationally in the OpAL model (Collins and Frank 2014; Maia and Frank 2017). We have used these ideas, albeit under a slightly different mathematical instantiation from that in prior formulations of OpAL, to suggest that increased phasic and tonic dopamine in TS—themselves due to dopaminergic hyperinnervation (figure 10.2; Maia and Conceição 2018)—may promote tic learning and expression (Maia and Conceição 2017).

a) The CBGTC-Inspired Reinforcement Learning Model   OpAL (Collins and Frank 2014) expands the *actor* component of the actor–critic model (see box 10.1; Barto 1995; Sutton and Barto 1998) to explicitly account for the existence of direct (Go) and indirect (NoGo) CBGTC pathways (box 10.1; figure 10.1). It does so by subdividing state-action preferences, $p(s,a)$ (where s and a denote a state and an action, respectively; see box 10.1), into two "subpreferences," $G(s,a)$ and $N(s,a)$, which denote positive and negative parts of the preference, respectively, and are coded by Go and NoGo pathways, respectively (Collins and Frank 2014). Loosely speaking, the preference then becomes equal to the difference between these two subpreferences: $p(s,a) = G(s,a) - N(s,a)$. As we will discuss next, however, these subpreferences are differentially modulated by dopamine.

Go and NoGo striatal medium spiny neurons (MSNs) express mostly D_1 and D_2 dopamine receptors, respectively, which are excitatory and inhibitory, respectively (Soares-Cunha et al. 2016). For this reason, dopamine modulates the excitability (or gain) of Go and NoGo striatal MSNs in opposite directions: higher striatal dopamine levels increase and decrease the excitability of Go and NoGo MSNs, respectively, and lower dopamine levels have the opposite effects (figure 10.1). The positive and negative action subpreferences (G and N, respectively) are therefore differentially modulated by dopamine. In OpAL, this differential modulation is captured by using different gains for the positive and negative action subpreferences: β_G and β_N, which represent the gains of the Go and NoGo pathways, respectively, and which are modulated by dopamine in opposite directions (Collins and Frank 2014; Maia and Frank 2017). This opposite modulation in OpAL is achieved in a simple formulation by making β_G and β_N depend on the level of dopamine, ω, with different signs:

$$\beta_G = \beta(1+\omega) \tag{10.10}$$

and

$$\beta_N = \beta(1-\omega), \tag{10.11}$$

where β is a constant. The dopamine-modulated preference then becomes: $p(s,a) = \beta_G G(s,a) - \beta_N N(s,a)$. Actions can then be selected, for example, with the softmax, as in other RL models (box 10.1), but using these dopamine-modulated preferences.

We previously associated mostly tonic dopamine with action selection (Maia and Conceição 2017), under the assumption that phasic firing of dopamine neurons occurs only in specific circumstances and its corresponding transients are short-lived (Venton et al. 2003). Tonic dopamine levels, which are in the nanomolar range (Sulzer, Cragg, and Rice 2016), likely act mostly on the NoGo pathway because, in the striatum, D_1 and D_2 receptors appear to be predominantly in low- and high-affinity states, respectively (Dreyer et al. 2010; Sulzer, Cragg, and Rice 2016). Thus, we had suggested that, in most cases, the gain parameters could be simplified to:

$$\beta_G = \beta,$$
$$\beta_N = \beta(1-\tau),$$

$$(10.12)$$

where τ represents tonic dopamine, which has a limited effect on β_G. On the other hand, we had already suggested that if action selection occurred shortly following phasic dopamine firing, it would be modulated by the corresponding dopamine transients (Maia and Frank 2017). In other words, we had suggested that $\omega = \tau + \rho$, where ρ represents phasic dopamine (Maia and Frank 2017), which could then affect β_G. Recent evidence (da Silva et al. 2018), added to other evidence (Howe and Dombeck 2016; Syed et al. 2016), suggests that phasic responses might commonly occur prior to self-initiated action, increasing the probability of, and invigorating, subsequent movement. Thus, we now favor the formulation in which action selection is commonly modulated by both tonic and phasic dopamine components, which can affect both β_N and, if there is a phasic dopamine component, β_G.

In addition to its effects during action selection, dopamine also has differential effects on plasticity (Lerner and Kreitzer 2011; Shen et al. 2008), and therefore learning, in the Go and NoGo pathways (Maia and Conceição 2017). Specifically, dopamine *increases* cause long-term potentiation (LTP) in corticostriatal projections to the Go pathway and may cause long-term depression (LTD) in corticostriatal projections to the NoGo pathway; dopamine *decreases* may have the opposite effects, causing LTP in corticostriatal projections to the NoGo pathway and possibly causing LTD in corticostriatal projections to the Go pathway (Lerner and Kreitzer 2011; Shen et al. 2008). Thus, in our formulation of the OpAL model, prediction errors affect learning in the Go and NoGo pathways in opposite directions:

$$G_{t+1}(s_t,a_t) = \begin{cases} G_t(s_t,a_t) + \alpha_{G,LTP}\delta_t, & \text{if } \delta_t \geq 0 \\ G_t(s_t,a_t) + \alpha_{G,LTD}\delta_t, & \text{if } \delta_t < 0 \end{cases}$$

$$(10.13)$$

and

$$N_{t+1}(s_t,a_t) = \begin{cases} N_t(s_t,a_t) - \alpha_{N,LTD}\delta_t, & \text{if } \delta_t \geq 0 \\ N_t(s_t,a_t) - \alpha_{N,LTP}\delta_t, & \text{if } \delta_t < 0 \end{cases} \tag{10.14}$$

where the parameters $\alpha_{G,LTP}$, $\alpha_{G,LTD}$, $\alpha_{N,LTP}$, and $\alpha_{N,LTD}$ are learning rates between 0 and 1, and the subpreferences $G(s_t,a_t)$ and $N(s_t,a_t)$ represent the strength of the corticostriatal synapses onto MSNs of the Go and NoGo pathways concerning the current state, s_t, and the selected action, a_t (Maia and Conceição 2017). Given that these subpreferences are meant to represent synaptic weights, they are constrained to be greater than, or equal to, 0 (Collins and Frank 2014).

The CBGTC loops have exactly the right anatomy to implement these computations (figure 10.1; Maia and Conceição 2017; Maia and Frank 2017).

b) Mechanistic Explanation of Behavioral Findings on Reinforcement Learning in Tourette Syndrome From the five RL studies reviewed above (section 10.2.1), two seem particularly consistent with the dopaminergic hyperinnervation hypothesis of TS (Palminteri et al. 2009; 2011). In one of these studies, which applied an RL task in which the cues were presented subliminally, unmedicated patients with TS learned from rewards, but they did not learn from punishments (Palminteri et al. 2009). Both of these effects are consistent with dopaminergic hyperinnervation: increased learning from rewards is consistent with increased phasic dopamine, given the role of increases in phasic dopamine in the learning from positive prediction errors (box 10.2); decreased learning from punishments is consistent with increased tonic dopamine, which might blunt the signaling of negative prediction errors by phasic decreases in dopamine. Furthermore, in that same study, the opposite pattern was found in unmedicated patients with Parkinson's disease (PD), who learned from punishments but not from rewards (Palminteri et al. 2009). The finding of opposite patterns in unmedicated patients with TS and PD is particularly relevant because PD is characterized by dopaminergic hypoinnervation, and we hypothesize that TS is characterized by dopaminergic hyperinnervation—hence, the two disorders are hypothesized to have the opposite dopaminergic disturbances. Further evidence for the dopaminergic-hyperinnervation hypothesis comes from the finding that patients with PD on levodopa and dopamine agonists became like unmedicated patients with TS, learning from rewards but not from punishments.

In the other study that supports the dopaminergic-hyperinnervation hypothesis, unmedicated patients with TS had higher internal reinforcement, R^+ (box 10.1), for a monetary reward as compared with healthy controls (Palminteri et al. 2011). Dopamine does not seem to be implicated in the hedonic value of the reinforcements (Berridge

2007), which, at first sight, relates more closely to R^+. However, unless the task is designed carefully and appropriate parameter-recovery simulations are conducted—see discussion in the supplemental materials in Maia and Conceição (2017)—the biological interpretation of RL parameters is often complex and can be misleading. Specifically, in the context of our discussion here, R^+ can potentially relate to the signaling of positive prediction errors, and hence to phasic dopamine, rather than to hedonic value—a possibility to which we now turn.

In tasks in which the only non-negligible reinforcement is a positive reward, r, prediction errors, δ, can be described by $\delta_t = R^+ - V(s_t)$, where R^+ is the internal value of r (box 10.1)[2]. We have noted that dopaminergic hyperinnervation is expected to lead to an increase in phasic dopamine release in TS. Suppose that such increase is additive; in other words, suppose that the increase in phasic dopamine release in TS is well captured by an additive parameter, a, that scales δ_t into $\delta_t^{TS} = \delta_t + a$. We can rewrite δ_t^{TS} as follows: $\delta_t^{TS} = \delta_t + a = R^+ - V(s_t) + a = (R^+ + a) - V(s_t)$. In other words, the change in phasic dopamine release would be well captured by a change in R^+ to $R^+ + a$ (i.e., the change in phasic dopamine release would be captured as a change in the R^+ parameter). Of course, we do not know if the increase in dopamine release is additive. In fact, the dopaminergic-hyperinnervation hypothesis may suggest that the increase is multiplicative, because more fibers would be available to release dopamine for the same signal. Even if the change is multiplicative, however, that may still lead to a change in R^+.[3]

We cannot overstate the importance of considering in detail the meaning of RL parameters and of conducting appropriate tests to ensure that, in a given task, parameters are identifiable and capture the intended meaning (Maia and Conceição 2017; see, in particular, the supplemental materials). For example, whereas one study found increased R^+ in unmedicated patients with TS, as discussed above, another found no alterations in R^+ (Worbe et al. 2011). We have shown through simulations, however, that the parameters in the latter study were not identifiable (Maia and Conceição 2017). Moreover, we also showed that blunted learning from negative prediction errors—that is, a reduced α^-—would, by following the model-fitting procedures in that study, erroneously be reflected in a reduced value for R^+ (Maia and Conceição 2017, supplemental materials). Now, note that dopaminergic hyperinnervation in TS would cause both (1) increased learning from positive prediction errors, which, as noted above, could be captured as an increase in R^+, and (2) reduced learning from negative prediction errors, which, as we have shown in simulations, could be captured as a decrease in R^+. These two opposing effects might therefore cancel each other out, leading to the observed finding of no alterations in R^+ in unmedicated patients with TS versus controls (Worbe et al. 2011).

In addition to these computational arguments, there is also empirical evidence that R^+ in these studies may have captured dopaminergic effects. Indeed, patients with TS on antipsychotics, which block dopamine, had reduced, rather than increased, values of R^+ in both studies (Palminteri et al. 2011; Worbe et al. 2011). Such reductions in R^+ values, like the finding that medicated patients with TS, contrary to unmedicated patients with TS, failed to learn from rewards in the aforementioned subliminal task (Palminteri et al. 2009), likely are explained, at least in part, by the fact that, when administered chronically, antipsychotics decrease the firing of dopaminergic neurons and decrease phasic and tonic dopamine (Maia and Conceição 2017). Antipsychotics also have other, more complex effects that further explain why they blunt Go learning (Maia and Conceição 2017).

Relatedly, the finding that medicated patients with TS, like unmedicated patients with PD, but unlike unmedicated patients with TS, learned from punishments in the subliminal task that we first discussed (Palminteri et al. 2009) may be explained by considering other effects of antipsychotic administration. Except for aripiprazole, antipsychotics seem to exert their beneficial effects in TS by blocking postsynaptic D_2 receptors (section 10.1.3). Computationally, the blockade of D_2 receptors in NoGo MSNs translates into an increase in the excitability (or gain, β_N) of the NoGo pathway, as well as into a tendency for strengthening of corticostriatal synapses onto NoGo MSNs, given that LTP and LTD in such synapses respectively depend on the lack of stimulation and stimulation of D_2 receptors (figure 10.1; Maia and Conceição 2017). Such effects therefore explain why patients with TS under antipsychotics learn better from punishments than unmedicated patients with TS do.[4]

c) Mechanistic Explanation of Behavioral Findings on Habits in Tourette Syndrome   As reviewed in section 10.2.2, unmedicated patients with TS seem to overrely on habitual, compared to goal-directed, behavioral control. As mentioned above, dopamine mediates habit learning and execution (section 10.1.2), with (1) increased phasic dopamine promoting excessive Go learning and (2) increased tonic dopamine, or increased phasic-dopamine release prior to action selection (da Silva et al. 2018), promoting excessive execution of the most ingrained motor actions (figure 10.1). Thus, dopamine hyperinnervation provides a natural explanation for the reported overreliance of unmedicated patients with TS on habits. In addition, the hypothesis that tics themselves are "exaggerated, maladaptive, and persistent motor habits" (Maia and Conceição 2017, 401) explains the observed positive correlation between the overreliance on habits and tic severity (Delorme et al. 2016).

As mentioned in section 10.2.2, two older studies found impaired habit learning in TS, but those studies did not disentangle learning from positive versus negative prediction errors (Kéri et al. 2002; Marsh et al. 2004). As mentioned above, under the dopaminergic-hyperinnervation hypothesis, one expects impaired learning from negative prediction errors because phasic dopamine decreases become blunted. The findings of those studies are therefore consistent with the dopaminergic-hyperinnervation hypothesis if they are driven mostly by impaired learning from negative prediction errors. A more recent study (Shephard, Groom, and Jackson 2019) lends further credence to this hypothesis. That study found that patients with TS, most of whom were unmedicated, were not impaired in a sequence-learning task. However, they were impaired in switching from a sequenced block to a nonsequenced one, arguably the process that most relied on negative prediction errors. Interestingly, patients with TS on that study were also faster overall, in both sequenced and nonsequenced blocks, without a decrement on accuracy, possibly due to increased tonic dopamine. Indeed, increased dopamine, by increasing the gain of the Go relative to the NoGo pathway, should lead to faster responses overall (Collins and Frank 2014).

d) Mechanistic Explanation of Tic Learning and Expression in Tourette Syndrome   As mentioned in section 10.1.2, dopaminergic hyperinnervation seems to explain why there is an increased propensity for tics to be learned and expressed in TS (figure 10.3a), via increased phasic and tonic dopamine. Indeed, tic learning may be driven either by maladaptive, aberrantly timed phasic-dopamine release or by phasic dopamine released following the cessation of premonitory urges by tic execution (Maia and Conceição 2017); thus, tic learning is likely facilitated by the higher striatal phasic-dopamine release that is predicted to occur under dopaminergic hyperinnervation.[5]

Furthermore, tic execution, like the execution of other well-learned motor actions, is likely facilitated by higher striatal dopamine levels—including both tonic and phasic dopamine—provided that the Go values of tics are considerable (figure 10.1). Considering the aforementioned evidence on the overlearning of habits in TS (Delorme et al. 2016; Shepherd, Groom, and Jackson 2019) and the association between tics and habits, the existence of tics with considerable Go values is likely generally the case in TS.

Tics, however, are not necessarily dependent on the existence of higher striatal dopamine levels, but rather on the existence of an overactivation of the Go compared to the NoGo motor pathway (figure 10.1). Consistent with this idea, chronic administration of quinpirole, which is a D_2/D_3 agonist and therefore suppresses the NoGo pathway, causes tics in a juvenile-rat model of TS (Nespoli et al. 2018). In that rat model, however, dopaminergic projections to the dorsal striatum had been lesioned previously, which in itself is sort of the opposite of dopaminergic hyperinnervation, so these findings have to be interpreted with care. Nonetheless, chronic quinpirole administration, without prior lesioning of the dopamine system, also induces compulsive checking in rats (Szechtman, Sulis, and Eilam 1998), which is interesting given the very high comorbidity of OCD in patients with TS.

e) Mechanistic Explanation of the Therapeutic Effects of Medication in Tourette Syndrome In addition to providing a mechanistic explanation for the role of dopaminergic hyperinnervation in tics, the proposed CBGTC-inspired RL model seems to explain both the fast (figure 10.3b) and cumulative (figure 10.3c) therapeutic effects of antipsychotics in TS (Maia and Conceição 2017), as well as possible increases in tic expression following withdrawal from antipsychotics (figure 10.3d). The proposed model, moreover, seems to explain the therapeutic effects of all other medications with well-established efficacy in TS because all such medications reduce phasic and/or tonic dopaminergic neurotransmission (Maia and Conceição 2018).

As we suggested previously, from the medications with proven efficacy in TS, ecopipam, a D_1 antagonist, could be particularly interesting from a scientific perspective because, given the lower affinity of D_1 receptors, it should mostly antagonize phasic dopamine (Maia and Conceição 2018). We had associated phasic dopamine with tic learning, but not necessarily with tic execution (Maia and Conceição 2017). The existence of novel, strong evidence implicating phasic dopamine in action execution (da Silva et al. 2018), however, indicates that ecopipam should target tic execution, in addition to tic learning, which further helps to explain its efficacy in TS (Gilbert et al. 2018).

The aforementioned mechanisms of TS medication also help to develop a rationale for the combination of pharmacological and behavioral treatments. Successful execution of tic-competing responses in HRT and successful tic suppression in ExRP (see section 10.1.3) both are conditional on the probability of tic execution not approximating 1. At least for the most severely affected patients (Ganos, Martino, and Pringsheim 2017), therefore, increasing NoGo relative to Go activation pharmacologically (e.g., through antipsychotic medications) may permit sufficient inhibition of the tic to allow the behavioral therapy to work. For other therapies, such as contingency management and massed negative practice, which work by assigning a negative value to tics, co-adjuvant medication may have a more direct therapeutic effect by increasing learning and expression of negative values (Maia and Frank 2011). Chronic antipsychotic administration, for example, shifts the plasticity of corticostriatal synapses onto (motor) NoGo MSNs toward LTP, compared to LTD (Maia and Conceição 2017), besides leading to an increased gain of NoGo MSNs. By facilitating the NoGo learning and

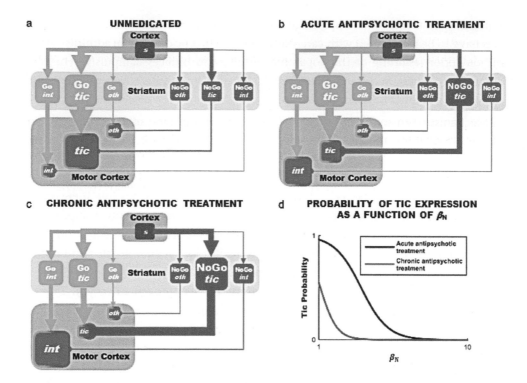

Figure 10.3

Effects of striatal dopamine levels and antipsychotic treatment on Tourette syndrome (TS). Panels (a)–(c) represent the Go and NoGo pathways (green and red, respectively) for three actions: an intended action (*int*), a tic (*tic*), and some other weakly supported action (*oth*). The pathways are represented schematically, through their ultimate effects on motor cortex, by omitting the globus pallidus and thalamus. Go and NoGo MSNs are therefore shown directly stimulating (or, more precisely, disinhibiting) and inhibiting the motor cortex, respectively, because activation in motor cortex ultimately reflects a subtraction of the outputs of the Go and NoGo pathways (section 10.3.2; figure 10.1). (In the figure, arrowheads represent excitation or disinhibition; circles represent inhibition.) The size of each square and the width of the arrow that departs from it represent the level of neuronal activity. Panels (a)–(c) differ in terms of patient medication status. (a) In unmedicated patients with TS, tics may have strong learned Go values, stored in corticostriatal synapses onto Go MSNs (see the thick green arrow from cortex to "Go tic" in the striatum); these Go values may be learned through ill-timed, exaggerated phasic dopamine responses or through negative reinforcement due to the temporary relief from the preceding premonitory urge (as mechanistically explained in section 10.3.3). Tics may also have relatively strong NoGo values, stored in corticostriatal synapses onto NoGo MSNs (see the relatively thick red arrow from cortex to "NoGo tic" in the striatum); these NoGo values may be learned through negative life experiences with tics (e.g., being embarrassed because of tics, feeling sore because of a tic, etc.).

Figure 10.3 (continued)

In unmedicated patients, however, the expression of these NoGo values is likely suppressed by the high striatal dopamine—predicted to occur under dopaminergic hyperinnervation (section 10.3.1; Hienert et al. 2018; Maia and Conceição 2018). Therefore, in an unmedicated patient with TS, the Go activity for tics overcomes the NoGo activity, making tic expression likely. (b) As soon as a patient begins antipsychotic treatment, or as soon as the antipsychotic reaches a sufficiently high dose, the antipsychotic blocks D_2 receptors in the NoGo pathway, disinhibiting that pathway, which then becomes stronger and better able to counteract the activity in the Go pathway. The tic thereby becomes less likely to be expressed. This very early effect of the antipsychotic may act mostly through this effect on excitability; the corticostriatal synapses representing Go and NoGo values may not yet be changed. (c) In addition to the effect on excitability, chronic antipsychotic treatment also increases NoGo values (by increasing the weight of corticostriatal synapses onto NoGo MSNs), decreases Go values (by decreasing the weight of corticostriatal synapses onto Go MSNs), or both (section 10.3.2; Maia and Conceição 2017). Thus, with the same level of D_2 occupancy as acute antipsychotic treatment, the tic becomes even less likely to be expressed [compare panels (b) and (c)]. [For illustrative purposes, panel (c) shows the case of both increased NoGo values and decreased Go values, but the same effect would be obtained with changes in just one or the other.] (d) Due to the fact that only chronic antipsychotic treatment is likely to strongly affect NoGo and/or Go values (i.e., to change synaptic weights rather than just excitability), acute and chronic antipsychotic treatment likely provide different levels of symptomatic control, as quantified by the probability of executing a given tic in each case. The x axis in the figure represents β_N as a proxy to the effect of the antipsychotic on excitability; larger values of β_N correspond to larger antipsychotic doses. The black and blue lines represent (qualitatively) the probabilities of tic execution following acute and chronic treatment, respectively. For a given dose of antipsychotic (i.e., for a given value of β_N), the probability of executing a tic is lower following chronic administration than following acute administration. This explains why antipsychotics may have a gradual cumulative effect and why, during chronic treatment, the dose may sometimes be reduced gradually without loss of efficacy (Maia and Conceição 2017). Still, if the dose is reduced too drastically or medication is completely stopped, tics that were completely absent may return. In the plot, this corresponds to moving left along the blue line, from a point in which the probability is nearly 0 to a point in which it becomes more substantial. Still, tics may be less severe than before treatment started (at least temporarily, until relearning occurs). In fact, tics may also be less severe right after stopping chronic treatment than they would be after a single acute dose of an antipsychotic wears off (compare the intercept of the blue vs. the black line). Figure reprinted from *Biological Psychiatry*, 82(6), Maia, T. V., and Conceição, V. A., The roles of phasic and tonic dopamine in tic learning and expression, pp. 332–344, 2017, with permission from Elsevier.

expression of tics (figure 10.3), chronic antipsychotic administration might therefore conceivably promote the success of contingency management or massed negative practice. Although these therapies have yet to present convincing results when administered as monotherapies (Fründt, Woods, and Ganos 2017), we are not aware of any systematic attempts to combine them with pharmacological therapies.

10.3.3 Premonitory Urges and Tics in Tourette Syndrome: Computational Mechanisms and Neural Correlates

Premonitory urges are aversive, distressful sensations that often precede, and are ceased by, tics (Brandt et al. 2016; Leckman, Walker, and Cohen 1993). Phasic dopamine is released following positive prediction errors (Schultz 2016; Maia 2009), including those elicited by the avoidance, and cessation, of aversive stimuli (Maia 2010; Navratilova and Porreca 2014; Seymour et al. 2005); thus, premonitory-urge cessation, via tic execution, may lead to phasic dopamine release. Such phasic release is possibly a key driver of tic learning (Conceição et al. 2017) via negative reinforcement (Capriotti et al. 2014)—that is, reinforcement due to escape from, or avoidance of, an aversive stimulus. However, as previously mentioned, aberrant, ill-timed phasic bursts may also reinforce tics.

a) **Computational Mechanisms of Premonitory-Urge-Driven Tic Learning and Execution** Two RL approaches may be used to describe how positive prediction errors may arise following premonitory-urge cessation (Conceição et al. 2017): an average-reward RL approach (Mahadevan 1996) and a standard RL approach (based on the actor–critic or similar state-value learning models—like OpAL models—but not on Q-learning models, which do not seem adequate to capture escape- or avoidance-learning behavior, as detailed in box 10.1). In average-reward RL, there is an ongoing computation of a recency-weighted average reinforcement, $\bar{r}_{t-1}$, which is used to evaluate the obtained reinforcements (Mahadevan 1996). Specifically, in average-reward RL, a positive reinforcement is not necessarily "rewarding" (nor is a negative reinforcement necessarily "punishing") unless it is higher (or lower, respectively) than the online estimate of the average reinforcement. Average-reward RL therefore attempts to optimize action policies by strengthening the associations between states and actions that yield a reinforcement higher than the average reinforcement at the time of action execution and by weakening those that yield a reinforcement lower than the average reinforcement. Given that, in this approach, all reinforcements are evaluated according to a mean reinforcement value, there is no mathematical reason to use a temporal discount factor γ (Mahadevan 1996), leading to the following equation for prediction-error calculation:

$$\delta_t = r(s_t) + \overline{r}_{t-1} + V_t(s_t) - V_t(s_{t-1}), \tag{10.15}$$

where $r(s_t)$ denotes the fact that the obtained reinforcement may be state-dependent. This equation has been shown to capture pain-termination-driven RL in humans (Seymour et al. 2005), which we have previously hypothesized to parallel tic learning due to premonitory-urge termination in patients with TS (Conceição et al. 2017), as described next.

Premonitory urges, U, are inherently aversive sensations $\left[r(U) < 0\right]$ that build up in time (Brandt et al. 2016); thus, immediately before premonitory-urge termination, $\overline{r}_{t-1}$ should typically be much lower than 0 ($\overline{r}_{t-1} \ll 0$). Therefore, unless premonitory-urge termination (via tic execution) is accompanied by a very negative reinforcement $\left[r(s_t) \ll 0\right]$, the term $r(s_t) - \overline{r}_{t-1}$ should be sufficiently positive to guarantee that, following premonitory-urge termination, $\delta_t > 0$, irrespective of the difference in state values at that time, $V_t(s_t) - V_t(s_{t-1})$, thereby strengthening the tic. Thus, under average-reward RL, state values are likely not necessary to explain tic learning, although they may certainly play a role (Conceição et al. 2017).

In standard RL (based on state-value learning models; see above), no average reinforcement is computed. Instead, prediction errors are calculated by

$$\delta_t = r(s_t) + \gamma V_t(s_t) - V_t(s_{t-1}), \tag{10.16}$$

where γ is the aforementioned temporal discount factor (box 10.1). The termination of an aversive premonitory urge does not per se result in a reward; in other words, $r(s_t)$ will not, in general, be positive. Thus, in standard RL, the elicitation of the positive prediction errors that may underlie tic learning is explained in terms of differences in state values (Conceição et al. 2017). Specifically, the combination of the aversive character of premonitory urges and the fact that they predict their own continuation means that the state of having a premonitory urge has a negative value $\left[V(U) < 0\right]$. Given that a tic terminates (even if only temporarily) a premonitory urge, the tic elicits a transition from a state with a negative value to a state with a neutral value, which produces a positive prediction error that reinforces the tic (Conceição et al. 2017). In other words, if it is assumed, for simplicity, that, on average, (1) $V_t(s_t)$ has no intrinsic value—because s_t is no longer characterized by the presence of a premonitory urge—and that (2) premonitory-urge termination is accompanied by a null, or no, primary reinforcement, $r(s_t)$, the prediction-error equation is therefore simplified into: $\delta_t = 0 - V_t(U) \Rightarrow \delta_t > 0$. Strikingly, however, δ_t would still be positive if premonitory-urge termination was accompanied by a negative $r(s_t)$ (e.g., social embarrassment) and/or by a negative $V_t(s_t)$, provided that $r(s_t) + \gamma V_t(s_t)$ is less negative than $V_t(U)$, which seems a reasonable assumption for most cases, given that premonitory urges are so aversive that they are often considered more distressing and life-impairing than tics themselves (Leckman, Walker, and Cohen 1993).

The positive prediction error elicited by premonitory-urge termination will tend to strengthen the association between the preceding state—having the premonitory urge—and the tic. Thus, the state of having a premonitory urge will come to elicit the tic, so premonitory urges will themselves come to elicit tic execution.

b) Neural Correlates of Premonitory-Urge-Driven Tic Learning and Execution   The insula and somatosensory cortices are strongly implicated in premonitory urges (figures 10.4 and 10.5; Cavanna et al. 2017; Conceição et al. 2017; Cox et al. 2018). In fact, the insula is also strongly implicated in natural urges (Jackson et al. 2011b) and in urges in addiction (Naqvi and Bechara 2010). Moreover, the insula is strongly implicated in interoceptive processing (Quadt, Critchley, and Garfinkel 2018), whose interaction with exteroceptive processing, in which the somatosensory cortices are strongly implicated, seems to underlie premonitory urges (figure 10.5; Cox et al. 2018). Abnormal interoceptive sensibility, in particular, correlates with both the severity of premonitory urges and tics in TS (Rae et al. 2019). Furthermore, the insula and somatosensory cortices are both structurally and functionally abnormal in TS, in addition to being aberrantly coupled structurally and functionally with regions from the motor CBGTC loop (figure 10.5; Conceição et al. 2017; Cox et al. 2018; Rae et al. 2018; Sigurdsson et al. 2018; Wen et al. 2018) that are implicated in tic learning and execution (Conceição et al. 2017; Maia and Conceição 2017). Like abnormal interoceptive sensibility, insular (structural and/or functional) connectivity has also been shown to correlate with both tic and premonitory urge severity (Conceição et al. 2017; Rae et al. 2018; Sigurdsson et al. 2018). The aforementioned abnormalities involving the insula and somatosensory cortices and their connections to the motor CBGTC loop are thereby likely to provide the substrate for premonitory urges and premonitory-urge-driven tic execution (figure 10.4; Conceição et al. 2017).

The insula, together with the ventral striatum (VS), is also strongly implicated in RL (Garrison, Erdeniz, and Done 2013; Palminteri and Pessiglione 2017; Seymour et al. 2004; Seymour et al. 2005)—particularly, in the case of the insula, with aversive outcomes (Garrison, Erdeniz, and Done 2013; Palminteri and Pessiglione 2017; Palminteri et al. 2012). Indeed, the insula has been strongly implicated in the coding of aversive state values $[V(s)<0]$ (Palminteri et al. 2012; Seymour et al. 2004), aversive prediction errors ($\delta < 0$) (Garrison, Erdeniz, and Done 2013; Seymour et al. 2004, Seymour et al. 2005), and aversive outcomes ($r < 0$), even when such outcomes are fully predicted and therefore do not elicit a prediction error (Conceição et al. 2017; Nitschke et al. 2006).

The insula is therefore a prime candidate to represent three of the tic-learning-related variables mentioned in the previous subsection: the intrinsic negative primary value of a premonitory urge $[r(U) < 0]$, its associated negative state value $[V(U) < 0]$, and the negative prediction errors ($\delta < 0$) associated with the onset of premonitory urges and their estimation over time (not to be confused with the *positive* prediction errors elicited by the *offset* of premonitory urges when a tic is executed; figure 10.4; Conceição et al. 2017).

More speculatively, the shell of the nucleus accumbens, which is a part of the VS, may be a good candidate to represent the average reinforcement, $\bar{r}$, over time (figure 10.4; Conceição et al. 2017; see also Niv et al. 2007 for a related proposal). Indeed, dopamine in the shell has a set of unique properties that should, in principle, allow the online computation of $\bar{r}$. Calculating $\bar{r}$ requires (1) inputs representing the (signed) primary reinforcers, r, and (2) a mechanism for the integration of those inputs over time. Dopamine in the shell might fulfill these two requirements: (1) appetitive and aversive stimuli have been shown to respectively cause phasic increases and decreases of dopamine in the shell, in a manner that does not seem to depend on how predictable or unpredictable such stimuli were (McCutcheon et al. 2012; Sackett, Saddoris, and Carelli 2017; see also Roitman et al. 2008)—thus, dopamine in the shell might represent the signed value of primary reinforcers; (2) DAT expression is comparatively low in the VS (Haber 2011), thereby permitting the slow integration of the shell's dopaminergic inputs over time, which would not be possible if the amount of DAT in the shell was such that phasic dopaminergic changes were always rapidly nullified via dopamine reuptake (Conceição et al. 2017).

The existence of direct and indirect projections from both the shell and the insula to the ventral tegmental area (VTA), in turn, explains how the VTA may have access to all variables that are necessary to calculate the prediction errors that are implicated in tic learning, as well as in the learning of related state values (figure 10.4; Conceição et al. 2017). Finally, striato-nigro-striatal spirals (Haber 2011) may allow the propagation of the prediction errors implicated in tic learning from the ventral to the dorsal striatum, where they can be used to update the Go and NoGo values of actions (in this case, the Go and NoGo values of tics) stored in the corticostriatal synapses onto D_1 and D_2 MSNs, respectively (figure 10.4; Conceição et al. 2017).

c) Premonitory Urges and Tics: Clinical Implications Considering the likely causal role of premonitory urges in tic learning and execution, we have previously suggested that optimal treatment strategies for TS would likely have to act upstream of tics, in premonitory-urge related processes, possibly by targeting the insula and/or the somatosensory cortices (Conceição et al. 2017). In line with such prediction, successful

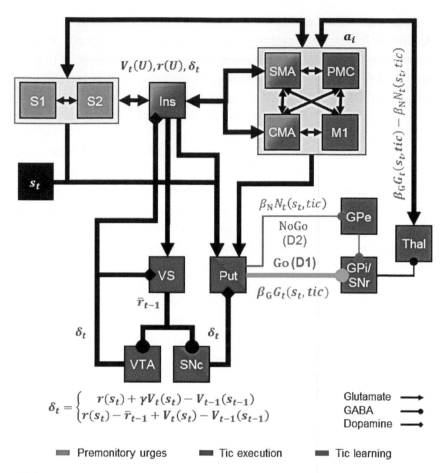

Figure 10.4

Regions and computations involved in premonitory urges, tic execution, and tic learning in Tourette syndrome (TS). The figure depicts the main regions involved in premonitory urges (gold), tic execution (gray), and tic learning (blue), and the most important connections between them, according to the framework that we have previously proposed (section 10.3.3; Conceição et al. 2017). This framework addresses both the computational roles of dopamine in motor-loop-mediated tic learning and execution (section 10.3.2; Maia and Conceição 2017) and the neural substrates and mechanistic roles of premonitory urges in tic learning and execution (Conceição et al. 2017). *Tic execution*: Cortical motor areas represent candidate actions (a_i), including tics, being considered for gating. Other cortical (and some subcortical) areas represent the current state or situation (s_t, where the subscript t denotes time). The putamen contains Go (direct-pathway, green) and NoGo (indirect-pathway, red) medium spiny neurons (MSNs; figure 10.1). Striatal hyperdopaminergia, due to dopaminergic hyperinnervation in TS (section 10.3.1; Hienert et al. 2018; Maia and Conceição 2018), increases the activation of the Go relative to the NoGo pathway

Figure 10.4 (continued)

(by increasing the value of β_G relative to β_N; figure 10.3). Such increase is disproportionately larger for actions with large Go (G) values, because β_G is a multiplicative gain parameter. Consequently, as tics become strongly learned behaviors (see below and sections 10.3.2–10.3.3), striatal hyperdopaminergia will make $\beta_G G_t(s_t, tic) \gg \beta_N N_t(s_t, tic)$ (compare the width of the green and red arrows leaving from the putamen; see section 10.3.2 and figures 10.1 and 10.3). As a consequence, there is strong inhibition of the tic representation in the basal ganglia output nuclei, the globus pallidus internal segment (GPi) and substantia nigra pars reticulata (SNr), by the direct pathway $[\beta_G G_t(s_t, tic)]$, with weak disinhibition by the NoGo pathway [with a value of $[\beta_N N_t(s_t, tic)]$. Given that $\beta_G G_t(s_t, tic) \gg \beta_N N_t(s_t, tic)$, tic execution is promoted (figure 10.3; Maia and Conceição 2017). Tic execution may also possibly be driven directly by cortico-cortical projections from somatosensory regions and the insula to motor cortices (Conceição et al. 2017). *Tic learning*: Tic execution commonly terminates a preceding premonitory urge, yielding a positive prediction error, δ_t, that promotes tic learning (Conceição et al. 2017). Like δ_t, $r(U)$ is a relevant variable to explain tic learning in the two reinforcement learning (RL) accounts that we have used to explain premonitory-urge-driven tic learning: standard RL and average-reward RL (Conceição et al. 2017). In contrast, $V_t(U)$ is necessary for the account using standard RL and optional for the account using average-reward RL, and $\bar{r}_{t-1}$ is only necessary for the account using average-reward RL (Conceição et al. 2017). In this figure, those variables are depicted near the regions and/or connections that we have hypothesized to subserve them (Conceição et al. 2017). The prediction errors represented in the insula, however, may be mostly aversive. *Additional figure details*: Some anatomical projections are omitted for simplicity. For clarity, both somatosensory cortical areas (primary [S1] and secondary [S2] somatosensory cortices) and motor cortical areas (cingulate motor area [CMA], supplementary motor area [SMA], premotor cortex [PMC], and primary motor cortex [M1]) are grouped. The distinct ways of calculating δ_t according to each of the proposed computational accounts are indicated in curly braces: $\delta_t = r(s_t) + \gamma V_t(s_t) - V_{t-1}(s_{t-1})$ (standard RL) and $\delta_t = r(s_t) + \bar{r}_{t-1} + V_t(s_t) - V_{t-1}(s_{t-1})$ (average-reward RL; section 10.3.3). *Additional abbreviations*: Ins: insula; Put: putamen; SNc: substantia nigra *pars compacta*; Thal: thalamus; VS: ventral striatum; VTA: ventral tegmental area. Figure reprinted, with minor alterations, from *Current Opinion in Neurobiology*, 46, Conceição, V. A., Dias, A., Farinha, A. C., and Maia, T. V., Premonitory urges and tics in Tourette syndrome: computational mechanisms and neural correlates, pp. 187–199, 2017, with permission from Elsevier.

---

tic reduction via high-frequency deep-brain stimulation of the thalamus was shown recently to correlate with changes in the activity of both the insula and sensorimotor regions (Jo et al. 2018). This prediction also has potential implications for repetitive transcranial magnetic stimulation (rTMS) treatment in TS (Conceição et al. 2017). Indeed, rTMS over the motor cortices has yet to prove better than sham stimulation in TS (Hsu, Wang, and Lin 2018), possibly because it is acting too downstream; it certainly seems that it would be worth trying rTMS over the insula or the somatosensory cortices to see if, by acting farther upstream, the effect would be better.

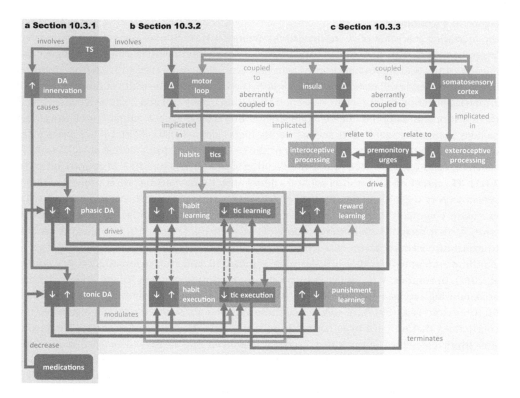

Figure 10.5

Concept map summarizing the main theoretical ideas in the chapter. The key brain regions that we discuss are shown in blue, the key cognitive processes are shown in gray, the key alterations in Tourette syndrome (TS) are shown in orange, and the key medication effects are shown in green. Upward- and downward-pointing arrows represent increases and decreases, respectively (due to TS or the medication if they are in orange or green boxes, respectively). Triangles show alterations. Each region shaded in a different color corresponds to a specific chapter section. (a) Section 10.3.1. As discussed in section 10.3.1 and depicted in the area shaded in gold, patients with TS likely suffer from dopaminergic hyperinnervation (Hienert et al. 2018; Maia and Conceição 2018), which causes increases in both phasic and tonic dopamine. Those dopaminergic increases help to explain why all medications with well-established efficacy for TS reduce phasic and/or tonic dopaminergic neurotransmission (Maia and Conceição 2018). (b) Section 10.3.2. As discussed in section 10.3.2 and depicted in the area shaded in medium-light gold, TS involves structural and functional disturbances in the motor loop (Maia and Conceição 2017; Worbe et al. 2015a; Worbe

Figure 10.5 (continued)

et al. 2015b), which is implicated in both habit learning and execution (Delorme et al. 2016; Horga et al. 2015; Yin and Knowlton 2006). Habit learning and habit execution are strongly mediated by phasic and tonic dopamine, respectively (Collins and Frank 2014; Maia and Conceição 2017), with some novel evidence also implicating phasic dopamine in habit execution (hence, the blue dashed arrow; da Silva et al. 2018). Tics seem to be pathological motor habits (hence, their depiction in the orange rectangle inside the blue "habits" rectangle), which explains why, in TS, phasic- and tonic-dopamine levels may play pathological roles in tic learning and execution that parallel the roles normally played by normal phasic- and tonic-dopamine levels in habit learning and execution (note the similarities between the respective orange and blue arrows; Maia and Conceição 2017). The latter associations help to explain mechanistically how medications may reduce tic severity in TS: by downregulating phasic and/or tonic dopaminergic neurotransmission, medication should reduce tic learning and/or execution (Maia and Conceição 2017). The role of phasic dopamine in signaling positive prediction errors explains why unmedicated patients with TS, with their likely increase in phasic dopamine, exhibit increased learning from rewards (Palminteri et al. 2009; Palminteri et al. 2011). The role of tonic dopamine in possibly blunting the signaling of negative prediction errors by phasic decreases in dopamine explains why TS involves reduced learning from punishments (Palminteri et al. 2009). In turn, the previously mentioned effects of TS medications on dopaminergic transmission—possibly along with other, more complex effects of the medication (Maia and Conceição 2017)—explain why patients with TS under antipsychotics (other than aripiprazole) are impaired at reward learning (Palminteri et al. 2009; Palminteri et al. 2011; Worbe et al. 2011). (c) Section 10.3.3. As discussed in section 10.3.3 and depicted in the area with the lightest gold shading, TS involves structural and/or functional abnormalities in the somatosensory cortices and insula, in addition to the motor loop. TS, moreover, involves structural and functional abnormalities in the connectivity between all those regions (Conceição et al. 2017; Neuner, Schneider, and Shah 2013; Sigurdsson et al. 2018). The somatosensory cortices are implicated in exteroception (Cox et al. 2018), and the insula is implicated in both (natural) urges (Naqvi and Bechara 2010; Jackson et al. 2011b) and interoception (Quadt, Critchley, and Garfinkel 2018; Cox et al. 2018). Premonitory urges, in turn, seem to be driven by the interplay between pathological exteroceptive and/or interoceptive processing (Cox et al. 2018), which explains the implication of the somatosensory cortices and insula in premonitory urges (figure 10.4; Conceição et al. 2017). Premonitory urges likely play a key role in tic learning, as the termination of premonitory urges, via tic execution, may elicit positive prediction errors, signaled by phasic dopamine, that reinforce tics (Conceição et al. 2017). Premonitory urges may also directly drive tic execution through the connections from somatosensory regions and the insula to motor cortices (Conceição et al. 2017).

10.4 Discussion

10.4.1 Strengths of the Proposed Theory-Driven Account: A Unified Account That Explains a Wide Range of Findings in Tourette Syndrome

The hypothesis that TS involves dopaminergic hyperinnervation provides a parsimonious and integrated explanation for extant neurochemical and pharmacological data in TS (Maia and Conceição 2018). Such a hypothesis, moreover, is supported by a recent meta-analysis that found significantly increased striatal DAT binding in patients with TS compared to controls (Hienert et al. 2018). Still, additional research on this issue is necessary because those meta-analytic findings became nonsignificant when controlling for age (Hienert et al. 2018), and most studies of the dopaminergic system in TS had very small samples and were subject to various other confounds (Maia and Conceição 2018).

Extensive evidence implicates phasic and tonic dopamine in action learning and selection, respectively (Collins and Frank 2014; Maia and Frank 2011, 2017), with recent evidence also implicating phasic dopamine in action selection (da Silva et al. 2018). Dopaminergic hyperinnervation would be expected to increase both phasic and tonic dopamine, which, in turn, would thereby increase both tic learning and expression (Maia and Conceição 2017). Hyperdopaminergia should also increase learning from rewards and increase habit learning, which are the main findings from RL and habit-learning studies in TS, respectively (Maia and Conceição 2017).

Finally, a ubiquitous clinical characteristic of TS is the presence of premonitory urges, which are alleviated temporarily by tics (Brandt et al. 2016; Leckman, Walker, and Cohen 1993). We have argued that the termination of premonitory urges likely elicits positive prediction errors, which reinforce tics (Conceição et al. 2017). These positive prediction errors likely elicit phasic firing of dopamine neurons, which again links to hyperdopaminergia in TS. A detailed consideration of the neural substrates of premonitory urges and their interactions with the motor system further explains how premonitory urges might play a role not only in tic learning but also in tic execution (Conceição et al. 2017). In short, our theoretical account, reviewed in section 10.3, provides a rigorous and comprehensive account of a wide range of findings in TS (figure 10.5).

10.4.2. Limitations and Extensions

a) Other Regions and Neurochemical Disturbances   We focused on the role of the motor CBGTC loop in tics and on the roles of the somatosensory cortices and insula in premonitory urges (as summarized in figures 10.4 and 10.5). Multiple other regions, however—among them, for example, the cerebellum (which is bidirectionally connected with the basal ganglia via disynaptic connections; Bostan, Dum, and Strick 2010) and the inferior frontal gyrus—have been strongly implicated in TS (Caligiore et al. 2017; Jo et al. 2018; Neuner, Schneider, and Shah 2013; Wen et al. 2017a; Wen et al. 2018; Wen et al. 2017b). We also did not address possible differences between the mechanisms and neural correlates underlying motor versus phonic tics, but some evidence suggests that phonic tics might be specifically related to limbic regions (Foltynie 2016; Jo et al. 2018).

We also focused on the involvement of the dopaminergic system, and specifically dopaminergic hyperinnervation, in TS. Multiple neurochemical abnormalities, however, have been implicated in TS (Cox, Seri, and Cavanna 2016; Kataoka et al. 2010; Lennington et al. 2016; Robertson et al. 2017), and some evidence suggests that targeting neuromodulators other than dopamine may also be beneficial for patients with TS (Augustine and Singer 2019; Thenganatt and Jankovic 2016). We should therefore emphasize that our focus on dopamine is not meant to imply that dopamine is the only or even the primary disturbance in TS. Other disturbances may also lead to TS if, like dopaminergic hyperinnervation, they have the same circuit-level effects: increased plasticity and excitability of the Go, relative to the NoGo, motor pathway (Conceição et al. 2017; Maia and Conceição 2017).

b) Inhibitory Control in Tourette Syndrome   There has been substantial interest in inhibitory control in TS due to the hypothesis that tics might result from impaired inhibitory control (Morand-Beaulieu et al. 2017). Alterations in inhibitory control in TS would be consistent with the implication of the inferior frontal gyrus in classification studies discriminating patients with TS from controls (section 10.2.1), because the inferior frontal gyrus is strongly implicated in inhibitory control (Aron, Robbins, and Poldrack 2014). Indeed, recent meta-analytic evidence seems to suggest that patients with TS have impairments in inhibitory control (Morand-Beaulieu et al. 2017). However, the same meta-analysis reported that inhibitory control was more impaired in patients with TS who had comorbid ADHD and in patients with TS under medication than in unmedicated patients with TS, who were themselves quite similar to controls. Thus, impaired inhibitory control in patients with TS may be a consequence of comorbid ADHD—indeed, inhibitory control is substantially impaired in ADHD (Brocki et al. 2007; Willcutt et al. 2005)—or of the medications. Some researchers, in fact, have even suggested that TS might involve enhanced (compensatory) cognitive control, including enhanced inhibitory control (Baym et al. 2008; Jackson et al. 2011a; Jung et al. 2013).

c) Appearance of Tics before Premonitory Urges in Development   We emphasized tic learning through negative reinforcement due to premonitory-urge termination, but children often develop tics before they start to report premonitory urges (Cavanna et al. 2017; Sambrani, Jakubovski, and Müller-Vahl 2016). One possible explanation for tic learning without premonitory-urge termination is that tics may also be learned due to excessive, "random" phasic dopamine transients. An alternative explanation for this seeming contradiction in timing during development is that children's failure to report premonitory urges does not mean that such premonitory urges are nonexistent; it may simply mean that children are impaired at reporting them (Conceição et al. 2017; Martino, Ganos, and Worbe 2018). In line with this statement, children with TS are even impaired at reporting tics themselves (Conceição et al. 2017), and the intensity of premonitory urges seems to be similar in children and youth of different ages (Raines et al. 2018; Steinberg et al. 2010; Woods et al. 2005). Also in line with the learning of tics through negative reinforcement, a recent report of two cases describes the onset of premonitory urges before tics and as early as the age of 5 (Li et al. 2019). Moreover, subliminal learning from rewards is increased in TS (Palminteri et al. 2009), which might imply that subliminal learning from positive prediction errors in general—including those due to negative reinforcement—might be increased in TS. Thus, it is certainly possible that negative reinforcement plays a role even when premonitory urges fail to be reported (Conceição et al. 2017).

A related consideration is that urges may only become especially notorious for the individual when the individual attempts to inhibit the corresponding behavior. A parallel might be drawn here to natural urges (e.g., to urinate, etc.). There, too, early in development, children might feel an urge that, however, is almost too fleeting to be noticed because it is immediately followed by the corresponding behavior (e.g., an urge to urinate, which leads immediately and necessarily to urination). It is only as children learn to inhibit the behavior that the urge may become more notorious and that the link between the urge and the behavior may become more apparent; prior to that, the urge and behavior may be linked into a single experiential unit that makes noticing the urge as a separate entity more difficult. The same thing may occur with tics: it may be only as children learn to inhibit tics that premonitory urges become more noticeable (even if they were there, and could support negative reinforcement, all along). In line with these ideas, premonitory-urge intensity is indeed higher during tic suppression (Brandt et al. 2016).

d) Feedback Connections and Oscillations in the Basal Ganglia   We focused on RL models formed by sets of equations that predominantly capture the feedforward functioning of CBGTC loops (section 10.3.2; box 10.1; figure 10.1). However, there are several phenomena, such as neuronal oscillations within CBGTC loops (Brittain and Brown 2014), that those models cannot capture due to the underlying circuit over-simplifications (see, e.g., Augustine and Singer 2019). Here, we address such oscillatory behavior because pathological, low-frequency neuronal oscillations have been implicated in hyperkinetic symptoms from several movement disorders (Ellens and Leventhal 2013; Neumann et al. 2018), including TS (Hashemiyoon, Kuhn, and Visser-Vandewalle 2017; Neumann et al. 2018). In TS, indeed, symptom severity has been shown to correlate with increased low-frequency oscillations, namely with pallidal and thalamic oscillations in the theta and beta bands (Neumann et al. 2018), and some authors now believe that prolonged theta bursts may be specifically implicated in involuntary movements (Neumann et al. 2018). Furthermore, in TS, reductions of tic severity induced by deep-brain stimulation have been shown to correlate with a relative increase of oscillations in the higher-frequency, gamma band (Hashemiyoon, Kuhn, and Visser-Vandewalle 2017).

The subthalamic nucleus (STN) and the globus pallidus external segment (GPe) seem to be centrally implicated in oscillatory behavior within CBGTC loops (Frank 2006; Gatev, Darbin, and Wichmann 2006). The STN and GPe are connected in a negative feedback loop, in which the STN stimulates the GPe, which in turn inhibits the STN. This negative feedback loop, driven by other inputs, may underlie the oscillatory behavior within CBGTC loops (Frank 2006; Gatev, Darbin, and Wichmann 2006). The projections from both the STN and GPe to the output nuclei of the basal ganglia, the globus pallidus internal segment/substantia nigra pars reticulata, in turn, allow the propagation of the aforementioned oscillations through CBGTC loops (Frank 2006). Simplified CBGTC-inspired RL models, like OpAL models (see section 10.3.2; Collins and Frank 2014; Maia and Conceição 2017; Maia and Frank 2017), do not explicitly account for STN-GPe bidirectional connectivity (see, e.g., figure 10.1), which explains why those models cannot be used to describe oscillatory behavior within CBGTC loops. These models also do not capture other phenomena that may similarly contribute to such oscillatory behavior (see, e.g., Llinás et al. 2005).

Although the models we have emphasized do not themselves exhibit oscillatory behavior, our main hypothesis that TS involves dopaminergic hyperinnervation is consistent with the observed increase of low-frequency oscillations in TS (Neumann et al. 2018). Indeed, these oscillations are present not only in TS but also in levodopa-induced dyskinesias in PD, where they arise specifically with levodopa administration (Alonso-Frech et al. 2006), which shows a clear association with dopamine. Moreover, these oscillations are also present in dystonia (Ellens and Leventhal 2013; Neumann et al. 2017), which, as hypothesized in Neumann et al. (2018), again might relate to dopamine because dystonia involves increased D_1 receptor availability (Simonyan et al. 2017)—which, like hyperdopaminergia, should increase Go pathway activation. Thus, dopaminergic hyperinnervation in TS, and the consequent hyperdopaminergia, might be the cause of the observed low-frequency oscillations.

10.5 Chapter Summary

TS, a disorder characterized by tics, seems to be associated with dopaminergic hyperin-nervation, which likely causes increases in both phasic and tonic dopamine (section 10.3.1; figure 10.5a). Given the roles of phasic and tonic dopamine in habit learn-ing and execution, these increases lead to an overactive habit system (figure 10.5b), with tics likely being persistent, maladaptive motor habits. This relation between tics and habits explains why the motor loop is centrally involved in both (figure 10.5b). The central role of hyperdopaminergia in the overactivity of the habit system in TS, with consequent tics, explains why all medications with well-established efficacy for TS reduce dopaminergic neurotransmission (section 10.3.2; figure 10.5a–b).

Tics are usually preceded by, and terminate, premonitory urges—aversive, distress-ful sensations in which the somatosensory cortices and insula seem to be strongly implicated (figure 10.5c). Premonitory-urge termination likely elicits positive predic-tion errors, which are signaled by phasic dopamine and reinforce tics (section 10.3.3; figure 10.5c). Under dopaminergic hyperinnervation, this signaling might be excessive, which, again, might contribute to tic learning.

In the context of this book, it is worth articulating briefly the overall strategy under-pinning the theoretical proposals in this chapter. We started with a well-motivated computational model of the function of CBGTC circuits and the role of dopamine therein, for which there is much evidence independent of TS; to understand dysfunc-tion computationally, it is fundamental to first understand function, to be able to understand how such function may be disrupted. We then used this model to inves-tigate the multiple implications of a simple and parsimonious hypothesis about an underlying disturbance in TS—dopaminergic hyperinnervation. We found that this simple hypothesis, when considered in light of the model, provided an explanation for a very broad range of experimental and clinical findings in TS—ranging from experi-mental findings about reinforcement and habit learning in TS to clinical findings about the medications that are used to treat TS. This body of work therefore showcases one of the key uses of theory-based computational psychiatry: developing a rigorous and integrated mechanistic understanding capable of explaining and bringing together a wide variety of seemingly disparate findings.

10.6 Further Study

Maia and Frank (2011) show how a biologically detailed model of RL in the basal ganglia, closely related to the models described in this chapter, sheds light on multiple neuropsychiatric disorders: TS, PD, attention-deficit/hyperactivity disorder, addiction, and schizophrenia. The article's proposals about TS are precursors for several of the ideas in this chapter. In addition, the article shows how a single model can help to understand not only TS but also multiple other disorders that similarly involve disturbances in the dopaminergic system and basal ganglia.

Maia and Frank (2017) reconcile evidence from studies of the dopaminergic system with behavioral and functional neuroimaging data from patients with schizophrenia, using a model and ideas akin to those that we later applied to TS and describe in this chapter. This interrelated treatment of TS and schizophrenia is particularly apt because, despite their very distinct clinical presentation, both are hyperdopaminergic disorders. Thus, for example, some of the insights on the effects of antipsychotics originally developed in Maia and Frank (2017) have close parallels in our account of the effects of antipsychotics in TS.

Maia (2010) shows how learning to (actively) avoid aversive outcomes relies on positive prediction errors, using an actor–critic framework. This link between negative reinforcement and positive prediction errors, which are signaled by phasic dopamine responses, provided much of the motivation for our suggestions linking the termination of premonitory urges with tic reinforcement in the context of hyperdopaminergia in TS.

Seymour et al. (2005) showed how average-reward learning can explain the relief signal that occurs when a painful stimulus is terminated. This account formed the basis for one of our accounts of how the termination of premonitory urges can reinforce tics (although the two accounts reviewed in this chapter are closely related, as they both imply that the termination of premonitory urges elicits positive prediction errors that strengthen tics).

Hienert et al. (2018) reports what is, to the best of our knowledge, the first and, to date, only meta-analysis of molecular-imaging studies of the dopaminergic system in TS—specifically, PET and SPECT studies of the dopamine transporter and D_2 receptor in the striatum. Consistent with the idea that TS involves dopaminergic hyperinnervation, the meta-analysis found significantly increased dopamine transporter binding in TS (although that finding was not entirely conclusive because it became nonsignificant after controlling for age).

10.7 Acknowledgments

The authors acknowledge funding from Fundação para a Ciência e a Tecnologia, Portugal (Ph.D. Fellowship PD/BD/105852/2014 to VAC) and from the Tourette Association of America (to TVM). The authors also thank João Antunes for assistance in searching the literature for relevant articles, as well as their participation in a twinning project (SynaNet) from the European Union Horizon 2020 Programme (project number: 692340).

11   Perspectives and Further Study in Computational Psychiatry

Peggy Seriès
University of Edinburgh

11.1 Processes and Disorders Not Covered in This Book

This book described examples of methods and questions that are currently at the forefront of research in computational psychiatry, and which have offered new insights into the mechanisms that underlie several psychiatric disorders. The examples we have covered describe multiple levels of analysis, from the biophysically detailed level (chapter 3) and network level (chapter 4) to algorithmic and normative models that are more abstract and use tools from reinforcement learning and Bayesian methods (chapter 5–10).

There are a number of important topics that have not been covered in the current volume, however.

In terms of processes as defined by RDoC (see chapter 1), chapter 3 and chapter 4 cover cognitive and reinforcement processes respectively, and chapter 10 touches on motor processes. However, social processes (affiliation and attachment, social communication, perception and understanding of self and others)—a domain where research has grown significantly in recent years (see Hackel and Amodio (2018) for a recent review)—would deserve a much better treatment. Arousal and regulatory systems (circadian rhythms, sleep, and wakefulness) are also absent from this volume, but very little research exists in this area in the context of computational psychiatry.

In terms of disorders, similarly, the book only covers a subset of disorders. Notably absent are bipolar disorder, and particularly mania; autism spectrum disorders (ASD); obsessive-compulsive disorders (OCD); attention deficit hyperactivity disorder (ADHD); eating disorders; personality disorders (e.g., borderline, paranoid, antisocial personality disorder); and post-traumatic stress disorder (PTSD).

In the following, we offer some pointers on research that exists in those domains as a starting point for the interested reader. This list is by no means exhaustive. While some of those topics are starting to attract a lot of interest from a computational point of view, others have only been addressed by a handful of studies to date. The idea we would like to convey is that understanding is still mostly lacking for those issues. Computational psychiatry is still in its infancy, and the field is wide open for interdisciplinary research progress.

11.1.1 Autistic Spectrum Disorder

There is a growing computational literature regarding autistic spectrum disorder (ASD).

A dominant theory is that ASD could be regarded as a disorder of prediction or Bayesian inference (Sinha et al. 2014; Palmer, Lawson, and Hohwy 2017). The general hypothesis is that the weight, also called "precision" (see section 2.4.6), ascribed to sensory evidence and prior expectations would be imbalanced in ASD, resulting in sensory evidence having a disproportionately strong influence on perception. This relatively stronger influence of sensory information could explain the hypersensitivity to sensory stimuli and extreme attention to details that are observed in ASD. The weaker influence of prior expectations would also result in more variability in sensory experiences. The desire for sameness and rigid behaviors could then be understood as an attempt to introduce more predictability in one's environment (Pellicano and Burr 2012). Furthermore, this could lead to prior expectations that are too specific and do not generalize across situations (Van de Cruys et al. 2014).

While all theories agree that the relative influence of prior expectations is weaker in ASD, the primary source of this imbalance has been debated: would it arise from increased sensory precision (i.e., sharper likelihood) or from reduced precision of prior expectations? While early authors argued for attenuated priors (Pellicano and Burr 2012), the hypothesis of increased sensory precision is currently gaining more traction (Lawson, Rees, and Friston 2014; Palmer, Lawson, and Hohwy 2017; Karvelis et al. 2018).

More recently, it has also been proposed that key differences in ASD could be in the extent to which participants can predict whether the environment is dynamically changing or whether it is relatively stable (Lawson et al. 2017). Participants with ASD would overestimate the volatility of the environment, thus failing to make use of relevant priors (but see Lieder et al. 2019).

Although the above theories have gained a lot of popularity, conclusive experimental evidence is still largely lacking.

The interested reader can consult Palmer, Lawson, and Hohwy (2017) and Haker, Schneebeli, and Stephan (2016) for recent reviews of the Bayesian approach.

At a more biological level, it has been proposed that deficits in prediction and inference could be related to an imbalance between excitation and inhibition in neural circuits (Rosenberg, Patterson, and Angelaki 2015). It is thought that, in the cortex, a key computation performed by neural circuits is that of "divisive normalization," which divides the net excitatory drive to a neuron by a measure of the local population activity. Alterations in divisive normalization, due to excitation/inhibition imbalances, may give rise to autism symptomatology (Rosenberg, Patterson, and Angelaki 2015). This is interesting because divisive normalization is thought to be a "canonical computation" (Carandini and Heeger 2011) that could implement the marginalization computations necessary for Bayesian inference (Beck, Latham, and Pouget 2011). To date, however, those levels of description have not been reconciled in the context of autism and more experimental support is still needed to confirm this model.

11.1.2 Bipolar Disorder

Recent computational theories propose that bipolar disorder may be related to the perception of reward and its interaction with mood (Eldar et al. 2016; Mason, Eldar, and Rutledge 2017). According to these theories, mood reflects the cumulative impact of differences between reward outcomes and expectations (Eldar et al. 2016). Moreover, when we are in a good mood, we may perceive rewards as better than they actually are. Reciprocally, when we are in a bad mood, we may perceive rewards as worse than they actually are. People whose moods bias their perception of rewards too strongly will be more likely to experience greater mood swings in reaction to the same sequence of good or bad events, potentially resulting in extreme behavior. Eldar et al. (2016) and Mason, Eldar, and Rutledge (2017) show that computational models based on such simple ideas can explain the mood oscillations and other symptoms specific to bipolar disorder.

Despite its prevalence, there have been only a handful of studies looking at bipolar disorder from a computational perspective (Mason, Eldar, and Rutledge 2017; Goldbeter 2011; Chang and Chou 2018; Steinacher and Wright 2013) and the disorder remains very poorly understood (Geddes and Miklowitz 2013). There is thus a huge potential for advances in this domain.

11.1.3 Obsessive-Compulsive Disorder

As described elsewhere in this book (section 2.3.3 and chapter 5), it is thought that decisions can arise from two distinct, parallel systems of instrumental control, called the goal-directed and habitual systems. In goal-directed control, choices are made depending on their likely affective outcomes as predicted by a model of the environment. In habitual control, on the contrary, choices aim to reproduce actions that were previously rewarded. Disorders of compulsivity have been associated with a bias toward model-free (habit) acquisition instead of toward the goal-directed system (Voon et al. 2015).

Additional insights into OCD might be gained by considering how beliefs and actions are coupled. For example, someone with OCD will tell you that they know their hands are clean, but nevertheless won't be able to stop washing them. Two things that are normally linked together—confidence and action—have become uncoupled. Using computational methods, it has been found that the degree to which action and confidence are uncoupled in a simple decision task correlates with OCD severity (Vaghi et al. 2017). Very recently, new models of OCD have been proposed (Fradkin et al. 2020) that suggest that the disorder could be related to excessive uncertainty regarding state transitions (transition uncertainty): a computational impairment in Bayesian inference leading to a reduced ability to use the past to predict the present and future, and to oversensitivity to feedback (i.e., prediction errors).

11.1.4 Attention-Deficit/Hyperactivity Disorder

Behaviorally, ADHD is best characterized by increased variability across multiple cognitive domains and time scales.

Ziegler et al. (2016) offers a detailed review of how drift-diffusion models (DDM; see section 2.2) of decision-making and reinforcement learning models (section 2.3) have been applied to understanding individual differences in ADHD. They conclude that empirical studies agree with theories' prediction for a lower DDM drift rate and reduced reinforcement learning choice sensitivity ("noisier" softmax parameter).

At a more neurobiological level, Hauser et al. (2016) propose that this reduced choice sensitivity could be explained by impairments in neural gain; that is, the degree to which neural signals are amplified or suppressed, a computation commonly associated with catecholaminergic neurotransmitter systems (i.e., dopamine and noradrenaline). They suggest that impaired gain modulation could then explain ADHD abnormalities, in particular increased variability, spanning from behavior to neural activity.

11.1.5 Post-Traumatic Stress Disorder

Computational psychiatry is a promising tool for understanding PTSD (Seriès 2019). Indeed, it is commonly believed that PTSD results from abnormalities in learning during and after the traumatic event. Fear conditioning could explain why neutral stimuli (people, places, sounds, etc.) that have been associated with the traumatic event acquire the capacity to trigger and maintain anxiety long after the trauma itself. Why this association doesn't weaken over time could be explained either by the fact that it was abnormally strong in the first place or—more likely—due to deficits in extinction processes; that is, a failure for the association to weaken when the same cues are reencountered without leading to the traumatic event. This could be a result of patients' avoidance strategies: individuals with PTSD avoid encountering such cues again and thus may never experience them as being safe. Other theories assume, on the contrary, that PTSD is related to basic deficits in acquiring associations between specific cues and the traumatic event. This would result in associating the trauma with the environment as a whole, causing heightened contextual anxiety and/or overgeneralization of fear to all cues resembling the initial cues.

Despite the popularity of the theories mentioned above, the specific components of anomalous learning in PTSD remain unclear. Recently, however, research studies associating behavioral avoidance-learning tasks, computational modeling, and fMRI have started to dissect how learning mechanisms could differ in PTSD. Homan et al. (2019) and Brown et al. (2018) found, for example, that combat-exposed veterans suffering from PTSD pay more attention to surprising aversive outcomes. The researchers could also identify the neural structures involved in these differences. This greater attention to perceived threat could, in turn, explain hypervigilant responses.

11.1.6 Personality Disorders

Computational perspectives in the fields of personality and personality disorders have been very limited. A recent review about the use of computational psychiatry methods in borderline personality disorder can be found in Fineberg, Stahl, and Corlett (2017). Lee (2017) offers a review of data and theories regarding paranoid personality disorder. Patzelt, Hartley, and Gershman (2018) also provide an interesting discussion of the concept and promise of a computational phenotype—a collection of mathematically derived parameters that precisely describe individual differences in personality, development, and psychiatric illness.

11.1.7 Eating Disorders

Computational approaches have yet to provide detailed theories and models of eating disorders. However, a growing body of evidence suggests that patients with anorexia nervosa have impairments in value-based learning and decision making (Verharen et al. 2019). Similarly, binge-eating disorders have been linked to impairments in making goal-directed decisions (Voon et al. 2015) and to biases toward exploratory behavior (Morris et al. 2016).

11.2 Data-Driven Approaches

This volume focused on theory-driven approaches, which, as described in chapter 1, employ mechanistic models to make explicit hypotheses at multiple levels of analysis.

On the other side of the spectrum, data-driven approaches use machine learning to make predictions from high-dimensional data and are generally agnostic as to underlying mechanisms. As the availability of large and multidimensional data sets is increasing through large neurophysiological studies, online behavioral studies, and the use of mobile devices like smartphones, data-driven approaches are currently getting a lot of attention. They are perceived as very promising ways to provide individual predictions of diagnosis, clinical outcome, and treatment response.

Readers interested in learning about the advances and challenges in the use of big data and machine learning approaches in psychiatry can refer to the recent review by Rutledge, Chekroud, and Huys (2019). Steele and Paulus (2019) also discuss how machine learning approaches applied to neuroscience data can impact clinical practice. Both reviews illustrate, based on recent studies, how objective and clinically useful predictions can be made for individual patients regarding diagnoses, illness severity, relapse, and psychotherapy or medication treatment outcomes. They also emphasize the fact that machine learning techniques can be misapplied, so care is needed in their use and interpretation.

It is important to note that data-driven and theory-driven approaches are not incompatible: theory-driven models can provide descriptions that efficiently summarize complex data, and these summaries can provide inputs for machine-learning algorithms. The combination of both methods has been found to outperform data-driven approaches alone (Huys et al. 2016b).

11.3 Realizing the Potential of Computational Psychiatry

As will hopefully be obvious from the previous chapters, computational psychiatry has already led to many insights into the neurobehavioral mechanisms that underlie several psychiatric disorders.

A number of tools have shown clinical potential (Paulus et al. 2016). For example, the development of theories and tasks related to model-free versus model-based learning has resulted in rich computational analyses and new insights into a variety of disorders, including substance abuse and OCD. Similarly, as described in many chapters of this book, theories about the role of dopamine in reinforcement learning have led to the development of tasks and models that have been applied to a wide range of disorders and can ultimately inform pharmacotherapy. It is often thought that computational assays, such as those based on Bayesian approaches, could help diagnostic tests (Haker, Schneebeli, and Stephan 2016). Computational psychiatry could also help psychotherapy: psychotherapy being a learning process, it may benefit from the rich computational understanding of learning processes (Moutoussis et al. 2018).

However, what is still lacking is a structured initiative to take computational psychiatry from the laboratory to the clinic.

As the field is maturing, there is a growing reflection about key developments required in the practice and infrastructure of computational psychiatry research to accelerate its clinical usefulness (Paulus et al. 2016; Browning et al. 2019; Teufel and Fletcher 2016).

These studies comment on the issue of measurement in computational psychiatry. Measurements usually involve choosing a behavioral task, to be modeled using an algorithm such as a reinforcement learning model, and potentially used also in fMRI. It is important that the reliability and validity of such a computational assay be assessed and iteratively optimized. As mentioned in section 2.5, parameter identifiability needs to be assessed through analysis of parameter recovery, model recovery, and model comparison. The reliability of the measurement also needs to be assessed; for example, whether measurements are consistent across time can be assessed by test-retest reliability. Other important measures of assessment include clinical utility (is the measurement related to clinically important outcomes such as symptom scores, treatment response, or illness course?) and convergent/divergent validity (does the measurement correlate with other measures of the same construct?). Meaningful measures for clinical purposes are then likely to consist not in one model parameter but in the relations between multiple such parameters within or across tasks. These relations can be obtained by collecting data from a range of related assays within a single population of participants and by using data-driven techniques such as clustering.

It is then crucial that the measured latent structures address clinically meaningful questions. This can be assessed by examining the predictive ability of the assay (e.g., can it predict response to treatment?) and/or the causal relationship between the process measured by the assay and clinically important outcomes such as symptoms. If causality can be established between the measurements and outcomes, the process measured by the assay can constitute a treatment target.

Related to this, an important issue is the recruitment of participants. For obvious practical reasons, emphasis has been in recruiting participants with mild and transient illness, rather than patients with severe and enduring illness or moderate-severe recurrent illness during periods of significant illness. Such bias in data collection could partly explain why progress in computational psychiatry has not yet been more significant.

Ideally, this process should be carried out at multiple sites involving individual laboratories that include a close collaboration between academic psychiatrists or psychologists and theoretical and computational neuroscientists. To be successful, the research environment must be developed to encourage large-scale, collaborative, interdisciplinary consortia.

11.4 Chapter Summary

Computational psychiatry is still in its infancy. While the potential of the field is clear, there is still much to do to take computational psychiatry from the laboratory to the clinic. As the field matures, improved and unified methodologies will be needed, as well as large-scale, collaborative, interdisciplinary consortia.

It is our hope that this book will inspire a generation of students who can make a difference.

Notes

Chapter 1

1. Effect size (d) is a statistical concept that measures the strength of the relationship between two variables on a numeric scale. Effect size is most commonly computed as the standardized difference between two means. The values of the effect size are in units of standard deviation. A small effect size ($d \leq 0.2$) indicates a difference that is somewhat trivial and probably not that important. A medium effect size ($0.4 \leq d \leq 0.6$) may have importance. A large effect size($d \geq 0.8$) is probably important.

Chapter 2

1. The XOR, or "exclusive or," is a digital logic gate that gives a true (1) output when the number of true inputs is odd. An XOR gate implements an exclusive or; that is, a true output results if one, and only one, of the inputs to the gate is true. If both inputs are false (0) or both are true, a false output results.

2. This subsection is loosely based on White et al. (2010b).

3. This section is partly inspired from Gershman and Daw (2017).

4. The section on Bayesian models is based on Seriès and Sprevak (2014).

5. This generalizes to Bayesian updates for all exponential families of likelihood distributions with conjugate prior.

6. A Gaussian random walk is a random walk that has a step size that varies according to a normal distribution.

7. This section is based on Leptourgos, Denève, and Jardri 2017.

Chapter 3

1. Parvalbumin is a calcium-binding protein involved in calcium-signaling. Alterations in the function of parvalbumin-expressing neurons have been implicated in various areas of

clinical interest such as Alzheimer's disease, age-related cognitive defects, and some forms of cancer.

2. The words "feedback," "lateral," and "recurrent" are here used interchangeably.

Chapter 5

1. There is a prominent exception in much of classical economics to the central role played by utility. There, preference between actions is considered to be primary (e.g., that the agent prefers reward A to reward B, without any necessary associated utility). Nevertheless, under certain regularity conditions, such as transitivity (such that if the agent prefers going left to right, and right to up, then it will also prefer going left to up), it is known to be possible to derive a possibly nonunique set of scalar utilities that are consistent with the preferences (Houthakker 1950; Samuelson 1938, 1948). Of course, human (and animal) choices rarely satisfy these conditions, even stochastically, leaving the link to be the subject of rich study. The primacy of preference also arises in policy-based RL algorithms such as policy gradient (Baxter and Bartlett 2001).

Chapter 7

1. How such psychological therapies can be applied successfully in real clinical environments is still debated, however.

2. One might wonder about the fact that the softmax function here does not include an (inverse) temperature parameter. However, it can be shown that such a parameter would be equivalent to ρ in these models (Huys et al. 2013).

Chapter 9

1. The dopamine signal is often described as a "reward-prediction error" signal, but this is a misnomer, as bursts also occur when unexpected value appears. Thus it is better referred to as a "value-prediction error" signal.

2. Although many studies have supported the hypothesis that the phasic bursting of dopamine signals positive value-prediction error, and that pauses in firing signal negative value-prediction error, recent experiments have suggested that the story may be more complex than previously thought. Such experiments have found that not all costs are reliably included in this calculation (Gan et al. 2010; Wanat, Kuhnen, and Phillips 2010). And recent experiments looking at tonic levels have suggested that dopamine is actually signaling value, so that value-prediction error would occur only from high-pass frequency filters of dopamine (Hamid et al. 2016).

3. Note that these equations use exponential discounting to reflect value decreases over observed delay. It is possible to construct consistent TDRL equations that express behaviors that reflect nonexponential discounting, but this requires additional complexities beyond what is necessary for this chapter (Kurth-Nelson and Redish 2009, 2010).

Chapter 10

1. In both studies, statistical tests did not reveal a statistically significant difference in the sex distribution between the groups, but failure to reject the null hypothesis cannot be construed as proof of no differences.

2. For simplicity, but without loss of generality, we focus our exposition on prediction errors as calculated by the critic in bandit tasks.

3. To see this, suppose that the increase in phasic dopamine release in TS is well captured by a multiplicative parameter, m, that scales δ_t into $\delta_t^{TS} = m\delta_t$. In RL equations (box 10.1), δ_t is multiplied by a learning rate (e.g., α), so this multiplicative transformation should in principle be better captured by a change in α such that $\alpha^{TS} = m\alpha$. However, in models with a single learning rate (α) for both positive and negative prediction errors—as was the case in the study under consideration (Palminteri et al. 2011)—this learning rate cannot adjust to increase only learning from positive prediction errors. In fact, if α increases, that will increase learning from both positive and negative prediction errors—and, as already discussed, learning from negative prediction errors might be blunted, rather than increased, in TS. Hence, it is not too surprising that the improved learning from positive prediction errors is captured, at least in part, by an increase in R^+.

4. Two other studies failed to find differences between unmedicated (Salvador et al. 2017) or mostly unmedicated (Shephard, Jackson, and Groom 2016) patients with TS and controls in RL tasks, but those studies suffered from confounds that were already discussed (section 10.2.1).

5. The mechanisms underlying tic learning following the cessation of premonitory urges are comprehensively explained in section 10.3.3 and in Conceição et al. (2017).

References

Abbott, L. F. 2008. Theoretical Neuroscience Rising. *Neuron* 60 (3): 489–495.

Abboud, R., J. P. Roiser, H. Khalifeh, S. Ali, I. Harrison, H. T. Killaspy, and E. M. Joyce. 2016. Are Persistent Delusions in Schizophrenia Associated with Aberrant Salience? *Schizophrenia Research: Cognition* 4 (June): 32–38.

Abramson, L. Y., M. E. Seligman, and J. D. Teasdale. 1978. Learned Helplessness in Humans: Critique and Reformulation. *Journal of Abnormal Psychology* 87 (1): 49–74.

Adams, C., and A. Dickinson. 1981. Actions and Habits: Variations in Associative Representations during Instrumental Learning. In *Information Processing in Animals: Memory Mechanisms*, edited by N. E. Spear and R. R. Miller, 143–165. Hillsdale, NJ: Lawrence Erlbaum Associates Inc.

Adams, R. A., Q. J. M. Huys, and J. P. Roiser. 2015. Computational Psychiatry: Towards a Mathematically Informed Understanding of Mental Illness. *Journal of Neurology, Neurosurgery & Psychiatry* 87 (1): 53–63.

Adams, R. A., G. Napier, J. P. Roiser, C. Mathys, and J. Gilleen. 2018. Attractor-like Dynamics in Belief Updating in Schizophrenia. *The Journal of Neuroscience* 38 (44): 9471–9485.

Adams, R. A., K. E. Stephan, H. R. Brown, C. D. Frith, and K. J. Friston. 2013. The Computational Anatomy of Psychosis. *Frontiers in Psychiatry* 4: 47.

Ahmed, S. H. 2010. Validation Crisis in Animal Models of Drug Addiction: Beyond Non-Disordered Drug Use toward Drug Addiction. *Neuroscience & Biobehavioral Reviews* 35 (2): 172–184.

Ainslie, G. 1992. *Picoeconomics: The Strategic Interaction of Successive Motivational States within the Person*. Cambridge, England: Cambridge University Press.

———. 2001. *Breakdown of Will*. Cambridge, England: Cambridge University Press.

Aitchison, L., and M. Lengyel. 2017. With or Without You: Predictive Coding and Bayesian Inference in the Brain. *Current Opinion in Neurobiology* 46 (October): 219–227.

Akbarian-Tefaghi, L., L. Zrinzo, and T. Foltynie. 2016. The Use of Deep Brain Stimulation in Tourette Syndrome. *Brain Sciences* 6 (3): 35.

Alexander, W. H., and J. W. Brown. 2011. Medial Prefrontal Cortex as an Action-Outcome Predictor. *Nature Neuroscience* 14 (10): 1338–1344.

Alexander, W. H., and J. W. Brown. 2014. A General Role for Medial Prefrontal Cortex in Event Prediction. *Frontiers in Computational Neuroscience* 8 (69): 1–11.

————. 2015. Hierarchical Error Representation: A Computational Model of Anterior Cingulate and Dorsolateral Prefrontal Cortex. *Neural Computation* 27 (11): 2354–2410.

Alonso, J., M. C. Angermeyer, S. Bernert, R. Bruffaerts, T. S. Brugha, H. Bryson, G. Girolamo, et al. 2004. Prevalence of Mental Disorders in Europe: Results from the European Study of the Epidemiology of Mental Disorders (ESEMeD) Project. *Acta Psychiatrica Scandinavica* 109 (s420): 21–27.

Alonso, J., J.-P. Lépine, and ESEMeD/MHEDEA 2000 Scientific Committee. 2007. Overview of Key Data from the European Study of the Epidemiology of Mental Disorders (ESEMeD). *The Journal of Clinical Psychiatry* 68 (Suppl. 2): 3–9.

Alonso-Frech, F., I. Zamarbide, M. Alegre, M.C. Rodríguez-Oroz, J. Guridi, M. Manrique, and J. A. Obeso. 2006. Slow Oscillatory Activity and Levodopa-Induced Dyskinesias in Parkinson's Disease. *Brain* 129 (7): 1748–1757.

Alpaydin, E. 2009. *Introduction to Machine Learning.* 2nd ed. Cambridge, MA: The MIT Press.

American Psychiatric Association. 1980. *Diagnostic and Statistical Manual of Mental Disorders.* 3rd edition. Washington, DC: American Psychiatric Association.

————. 2013. *Diagnostic and Statistical Manual of Mental Disorders: DSM-5.* 5th ed. Arlington, V. A.: American Psychiatric Association.

Amit, D., and N. Brunel. 1997. Model of Global Spontaneous Activity and Local Structured Activity during Delay Periods in the Cerebral Cortex. *Cerebral Cortex* 7 (3): 237–252.

Amit, D. J. 1995. The Hebbian Paradigm Reintegrated: Local Reverberations as Internal Representations. *Behavioral and Brain Sciences* 18 (4): 617–626.

Amit, D. J., H. Gutfreund, and H. Sompolinsky. 1985. Spin-Glass Models of Neural Networks. *Physical Review A: General Physics* 32 (2): 1007–1018.

Anderson, J. R. 1996. A.C.T.: A Simple Theory of Complex Cognition. *American Psychologist* 51 (4): 355–365.

Anderson, J. R., J. M. Fincham, Y. Qin, and A. Stocco. 2008. A Central Circuit of the Mind. *Trends in Cognitive Sciences* 12 (4): 136–143.

Anthony, J. C., L. A. Warner, and R. C. Kessler. 1994. Comparative Epidemiology of Dependence on Tobacco, Alcohol, Controlled Substances, and Inhalants: Basic Findings from the National Comorbidity Survey. *Experimental and Clinical Psychopharmacology* 2 (3): 244–268.

Anticevic, A., M. W. Cole, M. G. Repovs, J. D. Murray, M. S. Brumbaugh, A. M. Winkler, A. Savic, J. H. Krystal, G. D. Pearlson, and D. C. Glahn. 2014. Characterizing Thalamo-Cortical Disturbances in Schizophrenia and Bipolar Illness. *Cerebral Cortex* 24 (12): 3116–3130.

Anticevic, A., M. Gancsos, J. D. Murray, G. Repovs, N. R. Driesen, D. J. Ennis, M. J. Niciu, et al. 2012. NMDA Receptor Function in Large-scale Anticorrelated Neural Systems with Implications for Cognition and Schizophrenia. *Proceedings of the National Academy of Sciences* 109 (41): 16720–16725.

Anticevic, Alan, and J. D. Murray. 2017. *Computational Psychiatry: Mathematical Modeling of Mental Illness*. London: Academic Press.

Aragona, B. J., J. J. Day, M. F. Roitman, N. A. Cleaveland, R. Mark Wightman, and R. M. Carelli. 2009. Regional Specificity in the Real-Time Development of Phasic Dopamine Transmission Patterns during Acquisition of a Cue-Cocaine Association in Rats. *European Journal of Neuroscience* 30 (10): 1889–1899.

Aron, A. R., T. W. Robbins, and R. A. Poldrack. 2014. Inhibition and the Right Inferior Frontal Cortex: One Decade On. *Trends in Cognitive Sciences* 18 (4): 177–185.

Arrondo, G., N. Segarra, A. Metastasio, H. Ziauddeen, J. Spencer, N. R. Reinders, R. B. Dudas, T. W. Robbins, P. C. Fletcher, and G. K. Murray. 2015. Reduction in Ventral Striatal Activity When Anticipating a Reward in Depression and Schizophrenia: A Replicated Cross-Diagnostic Finding. *Frontiers in Psychology* 6 (August): 1280.

Aston-Jones, G., and J. D. Cohen. 2005. An Integrative Theory of Locus Coeruleus-Norepinephrine Function: Adaptive Gain and Optimal Performance. *Annual Review of Neuroscience* 28 (1): 403–450.

Atance, C. M., and D. K. O'Neill. 2001. Episodic Future Thinking. *Trends in Cognitive Sciences* 5 (12): 533–539.

Augustine, F., and H. S. Singer. 2019. Merging the Pathophysiology and Pharmacotherapy of Tics. *Tremor and Other Hyperkinetic Movements* 8: 595–619.

Averbeck, B. B., S. Evans, V. Chouhan, E. Bristow, and S. S. Shergill. 2011. Probabilistic Learning and Inference in Schizophrenia. *Schizophrenia Research* 127 (1–3): 115–122.

Aylward, J., C. Hales, E. Robinson, and O. J. Robinson. 2017. Back-Translating a Rodent Measure of Negative Bias into Humans: The Impact of Induced Anxiety and Unmedicated Mood and Anxiety Disorders. *BioRxiv*, May, 143453.

Aylward, J., V. Valton, W.-Y. Ahn, R. L. Bond, P. Dayan, J. P. Roiser, and O. J. Robinson. 2019. Altered Learning under Uncertainty in Unmedicated Mood and Anxiety Disorders. *Nature Human Behaviour*, June, 1–8.

Ayuso-Mateos, J. L., J. L. Vázquez-Barquero, C. Dowrick, V. Lehtinen, O. S. Dalgard, P. Casey, C. Wilkinson, et al. 2001. Depressive Disorders in Europe: Prevalence Figures from the ODIN Study. *British Journal of Psychiatry* 179 (4): 308–316.

Bach, D. R., and P. Dayan. 2017. Algorithms for Survival: A Comparative Perspective on Emotions. *Nature Reviews Neuroscience* 18 (5): 311–319.

Badcock, J. C., D. R. Badcock, C. Read, and A. Jablensky. 2008. Examining Encoding Imprecision in Spatial Working Memory in Schizophrenia. *Schizophrenia Research* 100 (1–3): 144–152.

Baddeley, A. 1986. *Working Memory*. Oxford, England: Oxford University Press.

Badre, D. 2008. Cognitive Control, Hierarchy, and the Rostro-Caudal Organization of the Frontal Lobes. *Trends in Cognitive Sciences* 12 (5): 193–200.

Badre, D., and M. D'Esposito. 2007. Functional Magnetic Resonance Imaging Evidence for a Hierarchical Organization of the Prefrontal Cortex. *Journal of Cognitive Neuroscience* 19 (12): 2082–2099.

———. 2009. Is the Rostro-Caudal Axis of the Frontal Lobe Hierarchical? *Nature Reviews Neuroscience* 10 (9): 659–669.

Baker, S. C., A. B. Konova, N. D. Daw, and G. Horga. 2019. A Distinct Inferential Mechanism for Delusions in Schizophrenia. *Brain* 142 (6): 1797–1812.

Baldermann, J. C., T. Schüller, D. Huys, I. Becker, L. Timmermann, F. Jessen, V. Visser-Vandewalle, and J. Kuhn. 2016. Deep Brain Stimulation for Tourette-Syndrome: A Systematic Review and Meta-Analysis. *Brain Stimulation* 9 (2): 296–304.

Balleine, B. W. 2005. Neural Bases of Food-Seeking: Affect, Arousal and Reward in Corticostriato-limbic Circuits. *Physiology & Behavior* 86 (5): 717–730.

Bansal, R., L. H. Staib, A. F. Laine, X. Hao, D. Xu, J. Liu, M. Weissman, and B. S. Peterson. 2012. Anatomical Brain Images Alone Can Accurately Diagnose Chronic Neuropsychiatric Illnesses. Edited by W. Zhan. *PLoS ONE* 7 (12): e50698.

Barch, D. M., C. S. Carter, T. S. Braver, F. W. Sabb, A. MacDonald, D. C. Noll, and J. D. Cohen. 2001. Selective Deficits in Prefrontal Cortex Function in Medication-Naive Patients With Schizophrenia. *Archives of General Psychiatry* 58 (3): 280.

Barch, D. M., and A. Ceaser. 2012. Cognition in Schizophrenia: Core Psychological and Neural Mechanisms. *Trends in Cognitive Sciences* 16 (1): 27–34.

Barch, D. M., A. Culbreth, and J. Sheffield. 2018. Systems Level Modeling of Cognitive Control in Psychiatric Disorders: A Focus on Schizophrenia. In *Computational Psychiatry: Mathematical Modeling of Mental Illness*, edited by Alan Anticevic and J. D. Murray, 145–173. Cambridge, MA: Academic Press.

Barlow, D. H. 2004. *Anxiety and Its Disorders: The Nature and Treatment of Anxiety and Panic*. Guilford Press.

Barlow, H. 1985. Cerebral Cortex as Model Builder. In *Models of Visual Cortex*, by David E. Rose and Vernon G. Dobson, 37–46. Chichester, England: Wiley.

Barto, A., M. Mirolli, and G. Baldassarre. 2013. Novelty or Surprise? *Frontiers in Psychology* 4.

Barto, A. G. 1995. Adaptive Critics and the Basal Ganglia. In *Computational Neuroscience: Models of Information Processing in the Basal Ganglia*, edited by J. C. Houk, J. L. Davis, and D. G. Beiser. Vol. 215–232. Cambridge, MA: The MIT Press.

Barto, A. G., R. S. Sutton, and C. W. Anderson. 1983. Neuronlike Adaptive Elements That Can Solve Difficult Learning Control Problems. *IEEE Transactions on Systems, Man, and Cybernetics* S. M. C.-13 (5): 834–846.

Bartos, D. C., E. Grandi, and C. M. Ripplinger. 2015. Ion Channels in the Heart. *Comprehensive Physiology* 5 (3): 1423–1464.

Bastos, A. M., W. M. Usrey, R. A. Adams, G. R. Mangun, P. Fries, and K. J. Friston. 2012. Canonical Microcircuits for Predictive Coding. *Neuron* 76 (4): 695–711.

Baxter, J. and P. L. Bartlett. 2001. Infinite-horizon policy-gradient estimation, *Journal of Artificial Intelligence Research*, 15, 319—350.

Baym, C. L., B. A. Corbett, S. B. Wright, and S. A. Bunge. 2008. Neural Correlates of Tic Severity and Cognitive Control in Children with Tourette Syndrome. *Brain* 131 (1): 165–179.

Bechtel, W. 1994. Levels of Description and Explanation in Cognitive Science. *Minds and Machines* 4 (1): 1–25.

Beck, A. T. 1991. Cognitive Therapy: A 30-Year Retrospective. *American Psychologist* 46 (4): 368–375.

———. 2008. The Evolution of the Cognitive Model of Depression and Its Neurobiological Correlates. *American Journal of Psychiatry* 165 (8): 969–977.

Beck, J.M., P.E. Latham, and A. Pouget. 2011. Marginalization in Neural Circuits with Divisive Normalization. *The Journal of Neuroscience* 31 (43): 15310–19.

Beck, A. T., C. H. Ward, M. Mendelson, and J. Erbaugh. 1961. An Inventory for Measuring Depression. *Archives of General Psychiatry* 4 (6): 561–571.

Becker, G. S., and K. M. Murphy. 1988. A Theory of Rational Addiction. *Journal of Political Economy* 96 (4): 675–700.

Beevers, C. G., D. A. Worthy, M. A. Gorlick, B. Nix, T. Chotibut, and W. Todd Maddox. 2013. Influence of Depression Symptoms on History-Independent Reward and Punishment Processing. *Psychiatry Research* 207 (1–2): 53–60.

Behrens, T. E. J., L. T. Hunt, M. W. Woolrich, and M. F. S. Rushworth. 2008. Associative Learning of Social Value. *Nature* 456 (7219): 245–249.

Behrens, T. E. J., M. W. Woolrich, M. E. Walton, and M. F. S. Rushworth. 2007. Learning the Value of Information in an Uncertain World. *Nature Neuroscience* 10 (9): 1214–1221.

Beierholm, U., M. Guitart-Masip, M. Economides, R. Chowdhury, E. Düzel, R. Dolan, and P. Dayan. 2013. Dopamine Modulates Reward-Related Vigor. *Neuropsychopharmacology* 38 (8): 1495–1503.

Bell, D. E. 1982. Regret in Decision Making under Uncertainty. *Operations Research* 30 (5): 961–981.

Belleville, S., H. Chertkow, and S. Gauthier. 2007. Working Memory and Control of Attention in Persons with Alzheimers Disease and Mild Cognitive Impairment. *Neuropsychology* 21 (4): 458–469.

Bellman, R. 1952. On the Theory of Dynamic Programming. *Proceedings of the National Academy of Sciences* 38 (8): 716–719.

Bernheim, B. D., and A. Rangel. 2004. Addiction and Cue-Triggered Decision Processes. *American Economic Review* 94 (5): 1558–1590.

Berridge, K. C. 1996. Food Reward: Brain Substrates of Wanting and Liking. *Neuroscience & Biobehavioral Reviews* 20 (1): 1–25.

———. 2007. The Debate over Dopamines Role in Reward: The Case for Incentive Salience. *Psychopharmacology* 191 (3): 391–431.

Berridge, K. C., and T. E. Robinson. 1998. What Is the Role of Dopamine in Reward: Hedonic Impact, Reward Learning, or Incentive Salience? *Brain Research Reviews* 28 (3): 309–369.

Berridge, K. C., and T. E. Robinson. 2003. Parsing Reward. *Trends in Neurosciences* 26 (9): 507–513.

Bickel, W. K., R. J. DeGrandpre, and S. T. Higgins. 1993. Behavioral Economics: A Novel Experimental Approach to the Study of Drug Dependence. *Drug and Alcohol Dependence* 33 (2): 173–192.

Bickel, W. K., R. D. Landes, Z. Kurth-Nelson, and A. D. Redish. 2014. A Quantitative Signature of Self-Control Repair: Rate-Dependent Effects Of Successful Addiction Treatment. *Clinical Psychological Science* 2 (6): 685–695.

Bickel, W. K., and L. A. Marsch. 2001. Toward a Behavioral Economic Understanding of Drug Dependence: Delay Discounting Processes. *Addiction* 96 (1): 73–86.

Bishop, S. J., and C. Gagne. 2018. Anxiety, Depression, and Decision Making: A Computational Perspective. *Annual Review of Neuroscience* 41 (1): 371–388.

Bitzer, S., H. Park, F. Blankenburg, and S. J. Kiebel. 2014. Perceptual Decision Making: Drift-Diffusion Model Is Equivalent to a Bayesian Model. *Frontiers in Human Neuroscience* 8: 102.

Blagys, M. D., and M. J. Hilsenroth. 2002. Distinctive Activities of Cognitive-Behavioral Therapy: A Review of the Comparative Psychotherapy Process Literature. *Clinical Psychology Review* 22 (5): 671–706.

Blanchard, D. C., and R. J. Blanchard. 1988. Ethoexperimental Approaches to the Biology of Emotion. *Annual Review of Psychology* 39 (1): 43–68.

Bogacz, R. 2017. A Tutorial on the Free-Energy Framework for Modeling Perception and Learning. *Journal of Mathematical Psychology* 76 (February): 198–211.

Bogacz, R., E. Brown, J. Moehlis, P. Holmes, and J. D. Cohen. 2006. The Physics of Optimal Decision Making: A Formal Analysis of Models of Performance in Two-Alternative Forced-Choice Tasks. *Psychological Review* 113 (4): 700–765.

Bogdan, R., and D. A. Pizzagalli. 2006. Acute Stress Reduces Reward Responsiveness: Implications for Depression. *Biological Psychiatry* 60 (10): 1147–1154.

Bolles, R. C. 1970. Species-Specific Defense Reactions and Avoidance Learning. *Psychological Review* 77 (1): 32–48.

Borsboom, D., and A. O. J. Cramer. 2013. Network Analysis: An Integrative Approach to the Structure of Psychopathology. *Annual Review of Clinical Psychology* 9 (1): 91–121.

Bostan, A. C., R. P. Dum, and P. L. Strick. 2010. The Basal Ganglia Communicate with the Cerebellum. *Proceedings of the National Academy of Sciences* 107 (18): 8452–8456.

Botvinick, M. M. 2008. Hierarchical Models of Behavior and Prefrontal Function. *Trends in Cognitive Sciences* 12 (5): 201–208.

Botvinick, M. M., T. S. Braver, D. M. Barch, C. S. Carter, and J. D. Cohen. 2001. Conflict Monitoring and Cognitive Control. *Psychological Review* 108 (3): 624–652.

Botvinick, M. M., and J. D. Cohen. 2014. The Computational and Neural Basis of Cognitive Control: Charted Territory and New Frontiers. *Cognitive Science* 38 (6): 1249–1285.

Botvinick, M. M., J. D. Cohen, and C. S. Carter. 2004. Conflict Monitoring and Anterior Cingulate Cortex: An Update. *Trends in Cognitive Sciences* 8 (12): 539–546.

Botvinick, M. M., Y. Niv, and A. C. Barto. 2009. Hierarchically Organized Behavior and Its Neural Foundations: A Reinforcement Learning Perspective. *Cognition* 113 (3): 262–280.

Boureau, Y.-L., and P. Dayan. 2010. Opponency Revisited: Competition and Cooperation Between Dopamine and Serotonin. *Neuropsychopharmacology* 36 (1): 74–97.

Brandt, V. C., C. Beck, V. Sajin, M. K. Baaske, T. Bäumer, C. Beste, S. Anders, and A. Münchau. 2016. Temporal Relationship between Premonitory Urges and Tics in Gilles de La Tourette Syndrome. *Cortex* 77 (April): 24–37.

Braver, T. S. 2012. The Variable Nature of Cognitive Control: A Dual Mechanisms Framework. *Trends in Cognitive Sciences* 16 (2): 106–113.

Braver, T. S, D. M. Barch, and J. D. Cohen. 1999. Cognition and Control in Schizophrenia: A Computational Model of Dopamine and Prefrontal Function. *Biological Psychiatry* 46 (3): 312–328.

Braver, T. S., and S. R. Bongiolatti. 2002. The Role of Frontopolar Cortex in Subgoal Processing during Working Memory. *NeuroImage* 15 (3): 523–536.

Braver, T.S., and J. D. Cohen. 1999. Dopamine, Cognitive Control, and Schizophrenia: The Gating Model. *Progress in Brain Research* 121 (2): 327–349.

———. 2000. On the Control of Control: The Role of Dopamine in Regulating Prefrontal Function and Working Memory. In *Control of Cognitive Processes: Attention and Performance XVIII*, edited by S. Monsell and J. Driver, 18:713–737. Cambridge, MA: The MIT Press.

Braver, T. S., J. D. Cohen, and D. M. Barch. 2002. The Role of Prefrontal Cortex in Normal and Disordered Cognitive Control: A Cognitive Neuroscience Perspective. In *Principles of Frontal Lobe Function*, edited by D. T. Stuss and R. T. Knight, 428–447. Oxford, England: Oxford University Press.

Braver, T. S, J. R. Reynolds, and D. I. Donaldson. 2003. Neural Mechanisms of Transient and Sustained Cognitive Control during Task Switching. *Neuron* 39 (4): 713–726.

Braver, T. S., and H. Ruge. 2006. Functional Neuroimaging of Executive Functions. In *Handbook of Functional Neuroimaging of Cognition*, edited by R. Cabeza and A. Kingstone, 307–348. Cambridge, MA: The MIT Press.

Breiter, H. C., I. Aharon, D. Kahneman, A. Dale, and P. Shizgal. 2001. Functional Imaging of Neural Responses to Expectancy and Experience of Monetary Gains and Losses. *Neuron* 30 (2): 619–639.

Breland, K., and M. Breland. 1961. The Misbehavior of Organisms. *American Psychologist* 16 (11): 681–684.

Brischoux, F., Chakraborty, S., Brierley, D. I., and Ungless, M. A. 2009. Phasic excitation of dopamine neurons in ventral VTA by noxious stimuli. Proc Natl Acad Sci U S A, 106(12):4894–4899.

Brittain, J.-S., and P. Brown. 2014. Oscillations and the Basal Ganglia: Motor Control and Beyond. *NeuroImage* 85 (January): 637–647.

Brocki, K. C., L. Nyberg, L. B. Thorell, and G. Bohlin. 2007. Early Concurrent and Longitudinal Symptoms of ADHD and O. D. D.: Relations to Different Types of Inhibitory Control and Working Memory. *Journal of Child Psychology and Psychiatry* 48 (10): 1033–1041.

Bromberg-Martin, E. S., and O. Hikosaka. 2009. Midbrain Dopamine Neurons Signal Preference for Advance Information about Upcoming Rewards. *Neuron* 63 (1): 119–126.

Brown, J. W., and T. S. Braver. 2005. Learned Predictions of Error Likelihood in the Anterior Cingulate Cortex. *Science* 307 (5712): 1110–21.

Brown, R. G., and C. D. Marsden. 1990. Cognitive Function in Parkinson's Disease: From Description to Theory. *Trends in Neurosciences* 13 (1): 21–29.

Brown, V. M., L. Zhu, J. M. Wang, B. C. Frueh, B. King-Casas, and P. H. Chiu. 2018. Associability-Modulated Loss Learning Is Increased in Posttraumatic Stress Disorder. Edited by M. J. Frank. *ELife* 7 (January): e30150.

Browning, M., T. E. Behrens, G. Jocham, J. X. O'Reilly, and S. J. Bishop. 2015. Anxious Individuals Have Difficulty Learning the Causal Statistics of Aversive Environments. *Nature Neuroscience* 18 (4): 590–596.

Browning, M., C. Carter, C. H. Chatham, H. den Ouden, C. Gillan, J. T. Baker, A. Chekroud, et al. 2019. Realizing the Clinical Potential of Computational Psychiatry: Report from the Banbury Center Meeting, February 2019. *PsyArXiv*, August.

Browning, M., E. A. Holmes, M. Charles, P. J. Cowen, and C. J. Harmer. 2012. Using Attentional Bias Modification as a Cognitive Vaccine against Depression. *Biological Psychiatry* 72 (7): 572–579.

Brunel, N., and X.-J. Wang. 2001. Effects of Neuromodulation in a Cortical Network Model of Object Working Memory Dominated by Recurrent Inhibition. *Journal of Computational Neuroscience* 11 (1): 63–85.

Bruner, N. R., and M. W. Johnson. 2014. Demand Curves for Hypothetical Cocaine in Cocaine-Dependent Individuals. *Psychopharmacology* 231(5): 889–897.

Buck, R. 2014. *Emotion: A Biosocial Synthesis*. Cambridge: Cambridge University Press.

Buse, J., K. Schoenefeld, A. Münchau, and V. Roessner. 2013. Neuromodulation in Tourette Syndrome: Dopamine and Beyond. *Neuroscience & Biobehavioral Reviews* 37 (6): 1069–1084.

Butler, P. D., S. M. Silverstein, and S. C. Dakin. 2008. Visual Perception and Its Impairment in Schizophrenia. *Biological Psychiatry* 64 (1): 40–47.

Buzsáki, G., and X.-J. Wang. 2012. Mechanisms of Gamma Oscillations. *Annual Review of Neuroscience* 35 (1): 203–225.

Caligiore, D., F. Mannella, M. A. Arbib, and G. Baldassarre. 2017. Dysfunctions of the Basal Ganglia-Cerebellar-Thalamo-Cortical System Produce Motor Tics in Tourette Syndrome. Edited by A. M. Haith. *PLOS Computational Biology* 13 (3): e1005395.

Camerer, C. F., T.-H. Ho, and J.-K. Chong. 2004. A Cognitive Hierarchy Model of Games. *The Quarterly Journal of Economics* 119 (3): 861–898.

Camerer, C., and T. Hua Ho. 1999. Experience-Weighted Attraction Learning in Normal Form Games. *Econometrica* 67 (4): 827–874.

Camerer, Colin F. 2003. *Behavioral Game Theory: Experiments in Strategic Interaction*. Princeton NJ: Princeton University Press.

Camille, N., G. Coricelli, J. Sallet, P. Pradat-Diehl, J.-R. Duhamel, and A. Sirigu. 2004. The Involvement of the Orbitofrontal Cortex in the Experience of Regret. *Science (New York, N. Y.)* 304 (5674): 1167.

Capriotti, M. R., B. C. Brandt, J. E. Turkel, H.-J. Lee, and D. W. Woods. 2014. Negative Reinforcement and Premonitory Urges in Youth With Tourette Syndrome: An Experimental Evaluation. *Behavior Modification* 38 (2): 276–296.

Carandini, M., and D.J. Heeger. 2011. Normalization as a Canonical Neural Computation. *Nature Reviews Neuroscience* 13 (1): 51–62.

Carter, C. S., T. S. Braver, D. M. Barch, M. M. Botvinick, D. C. Noll, and J. D. Cohen. 1998. Anterior Cingulate Cortex, Error Detection, and the Online Monitoring of Performance. *Science* 280 (5364): 747–749.

Cartoni, E., B. Balleine, and G. Baldassarre. 2016. Appetitive Pavlovian-Instrumental Transfer: A Review. *Neuroscience & Biobehavioral Reviews* 71 (December): 829–848.

Casey, A. B., and C. E. Canal. 2017. Classics in Chemical Neuroscience: Aripiprazole. *ACS Chemical Neuroscience* 8 (6): 1135–1146.

Cassidy, C. M., P. D. Balsam, J. J. Weinstein, R. J. Rosengard, M. Slifstein, N. D. Daw, A. Abi-Dargham, and G. Horga. 2018. A Perceptual Inference Mechanism for Hallucinations Linked to Striatal Dopamine. *Current Biology* 28 (4): 503–514.e4.

Castellanos, F. X., E. J. S. Sonuga-Barke, M. P. Milham, and R. Tannock. 2006. Characterizing Cognition in ADHD: Beyond Executive Dysfunction. *Trends in Cognitive Sciences* 10 (3): 117–123.

Cavanna, A. E., K. J. Black, M. Hallett, and V. Voon. 2017. Neurobiology of the Premonitory Urge in Tourette's Syndrome: Pathophysiology and Treatment Implications. *The Journal of Neuropsychiatry and Clinical Neurosciences* 29 (2): 95–104.

Chalk, M., A. Seitz, and P. Seriès. 2010. Rapidly Learned Expectations Alter Perception of Motion. *Journal of Vision* 10 (7): 237–237.

Chambon, V., N. Franck, E. Koechlin, E. Fakra, G. Ciuperca, J.-M. Azorin, and C. Farrer. 2008. The Architecture of Cognitive Control in Schizophrenia. *Brain* 131 (4): 962–970.

Chang, S.-S., and T. Chou. 2018. A Dynamical Bifurcation Model of Bipolar Disorder Based on Learned Expectation and Asymmetry in Mood Sensitivity. *Computational Psychiatry* 2: 205–22.

Changeux, J.-P., and S. Dehaene. 1989. Neuronal Models of Cognitive Functions. *Cognition* 33 (1–2): 63–109.

Charpentier, C. J., J. Aylward, J. P. Roiser, and O. J. Robinson. 2017. Enhanced Risk Aversion, But Not Loss Aversion, in Unmedicated Pathological Anxiety. *Biological Psychiatry* 81 (12): 1014–1022.

Chase, H. W., M. J. Frank, A. Michael, E. T. Bullmore, B. J. Sahakian, and T. W. Robbins. 2010. Approach and Avoidance Learning in Patients with Major Depression and Healthy Controls: Relation to Anhedonia. *Psychological Medicine* 40 (3): 433–440.

Chase, H. W., P. Kumar, S. B. Eickhoff, and A. Y. Dombrovski. 2015. Reinforcement Learning Models and Their Neural Correlates: An Activation Likelihood Estimation Meta-Analysis. *Cognitive, Affective, & Behavioral Neuroscience* 15 (2): 435–459.

Chaudhuri, R., K. Knoblauch, M.-A. Gariel, H. Kennedy, and X.-J. Wang. 2015. A Large-Scale Circuit Mechanism for Hierarchical Dynamical Processing in the Primate Cortex. *Neuron* 88 (2): 419–431.

Chekroud, A. M., R. J. Zotti, Z. Shehzad, R. Gueorguieva, M. K. Johnson, M. H. Trivedi, T. D. Cannon, J. H. Krystal, and P. R. Corlett. 2016. Cross-Trial Prediction of Treatment Outcome in Depression: A Machine Learning Approach. *The Lancet Psychiatry* 3 (3): 243–250.

Chen, Y., L. C. Bidwell, and P. S. Holzman. 2005. Visual Motion Integration in Schizophrenia Patients, Their First-Degree Relatives, and Patients with Bipolar Disorder. *Schizophrenia Research* 74 (2–3): 271–281.

Chen, Y., D. L. Levy, S. Sheremata, and P. S. Holzman. 2004. Compromised Late-Stage Motion Processing in Schizophrenia. *Biological Psychiatry* 55 (8): 834–841.

Chen, Y., K. Nakayama, D. Levy, S. Matthysse, and P. Holzman. 2003. Processing of Global, but Not Local, Motion Direction Is Deficient in Schizophrenia. *Schizophrenia Research* 61 (2–3): 215–227.

Chen, C., T. Takahashi, S. Nakagawa, T. Inoue, and I. Kusumi. 2015. Reinforcement Learning in Depression: A Review of Computational Research. *Neuroscience & Biobehavioral Reviews* 55 (August): 247–267.

Choi, E. Y., B. T. T. Yeo, and R. L. Buckner. 2012. The Organization of the Human Striatum Estimated by Intrinsic Functional Connectivity. *Journal of Neurophysiology* 108 (8): 2242–2263.

Christophel, T. B., P. C. Klink, B. Spitzer, P. R. Roelfsema, and J.-D. Haynes. 2017. The Distributed Nature of Working Memory. *Trends in Cognitive Sciences* 21 (2): 111–124.

Churchland, P. S., and T. J. Sejnowski. 1994. *The Computational Brain*. Cambridge, MA: The MIT Press.

Cléry-Melin, M.-L., F. Jollant, and P. Gorwood. 2018. Reward Systems and Cognitions in Major Depressive Disorder. *CNS Spectrums* 24 (1): 64–77.

Cléry-Melin, M.-L., L. Schmidt, G. Lafargue, N. Baup, P. Fossati, and M. Pessiglione. 2011. Why Don't You Try Harder? An Investigation of Effort Production in Major Depression. *PLoS ONE* 6 (8): e23178.

Cohen, J. D., T. S. Braver, and J. W. Brown. 2002. Computational Perspectives on Dopamine Function in Prefrontal Cortex. *Current Opinion in Neurobiology* 12 (2): 223–229.

Cohen, J. D., T. S. Braver, and R. C. O'Reilly. 1996. A Computational Approach to Prefrontal Cortex, Cognitive Control and Schizophrenia: Recent Developments and Current Challenges. *Philosophical Transactions of the Royal Society of London. Series B: Biological Sciences* 351 (1346): 1515–1527.

Cohen, J. D., N. Daw, B. Engelhardt, U. Hasson, K. Li, Y. Niv, K. A. Norman, et al. 2017. Computational Approaches to FMRI Analysis. *Nature Neuroscience* 20 (3): 304–313.

Cohen, J. D., K. Dunbar, and J. L. McClelland. 1990. On the Control of Automatic Processes: A Parallel Distributed Processing Account of the Stroop Effect. *Psychological Review* 97 (3): 332–361.

Cohen, J. D., and D. Servan-Schreiber. 1992. Context, Cortex, and Dopamine: A Connectionist Approach to Behavior and Biology in Schizophrenia. *Psychological Review* 99 (1): 45–77.

Cohen, J. Y., S. Haesler, L. Vong, B. B. Lowell, and N. Uchida. 2012. Neuron-Type-Specific Signals for Reward and Punishment in the Ventral Tegmental Area. *Nature* 482 (7383): 85–88.

Collins, A. G. E. 2017. The Cost of Structure Learning. *Journal of Cognitive Neuroscience* 29 (10): 1646–1655.

Collins, A. G. E., J. K. Brown, J. M. Gold, J. A. Waltz, and M. J. Frank. 2014. Working Memory Contributions to Reinforcement Learning Impairments in Schizophrenia. *The Journal of Neuroscience* 34 (41): 13747–13756.

Collins, A. G. E., and M. J. Frank. 2013. Cognitive Control over Learning: Creating, Clustering, and Generalizing Task-Set Structure. *Psychological Review* 120 (1): 190–229.

———. 2014. Opponent Actor Learning (OpAL): Modeling Interactive Effects of Striatal Dopamine on Reinforcement Learning and Choice Incentive. *Psychological Review* 121 (3): 337–366.

Compte, A., N. Brunel, P. S. Goldman-Rakic, and X.-J. Wang. 2000. Synaptic Mechanisms and Network Dynamics Underlying Spatial Working Memory in a Cortical Network Model. *Cerebral Cortex* 10 (9): 910–923.

Conceição, V. A., Â. Dias, A. C. Farinha, and T. V. Maia. 2017. Premonitory Urges and Tics in Tourette Syndrome: Computational Mechanisms and Neural Correlates. *Current Opinion in Neurobiology* 46 (October): 187–199.

Cooper, R. P., and T. Shallice. 2006. Hierarchical Schemas and Goals in the Control of Sequential Behavior. *Psychological Review* 113 (4): 887–916.

Corbit, L. H., and B. W. Balleine. 2011. The General and Outcome-Specific Forms of Pavlovian-Instrumental Transfer Are Differentially Mediated by the Nucleus Accumbens Core and Shell. *Journal of Neuroscience* 31 (33): 11786–11794.

Corbit, L. H., S. C. Fischbach, and P. H. Janak. 2016. Nucleus Accumbens Core and Shell Are Differentially Involved in General and Outcome-Specific Forms of Pavlovian-Instrumental Transfer with Alcohol and Sucrose Rewards. *European Journal of Neuroscience* 43 (9): 1229–1236.

Coricelli, G., R. J. Dolan, and A. Sirigu. 2007. Brain, Emotion and Decision Making: The Paradigmatic Example of Regret. *Trends in Cognitive Sciences* 11 (6): 258–265.

Corlett, P. R., G. K. Murray, G. D. Honey, M. R. F. Aitken, D. R. Shanks, T. W. Robbins, E. T. Bullmore, A. Dickinson, and P. C. Fletcher. 2007. Disrupted Prediction-Error Signal in Psychosis: Evidence for an Associative Account of Delusions. *Brain* 130 (9): 2387–2400.

Costa-Gomes, M., V. P. Crawford, and B. Broseta. 2001. Cognition and Behavior in Normal-Form Games: An Experimental Study. *Econometrica* 69 (5): 1193–1235.

Cox, A. 1986. *Sid and Nancy*. Film. Palace Pictures, London.

Cox, J. H., S. Seri, and A. E. Cavanna. 2016. Histaminergic Modulation in Tourette Syndrome. *Expert Opinion on Orphan Drugs* 4 (2): 205–213.

———. 2018. Sensory Aspects of Tourette Syndrome. *Neuroscience & Biobehavioral Reviews* 88 (May): 170–176.

Cox, J. R., R. G. Martinez, and M. A. Southam-Gerow. 2019. Treatment Integrity in Psychotherapy Research and Implications for the Delivery of Quality Mental Health Services. *Journal of Consulting and Clinical Psychology* 87 (3): 221–233.

Craske, M. G., M. B. Stein, T. C. Eley, M. R. Milad, A. Holmes, R. M. Rapee, and H.-U. Wittchen. 2017. Anxiety Disorders. *Nature Reviews Disease Primers* 3 (1): 17024.

Crockett, M. J., J. Z. Siegel, Z. Kurth-Nelson, P. Dayan, and R. J. Dolan. 2017. Moral Transgressions Corrupt Neural Representations of Value. *Nature Neuroscience* 20 (6): 879–885.

Cross-Disorder Group of the Psychiatric Genomics Consortium. 2013. Identification of Risk Loci with Shared Effects on Five Major Psychiatric Disorders: A Genome-Wide Analysis. *The Lancet* 381 (9875): 1371–1379.

Crossley, N. A., M. Constante, P. McGuire, and P. Power. 2010. Efficacy of Atypical v. Typical Antipsychotics in the Treatment of Early Psychosis: Meta-Analysis. *British Journal of Psychiatry* 196 (6): 434–439.

Custer, R. L. 1984. Profile of the Pathological Gambler. *The Journal of Clinical Psychiatry* 45 (1): 35–38.

Cytowic, R. E. 1998. *The Man Who Tasted Shapes*. Cambridge, MA: The MIT Press.

Da Silva, J. A., F. Tecuapetla, V. Paixão, and R. M. Costa. 2018. Dopamine Neuron Activity before Action Initiation Gates and Invigorates Future Movements. *Nature* 554 (7691): 244–248.

Damasio, A. R. 2010. *Self Comes to Mind: Constructing the Conscious Brain*. London, England: W. Heinemann.

D'Ardenne, K., N. Eshel, J. Luka, A. Lenartowicz, L. E. Nystrom, and J. D. Cohen. 2012. Role of Prefrontal Cortex and the Midbrain Dopamine System in Working Memory Updating. *Proceedings of the National Academy of Sciences* 109 (49): 19900–19909.

Davey, G. C. L., J. H. Phillips, and S. Witty. 1989. Signal-Directed Behavior in the Rat: Interactions between the Nature of the CS and the Nature of the UCS. *Animal Learning & Behavior* 17 (4): 447–456.

Daw, N. D. 2011. Trial-by-Trial Data Analysis Using Computational Models. In *Decision Making, Affect, and Learning XXIII*, 3–38. Decision Making, Affect, and Learning 23. Oxford, England: Oxford University Press.

Daw, N. D., and P. Dayan. 2014. The Algorithmic Anatomy of Model-Based Evaluation. *Philosophical Transactions of the Royal Society B: Biological Sciences* 369 (1655): 20130478.

Daw, N. D., S. J. Gershman, B. Seymour, P. Dayan, and R. J. Dolan. 2011. Model-Based Influences on Humans Choices and Striatal Prediction Errors. *Neuron* 69 (6): 1204–1215.

Daw, N. D., S. Kakade, and P. Dayan. 2002. Opponent Interactions between Serotonin and Dopamine. *Neural Networks* 15 (4–6): 603–616.

Daw, N. D., Y. Niv, and P. Dayan. 2005. Uncertainty-Based Competition between Prefrontal and Dorsolateral Striatal Systems for Behavioral Control. *Nature Neuroscience* 8 (12): 1704–1711.

Daw, N. D., Y. Niv, and P. Dayan. 2006. Actions, Policies, Values and the Basal Ganglia. *Recent Breakthroughs in Basal Ganglia Research* 10 (9): 1214–1221.

Daw, N. D. and P. Tobler. 2013. Value learning through reinforcement: The basics of dopamine and reinforcement learning, in Glimcher, P. and Fehr, E., eds, Neuroeconomics: Decision making and the brain, 2nd edition, Elsevier.

Daw, N. D., and D. S. Touretzky. 2000. Behavioral Considerations Suggest an Average Reward TD Model of the Dopamine System. *Neurocomputing* 32–33 (June): 679–684.

Dayan, P. 2006. Levels of Analysis in Neural Modeling. In *Encyclopedia of Cognitive Science*, edited by L. Nadel. London, England: MacMillan Press.

———. 2012a. Instrumental Vigour in Punishment and Reward. *European Journal of Neuroscience* 35 (7): 1152–1168.

———. 2012b. Exploration from Generalization Mediated by Multiple Controllers. In *Intrinsically Motivated Learning in Natural and Artificial Systems*, edited by G. Baldassarre and M. Mirolli, 73–91. Berlin: Springer.

———. 2012c. How to Set the Switches on This Thing. *Current Opinion in Neurobiology* 22 (6): 1068–1074.

Dayan, P., and L. F. Abbott. 2000. *Theoretical Neuroscience: Computational and Mathematical Modeling of Neural Systems*. Cambridge, MA: MIT Press.

Dayan, P., and K. C. Berridge. 2014. Model-Based and Model-Free Pavlovian Reward Learning: Revaluation, Revision, and Revelation. *Cognitive, Affective, & Behavioral Neuroscience* 14 (2): 473–492.

Dayan, P., and Q. J. M. Huys. 2009. Serotonin in Affective Control. *Annual Review of Neuroscience* 32 (1): 95–126.

Dayan, P., Y. Niv, B. Seymour, and N. D. Daw. 2006. The Misbehavior of Value and the Discipline of the Will. *Neural Networks* 19 (8): 1153–1160.

De Wit, S., P. Watson, H. A. Harsay, M. X. Cohen, I. van de Vijver, and K. R. Ridderinkhof. 2012. Corticostriatal Connectivity Underlies Individual Differences in the Balance between Habitual and Goal-Directed Action Control. *Journal of Neuroscience* 32 (35): 12066–12075.

Deakin, J. 2013. The Origins of "5-HT and Mechanisms of Defence" by Deakin and Graeff: A Personal Perspective. *Journal of Psychopharmacology* 27 (12): 1084–1089.

Deakin, J. F. W. 1983. Roles of Brain Serotonergic Neurons in Escape, Avoidance and Other Behaviors. *Journal of Psychopharmacology* 43: 563–577.

Deakin, J. F. William, and F. G. Graeff. 1991. 5-HT and Mechanisms of Defence. *Journal of Psychopharmacology* 5 (4): 305–315.

De Jong, J.W, S. A. Afjei, I. Pollak Dorocic, J. R. Peck, C. Liu, C. K. Kim, L. Tian, K. Deisseroth, S. Lammel. 2019. A Neural Circuit Mechanism for Encoding Aversive Stimuli in the Mesolimbic Dopamine System. *Neuron* 101(1): 133–151.

Deco, G., and E. T. Rolls. 2003. Attention and Working Memory: A Dynamical Model of Neuronal Activity in the Prefrontal Cortex. *European Journal of Neuroscience* 18 (8): 2374–2390.Delorme, C., A. Salvador, R. Valabrègue, E. Roze, S. Palminteri, M. Vidailhet, S. de Wit, T. Robbins, A. Hartmann, and Y. Worbe. 2016. Enhanced Habit Formation in Gilles de La Tourette Syndrome. *Brain* 139 (2): 605–615.

Demjaha, A., A. Egerton, R. M. Murray, S. Kapur, O. D. Howes, J. M. Stone, and P. K. McGuire. 2014. Antipsychotic Treatment Resistance in Schizophrenia Associated with Elevated Glutamate Levels but Normal Dopamine Function. *Biological Psychiatry* 75 (5): e11–13.

Deroche-Gamonet, V. 2004. Evidence for Addiction-like Behavior in the Rat. *Science* 305 (5686): 1014–1017.

Deserno, L., R. Boehme, A. Heinz, and F. Schlagenhauf. 2013. Reinforcement Learning and Dopamine in Schizophrenia: Dimensions of Symptoms or Specific Features of a Disease Group? *Frontiers in Psychiatry* 4: 172.

Devauges, V., and S. J. Sara. 1990. Activation of the Noradrenergic System Facilitates an Attentional Shift in the Rat. *Behavioural Brain Research* 39 (1): 19–28.

Dezfouli, A., P. Piray, M. M. Keramati, H. Ekhtiari, C. Lucas, and A. Mokri. 2009. A Neurocomputational Model for Cocaine Addiction. *Neural Computation* 21 (10): 2869–2893.

Di Chiara, G. 1999. Drug Addiction as Dopamine-Dependent Associative Learning Disorder. *European Journal of Pharmacology* 375 (1–3): 13–30.

Diamond, J. 2006. *The Third Chimpanzee*. New York, NY: HarperCollins.

Dickinson, A. 1985. Actions and Habits: The Development of Behavioural Autonomy. *Philosophical Transactions of the Royal Society B: Biological Sciences* 308 (1135): 67–78.

Dickinson, Anthony, and B. Balleine. 2002. The Role of Learning in the Operation of Motivational Systems. In *Stevens Handbook of Experimental Psychology*, edited by H. E. Pashler, 497–533. New York, NY: John Wiley & Sons, Inc.

Dillon, D. G., and D. A. Pizzagalli. 2018. Mechanisms of Memory Disruption in Depression. *Trends in Neurosciences* 41 (3): 137–149.

Dillon, D. G., T. Wiecki, P. Pechtel, C. Webb, F. Goer, L. Murray, M. Trivedi, et al. 2015. A Computational Analysis of Flanker Interference in Depression. *Psychological Medicine* 45 (11): 2333–2344.

Dinsmoor, J. A. 1983. Observing and Conditioned Reinforcement. *Behavioral and Brain Sciences* 6 (04): 693–728.

Dixon, M. L., and K. Christoff. 2012. The Decision to Engage Cognitive Control Is Driven by Expected Reward-Value: Neural and Behavioral Evidence. *PLoS ONE* 7 (12): e51637.

Dolan, R. J., and P. Dayan. 2013. Goals and Habits in the Brain. *Neuron* 80 (2): 312–325.

Dombrovski, A. Y., L. Clark, G. J. Siegle, M. A. Butters, N. Ichikawa, B. J. Sahakian, and K. Szanto. 2010. Reward/Punishment Reversal Learning in Older Suicide Attempters. *American Journal of Psychiatry* 167 (6): 699–707.

Doya, K. 1999. What Are the Computations of the Cerebellum, the Basal Ganglia and the Cerebral Cortex? *Neural Networks* 12 (7–8): 961–974.

Dreyer, J. K., K. F. Herrik, R. W. Berg, and J. D. Hounsgaard. 2010. Influence of Phasic and Tonic Dopamine Release on Receptor Activation. *Journal of Neuroscience* 30 (42): 14273–14283.

Dudley, R., P. Taylor, S. Wickham, and P. Hutton. 2016. Psychosis, Delusions and the "Jumping to Conclusions" Reasoning Bias: A Systematic Review and Meta-Analysis. *Schizophrenia Bulletin* 42 (3): 652–665.

Duits, P., D. C. Cath, S. Lissek, J. J. Hox, A. O. Hamm, I. M. Engelhard, M. A. van den Hout, and J. M. P. Baas. 2015. Updated Meta-Analysis of Classical Fear Conditioning in the Anxiety Disorders. *Depression and Anxiety* 32 (4): 239–253.

Duncan, J. 2010. The Multiple-Demand (MD) System of the Primate Brain: Mental Programs for Intelligent Behaviour. *Trends in Cognitive Sciences* 14 (4): 172–179.

Duncan, J., and A. M. Owen. 2000. Common Regions of the Human Frontal Lobe Recruited by Diverse Cognitive Demands. *Trends in Neurosciences* 23 (10): 475–483.

Dunlop, B. W., and C. B. Nemeroff. 2007. The Role of Dopamine in the Pathophysiology of Depression. *Archives of General Psychiatry* 64 (3): 327–337.

Durstewitz, D., Q. J. Huys, and G. Koppe. 2018. Psychiatric Illnesses as Disorders of Network Dynamics. *ArXiv Preprint ArXiv:1809.06303*.

Durstewitz, D., and J. K. Seamans. 2008. The Dual-State Theory of Prefrontal Cortex Dopamine Function with Relevance to Catechol-O-Methyltransferase Genotypes and Schizophrenia. *Biological Psychiatry* 64 (9): 739–749.

Durstewitz, D., J. K. Seamans, and T. J. Sejnowski. 2000. Neurocomputational Models of Working Memory. *Nature Neuroscience* 3 (S11): 1184–1191.

Duvarci, S., and D. Paré. 2014. Amygdala Microcircuits Controlling Learned Fear. *Neuron* 82 (5): 966–980.

Duverne, S., and E. Koechlin. 2017. Rewards and Cognitive Control in the Human Prefrontal Cortex. *Cerebral Cortex* 27 (10): 5024–5039.

Dymond, S., J. E. Dunsmoor, B. Vervliet, B. Roche, and D. Hermans. 2015. Fear Generalization in Humans: Systematic Review and Implications for Anxiety Disorder Research. *Behavior Therapy* 46 (5): 561–582.

Egner, T. 2009. Prefrontal Cortex and Cognitive Control: Motivating Functional Hierarchies. *Nature Neuroscience* 12 (7): 821–822.

Eldar, E., R. B. Rutledge, R. J. Dolan, and Y. Niv. 2016. Mood as Representation of Momentum. *Trends in Cognitive Sciences* 20 (1): 15–24.

Eliasmith, C., T. C. Stewart, X. Choo, T. Bekolay, T. DeWolf, Y. Tang, and D. Rasmussen. 2012. A Large-Scale Model of the Functioning Brain. *Science* 338 (6111): 1202–1205.

Ellens, D. J., and D. K. Leventhal. 2013. Electrophysiology of Basal Ganglia and Cortex in Models of Parkinson Disease. *Journal of Parkinson's Disease* 3 (3): 241–254.

Ellis, A. 1957. Rational Psychotherapy and Individual Psychology. *Journal of Individual Psychology* 13 (1): 38–44.

Ellsberg, D. 1961. Risk, Ambiguity, and the Savage Axioms. *The Quarterly Journal of Economics* 75 (4): 643.

Engle, R. W., and M. J. Kane. 2004. Executive Attention, Working Memory Capacity, and a Two-Factor Theory of Cognitive Control. *The Psychology of Learning and Motivation: Advances in Research and Theory* 44: 145–199.

Ermakova, A. O., N. Gileadi, F. Knolle, A. Justicia, R. Anderson, P. C. Fletcher, M. Moutoussis, and G. K. Murray. 2019. Cost Evaluation during Decision-Making in Patients at Early Stages of Psychosis. *Computational Psychiatry* 3 (February): 18–39.

Eshel, N., and J. P. Roiser. 2010. Reward and Punishment Processing in Depression. *Biological Psychiatry* 68 (2): 118–124.

Eshel, N., J. Tian, and N. Uchida. 2013. Opening the Black Box: Dopamine, Predictions, and Learning. *Trends in Cognitive Sciences* 17 (9): 430–431.

Estes, W. K. 1943. Discriminative Conditioning. I. A Discriminative Property of Conditioned Anticipation. *Journal of Experimental Psychology* 32 (2): 150–155.

Evans, K. L., and E. Hampson. 2015. Sex-Dependent Effects on Tasks Assessing Reinforcement Learning and Interference Inhibition. *Frontiers in Psychology* 6 (July).

Evenden, J. L. 1999. Varieties of Impulsivity. *Psychopharmacology* 146 (4): 348–361.

Everitt, B. J., and T. W. Robbins. 2005. Neural Systems of Reinforcement for Drug Addiction: From Actions to Habits to Compulsion. *Nature Neuroscience* 8 (11): 1481–1489.

Fales, C. L., D. M. Barch, M. M. Rundle, M. A. Mintun, A. Z. Snyder, J. D. Cohen, J. Mathews, and Y. I. Sheline. 2008. Altered Emotional Interference Processing in Affective and Cognitive-Control Brain Circuitry in Major Depression. *Biological Psychiatry* 63 (4): 377–384.

Farah, M. J., and S. J. Gillihan. 2012. The Puzzle of Neuroimaging and Psychiatric Diagnosis: Technology and Nosology in an Evolving Discipline. *AJOB Neuroscience* 3 (4): 31–41.

Faulkner, P., and J. F. W. Deakin. 2014. The Role of Serotonin in Reward, Punishment and Behavioural Inhibition in Humans: Insights from Studies with Acute Tryptophan Depletion. *Neuroscience & Biobehavioral Reviews* 46 (3): 365–378.

Faure, A., S. M. Reynolds, J. M. Richard, and K. C. Berridge. 2008. Mesolimbic Dopamine in Desire and Dread: Enabling Motivation to Be Generated by Localized Glutamate Disruptions in Nucleus Accumbens. *Journal of Neuroscience* 28 (28): 7184–7192.

Fear, C. F., and D. Healy. 1997. Probabilistic Reasoning in Obsessive-Compulsive and Delusional Disorders. *Psychological Medicine* 27 (1): 199–208.

Fehr, E., and K. M. Schmidt. 1999. A Theory of Fairness, Competition, and Cooperation. *The Quarterly Journal of Economics* 114 (3): 817–868.

Fernando, A. B. P., G. P. Urcelay, A. C. Mar, A. Dickinson, and T. W. Robbins. 2014. Safety Signals as Instrumental Reinforcers during Free-Operant Avoidance. *Learning & Memory* 21 (9): 488–497.

Ferrante, M., C. F. Shay, Y. Tsuno, G. William Chapman, and M. E. Hasselmo. 2016. Post-Inhibitory Rebound Spikes in Rat Medial Entorhinal Layer II/III Principal Cells: In Vivo, In Vitro, and Computational Modeling Characterization. *Cerebral Cortex*, March, bhw058.

Fibiger, H. C. 2012. Psychiatry, the Pharmaceutical Industry, and the Road to Better Therapeutics. *Schizophrenia Bulletin* 38 (4): 649–650.

Fineberg, N. A., A. M. Apergis-Schoute, M. M. Vaghi, P. Banca, C. M. Gillan, V. Voon, S. R. Chamberlain, et al. 2018. Mapping Compulsivity in the DSM-5 Obsessive Compulsive and Related Disorders: Cognitive Domains, Neural Circuitry, and Treatment. *International Journal of Neuropsychopharmacology* 21 (1): 42–58.

Fineberg, S. K., D. Stahl, and P. Corlett. 2017. Computational Psychiatry in Borderline Personality Disorder. *Current Behavioral Neuroscience Reports* 4 (1): 31–40.

Fiorillo, C. D. 2013. Two Dimensions of Value: Dopamine Neurons Represent Reward But Not Aversiveness. *Science* 341 (6145): 546–549.

Fischer, B. A. 2012. A Review of American Psychiatry through Its Diagnoses. *The Journal of Nervous and Mental Disease* 200 (12): 1022–1030.

Fischer, B. J., and J. L. Peña. 2011. Owl's Behavior and Neural Representation Predicted by Bayesian Inference. *Nature Neuroscience* 14 (8): 1061–1066.

Foa, E. B. 2011. Prolonged Exposure Therapy: Past, Present, and Future. *Depression and Anxiety* 28 (12): 1043–1047.

Foa, E. B., and M. J. Kozak. 1986. Emotional Processing of Fear: Exposure to Corrective Information. *Psychological Bulletin* 99 (1): 20–35.

Foltynie, T. 2016. Vocal Tics in Tourette's Syndrome. *The Lancet Neurology* 15 (3): e1.

Fox, C. R., and A. Tversky. 1995. Ambiguity Aversion and Comparative Ignorance. *The Quarterly Journal of Economics* 110 (3): 585–603.

Fradkin, I., C. Ludwig, E. Eldar, and J. D. Huppert. 2020. Doubting What You Already Know: Uncertainty Regarding State Transitions Is Associated with Obsessive Compulsive Symptoms. *PLoS Computational Biology* 16 (2): e1007634.

Frank, M. J. 2006. Hold Your Horses: A Dynamic Computational Role for the Subthalamic Nucleus in Decision Making. *Neural Networks* 19 (8): 1120–1136.

Frank, M. J., and D. Badre. 2012. Mechanisms of Hierarchical Reinforcement Learning in Cortico-striatal Circuits 1: Computational Analysis. *Cerebral Cortex* 22 (3): 509–526.

Frank, M. J., and E. D. Claus. 2006. Anatomy of a Decision: Striato-Orbitofrontal Interactions in Reinforcement Learning, Decision Making, and Reversal. *Psychological Review* 113 (2): 300–326.

Frank, M. J., B. Loughry, and R. C. O'Reilly. 2001. Interactions between Frontal Cortex and Basal Ganglia in Working Memory: A Computational Model. *Cognitive, Affective, & Behavioral Neuroscience* 1 (2): 137–160.

Frank, M. J., A. A. Moustafa, H. M. Haughey, T. Curran, and K. E. Hutchison. 2007. Genetic Triple Dissociation Reveals Multiple Roles for Dopamine in Reinforcement Learning. *Proceedings of the National Academy of Sciences* 104 (41): 16311–16316.

Frank, M. J., Seeberger, L. C., and R. C. O'Reilly. 2004. By carrot or by stick: cognitive reinforcement learning in Parkinsonism. *Science*, 306(5703): 1940–1943.

Freud, S. 1966. *The Complete Introductory Lectures on Psychoanalysis*. Edited by J. Strachey. New York, NY: Norton.

Fried, E. I., R. M. Nesse, K. Zivin, C. Guille, and S. Sen. 2014. Depression Is More than the Sum Score of Its Parts: Individual DSM Symptoms Have Different Risk Factors. *Psychological Medicine* 44 (10): 2067–2076.

Fried, E. I., and R. M. Nesse. 2015. Depression Is Not a Consistent Syndrome: An Investigation of Unique Symptom Patterns in the STAR*D Study. *Journal of Affective Disorders* 172 (February): 96–102.

Friedrich, J., and M. Lengyel. 2016. Goal-Directed Decision Making with Spiking Neurons. *The Journal of Neuroscience* 36 (5): 1529–1546.

Friston, K. J., K. E. Stephan, R. Montague, and R. J. Dolan. 2014. Computational Psychiatry: The Brain as a Phantastic Organ. *The Lancet Psychiatry* 1 (2): 148–158.

Fründt, O., D. Woods, and C. Ganos. 2017. Behavioral Therapy for Tourette Syndrome and Chronic Tic Disorders. *Neurology: Clinical Practice* 7 (2): 148–156.

Funahashi, S., C. J. Bruce, and P. S. Goldman-Rakic. 1989. Mnemonic Coding of Visual Space in the Monkey's Dorsolateral Prefrontal Cortex. *Journal of Neurophysiology* 61 (2): 331–349.

Furman, M., and X.-J. Wang. 2008. Similarity Effect and Optimal Control of Multiple-Choice Decision Making. *Neuron* 60 (6): 1153–1168.

Fuster, J. M. 2001. The Prefrontal Cortex—An Update: Time Is of the Essence. *Neuron* 30 (2): 319–333.

Gabbard, G. 2011. Psychotherapies. In *Kaplan and Sadock's Synopsis of Psychiatry: Behavioral Sciences/Clinical Psychiatry*, edited by B. J. Sadock, V. A. Sadock, and H. I. Kaplan. Philadelphia, PA: Wolter Kluwer/Lippincott Williams & Wilkins.

Gan, J. O., M. E. Walton, and P. E. M. Phillips. 2010. Dissociable Cost and Benefit Encoding of Future Rewards by Mesolimbic Dopamine. *Nature Neuroscience* 13 (1): 25–27.

Ganos, C., D. Martino, and T. Pringsheim. 2017. Tics in the Pediatric Population: Pragmatic Management. *Movement Disorders Clinical Practice* 4 (2): 160–172.

Garety, P. A., D. R. Hemsley, and S. Wessely. 1991. Reasoning in Deluded Schizophrenic and Paranoid Patients. *The Journal of Nervous and Mental Disease* 179 (4): 194–201.

Garrison, J., B. Erdeniz, and J. Done. 2013. Prediction Error in Reinforcement Learning: A Meta-Analysis of Neuroimaging Studies. *Neuroscience & Biobehavioral Reviews* 37 (7): 1297–1310.

Gasnier, L. J. 1936. *Reefer Madness*. Film. Motion Picture Ventures, Los Angeles, CA.

Gatev, P., O. Darbin, and T. Wichmann. 2006. Oscillations in the Basal Ganglia under Normal Conditions and in Movement Disorders. *Movement Disorders* 21 (10): 1566–1577.

Geddes, J., N. Freemantle, P. Harrison, and P. Bebbington. 2000. Atypical Antipsychotics in the Treatment of Schizophrenia: Systematic Overview and Meta-Regression Analysis. *B. M. J.: British Medical Journal* 321 (7273): 1371–1376.

Gehring, W. J., B. Goss, M. G. H. Coles, D. E. Meyer, and E. Donchin. 1993. A Neural System for Error Detection and Compensation. *Psychological Science* 4 (6): 385–390.

Geddes, J.R., and D.J. Miklowitz. 2013. Treatment of Bipolar Disorder. *Lancet* 381 (9878): 1672–82.

Gershman, S. J., D. M. Blei, and Y. Niv. 2010. Context, Learning, and Extinction. *Psychological Review* 117 (1): 197–209.

Gershman, S., J. Cohen, and Y. Niv. 2010. Learning to Selectively Attend. In *Proceedings of the Annual Meeting of the Cognitive Science Society*, 32:1270–1275. Cognitive Science Society.

Gershman, S. J., and N. D. Daw. 2017. Reinforcement Learning and Episodic Memory in Humans and Animals: An Integrative Framework. *Annual Review of Psychology* 68 (1): 101–128.

Gilbert, D. L., T. K. Murphy, J. Jankovic, C. L. Budman, K. J. Black, R. M. Kurlan, K. A. Coffman, et al. 2018. Ecopipam, a D_1 Receptor Antagonist, for Treatment of Tourette Syndrome in Children: A Randomized, Placebo-Controlled Crossover Study: Selective D_1 Receptor Antagonism: Novel TS Treatment. *Movement Disorders* 33 (8): 1272–1280.

Gillan, C. M., M. Kosinski, R. Whelan, E. A. Phelps, and N. D. Daw. 2016. Characterizing a Psychiatric Symptom Dimension Related to Deficits in Goal-Directed Control. *ELife* 5 (March).

Gittins, J. C. 1979. Bandit Processes and Dynamic Allocation Indices. *Journal of the Royal Statistical Society: Series B (Methodological)* 41 (2): 148–164.

Gläscher, J., N. Daw, P. Dayan, and J. P. O'Doherty. 2010. States versus Rewards: Dissociable Neural Prediction Error Signals Underlying Model-Based and Model-Free Reinforcement Learning. *Neuron* 66 (4): 585–595.

Gmytrasiewicz, P. J., and P. Doshi. 2005. A Framework for Sequential Planning in Multi-Agent Settings. *Journal of Artificial Intelligence Research* 24 (July): 49–79.

Gold, J. I., and M. N. Shadlen. 2007. The Neural Basis of Decision Making. *Annual Review of Neuroscience* 30 (1): 535–574.

Gold, J. M., B. Hahn, W. W. Zhang, B. M. Robinson, E. S. Kappenman, V. M. Beck, and S. J. Luck. 2010. Reduced Capacity but Spared Precision and Maintenance of Working Memory Representations in Schizophrenia. *Archives of General Psychiatry* 67 (6): 570.

Gold, J. M., G. P. Strauss, J. A. Waltz, B. M. Robinson, J. K. Brown, and M. J. Frank. 2013. Negative Symptoms of Schizophrenia Are Associated with Abnormal Effort-Cost Computations. *Biological Psychiatry* 74 (2): 130–136.

Gold, J. M., J. A. Waltz, T. Matveeva, Z. Kasanova, G. P. Strauss, E. S. Herbener, A. G. E. Collins, and M. J. Frank. 2012. Negative Symptoms and the Failure to Represent the Expected Reward Value of Actions. *Archives of General Psychiatry* 69 (2): 129–138.

Goldbeter, A. 2011. A Model for the Dynamics of Bipolar Disorders. Progress in Biophysics and Molecular Biology, BrainModes: The role of neuronal oscillations in health and disease, 105 (1): 119–27.

Goldman-Rakic, P. S. 1995. Cellular Basis of Working Memory. *Neuron* 14 (3): 477–485.

Goldstein, A. 2001. *Addiction: From Biology to Drug Policy*. Oxford, England: Oxford University Press.

Gomez, J. F., K. Cardona, and B. Trenor. 2015. Lessons Learned from Multi-Scale Modeling of the Failing Heart. *Journal of Molecular and Cellular Cardiology* 89 (December): 146–159.

Gonzalez-Burgos, G., and D. A. Lewis. 2008. GABA Neurons and the Mechanisms of Network Oscillations: Implications for Understanding Cortical Dysfunction in Schizophrenia. *Schizophrenia Bulletin* 34 (5): 944–961.

———. 2012. NMDA Receptor Hypofunction, Parvalbumin-Positive Neurons, and Cortical Gamma Oscillations in Schizophrenia. *Schizophrenia Bulletin* 38 (5): 950–957.

Gotlib, I. H., and J. Joormann. 2010. Cognition and Depression: Current Status and Future Directions. *Annual Review of Clinical Psychology* 6 (1): 285–312.

Gottlieb, J., and P. Balan. 2010. Attention as a Decision in Information Space. *Trends in Cognitive Sciences* 14 (6): 240–248.

Grabli, D. McCairn, K. Hirsch, E. C. Agid, Y. Féger, J. François, C. and L. Tremblay. 2004. Behavioural Disorders Induced by External Globus Pallidus Dysfunction in Primates: I. Behavioural Study. *Brain* 127 (9): 2039–2054.

Grace, A., and B. Bunney. 1984a. The Control of Firing Pattern in Nigral Dopamine Neurons: Burst Firing. *The Journal of Neuroscience* 4 (11): 2877–2890.

———. 1984b. The Control of Firing Pattern in Nigral Dopamine Neurons: Single Spike Firing. *The Journal of Neuroscience* 4 (11): 2866–2876.

Gradin, V. B., P. Kumar, G. Waiter, T. Ahearn, C. Stickle, M. Milders, I. Reid, J. Hall, and J. D. Steele. 2011. Expected Value and Prediction Error Abnormalities in Depression and Schizophrenia. *Brain* 134 (6): 1751–1764.

Greene, D. J., J. A. Church, N. U. F. Dosenbach, A. N. Nielsen, B. Adeyemo, B. Nardos, S. E. Petersen, K. J. Black, and B. L. Schlaggar. 2016. Multivariate Pattern Classification of Pediatric Tourette Syndrome Using Functional Connectivity MRI. *Developmental Science* 19 (4): 581–598.

Greene, R. 2001. Circuit Analysis of NMDAR Hypofunction in the Hippocampus, in Vitro, and Psychosis of Schizophrenia. *Hippocampus* 11 (5): 569–577.

Greisberg, S., and D. McKay. 2003. Neuropsychology of Obsessive-Compulsive Disorder: A Review and Treatment Implications. *Clinical Psychology Review* 23 (1): 95–117.

Griffiths, M. D. 1994. The Role of Cognitive Bias and Skill in Fruit Machine Gambling. *British Journal of Psychology* 85 (3): 351–369.

Grossman, M., and F. J. Chaloupka. 1998. The Demand for Cocaine by Young Adults: A Rational Addiction Approach. *Journal of Health Economics* 17 (4): 427–474.

Grupe, D. W. 2017. Decision-Making in Anxiety and Its Disorders. In *Decision Neuroscience: An Integrative Perspective*, edited by J.-C. Dreher and L. Tremblay, 327–338. Amsterdam, Netherlands: Elsevier Science.

Guitart-Masip, M., E. Duzel, R. Dolan, and P. Dayan. 2014. Action versus Valence in Decision Making. *Trends in Cognitive Sciences* 18 (4): 194–202.

Guitart-Masip, M., Q. J. M. Huys, L. Fuentemilla, P. Dayan, E. Duzel, and R. J. Dolan. 2012. Go and No-Go Learning in Reward and Punishment: Interactions between Affect and Effect. *NeuroImage* 62 (1): 154–166.

Gutenkunst, R. N., J. Waterfall, F. Casey, K. Brown, C. R. Myers, and J. P. Sethna. 2007. Universally Sloppy Parameter Sensitivities in Systems Biology Models. *PLoS Computational Biology* preprint: e189.

Gutkin, B. S., S. Dehaene, and J.-P. Changeux. 2006. A Neurocomputational Hypothesis for Nicotine Addiction. *Proceedings of the National Academy of Sciences* 103 (4): 1106–1111.

Haber, S. 2011. Neuroanatomy of Reward: A View from the Ventral Striatum. In *Neurobiology of Sensation and Reward*, edited by J. A. Gottfried, 235–261. Boca Raton, FL: Taylor & Francis.

Haber, S. N., J. L. Fudge, and N. R. McFarland. 2000. Striatonigrostriatal Pathways in Primates Form an Ascending Spiral from the Shell to the Dorsolateral Striatum. *The Journal of Neuroscience* 20 (6): 2369–2382.

Hackel, L. M., and D. M. Amodio. 2018. Computational Neuroscience Approaches to Social Cognition. Current Opinion in Psychology 24: 92–97.

Haker, H., M. Schneebeli, and K. E. Stephan. 2016. Can Bayesian Theories of Autism Spectrum Disorder Help Improve Clinical Practice? *Frontiers in Psychiatry* 7 (June).

Halari, R., M. Simic, C. M. Pariante, A. Papadopoulos, A. Cleare, M. Brammer, E. Fombonne, and K. Rubia. 2009. Reduced Activation in Lateral Prefrontal Cortex and Anterior Cingulate during Attention and Cognitive Control Functions in Medication-Naïve Adolescents with Depression Compared to Controls. *Journal of Child Psychology and Psychiatry* 50 (3): 307–316.

Hamid, A. A., J. R. Pettibone, O. S. Mabrouk, V. L. Hetrick, R. Schmidt, C. M. Vander Weele, R. T. Kennedy, B. J. Aragona, and J. D. Berke. 2016. Mesolimbic Dopamine Signals the Value of Work. *Nature Neuroscience* 19 (1): 117–126.

Hanson, K., S. Allen, S. Jensen, and D. Hatsukami. 2003. Treatment of Adolescent Smokers with the Nicotine Patch. *Nicotine & Tobacco Research* 5 (4): 515–526.

Hare, T. A., C. F. Camerer, D. T. Knoepfle, J. P. O'Doherty, and A. Rangel. 2010. Value Computations in Ventral Medial Prefrontal Cortex during Charitable Decision Making Incorporate Input from Regions Involved in Social Cognition. *Journal of Neuroscience* 30 (2): 583–590.

Hare, T. A., C. F. Camerer, and A. Rangel. 2009. Self-Control in Decision-Making Involves Modulation of the VmP. F. C. Valuation System. *Science* 324 (5927): 646–648.

Hare, T. A., J. Malmaud, and A. Rangel. 2011. Focusing Attention on the Health Aspects of Foods Changes Value Signals in vmPFC and Improves Dietary Choice. *Journal of Neuroscience* 31 (30): 11077–11087.

Hare, T. A., J. O'Doherty, C. F. Camerer, W. Schultz, and A. Rangel. 2008. Dissociating the Role of the Orbitofrontal Cortex and the Striatum in the Computation of Goal Values and Prediction Errors. *Journal of Neuroscience* 28 (22): 5623–5630.

Harmer, C. J., G. M. Goodwin, and P. J. Cowen. 2009. Why Do Antidepressants Take So Long to Work? A Cognitive Neuropsychological Model of Antidepressant Drug Action. *British Journal of Psychiatry* 195 (2): 102–108.

Harrison, P. J., A. Cipriani, C. J. Harmer, A. C. Nobre, K. Saunders, G. M. Goodwin, and J. R. Geddes. 2016. Innovative Approaches to Bipolar Disorder and Its Treatment. *Annals of the New York Academy of Sciences* 1366 (1): 76–89.

Harsanyi, J. C. 1967. Games with Incomplete Information Played by "Bayesian" Players, I–III Part I. The Basic Model. *Management Science* 14 (3): 159–182.

Hart, A. S., R. B. Rutledge, P. W. Glimcher, and P. E. M. Phillips. 2014. Phasic Dopamine Release in the Rat Nucleus Accumbens Symmetrically Encodes a Reward Prediction Error Term. *The Journal of Neuroscience* 34 (3): 698–704.

Hart, C. 2013. *High Price: Drugs, Neuroscience, and Discovering Myself.* New York, NY: Harper-Collins.

Haruno, M., and M. Kawato. 2006. Heterarchical Reinforcement-Learning Model for Integration of Multiple Cortico-Striatal Loops: FMRI Examination in Stimulus-Action-Reward Association Learning. *Neural Networks* 19 (8): 1242–1254.

Hashemiyoon, R., J. Kuhn, and V. Visser-Vandewalle. 2017. Putting the Pieces Together in Gilles de La Tourette Syndrome: Exploring the Link Between Clinical Observations and the Biological Basis of Dysfunction. *Brain Topography* 30 (1): 3–29.

Hauser, T. U., R. Iannaccone, J. Ball, C. Mathys, D. Brandeis, S. Walitza, and S. Brem. 2014. Role of the Medial Prefrontal Cortex in Impaired Decision Making in Juvenile Attention-Deficit/ Hyperactivity Disorder. *JAMA Psychiatry* 71 (10): 1165–1173.

Hauser, T. U., V. G. Fiore, M. Moutoussis, and R. J. Dolan. 2016. Computational Psychiatry of ADHD: Neural Gain Impairments across Marrian Levels of Analysis. *Trends in Neurosciences* 39 (2): 63–73.

Hazy, T. E., M. J. Frank, and R. C. O'Reilly. 2007. Towards an Executive without a Homunculus: Computational Models of the Prefrontal Cortex/Basal Ganglia System. *Philosophical Transactions of the Royal Society B: Biological Sciences* 362 (1485): 1601–1613.

Heath, R. G. 1963. Electrical Self-Stimulation of the Brain in Man. *American Journal of Psychiatry* 120 (6): 571–577.

Hebb, D. O. 1949. *The Organization of Behavior: A Neuropsychological Theory*. Hoboken, NJ: Wiley.

Heinz, A. 2017. *A New Understanding of Mental Disorders: Computational Models for Dimensional Psychiatry*. Cambridge, MA: The MIT Press.

Hertz, J., A. Krogh, and R. G. Palmer. 1991. *Introduction to the Theory of Neural Computation*. Reading, MA: Addison-Wesley.

Herwig, A., M. Beisert, and W. X. Schneider. 2010. On the Spatial Interaction of Visual Working Memory and Attention: Evidence for a Global Effect from Memory-Guided Saccades. *Journal of Vision* 10 (5): 8–8.

Heyman, G. M. 2009. *Addiction: A Disorder of Choice*. Cambridge, MA: Harvard University Press.

Hienert, M., G. Gryglewski, M. Stamenkovic, S. Kasper, and R. Lanzenberger. 2018. Striatal Dopaminergic Alterations in Tourette's Syndrome: A Meta-Analysis Based on 16 PET and SPECT Neuroimaging Studies. *Translational Psychiatry* 8 (1): 143.

Higgins, S. T., S. M. Alessi, and R. L. Dantona. 2002. Voucher-Based Incentives. *Addictive Behaviors* 27 (6): 887–910.

Hikosaka, O., H. Nakahara, M. K. Rand, K. Sakai, X. Lu, K. Nakamura, S. Miyachi, and K. Doya. 1999. Parallel Neural Networks for Learning Sequential Procedures. *Trends in Neurosciences* 22 (10): 464–471.

Hinton, G. E. 1984. Distributed Representations. Technical Report CMU-C S.-84–157. Computer Science Technical Reports. Pittsburgh, PA: Department of Computer Science, Carnegie-Mellon University.

Hitchcock, P., Y. Niv, A. Radulescu, and C. R. Sims. 2017. Translating a Reinforcement Learning Task into a Computational Psychiatry Assay: Challenges and Strategies. In *Proceedings of the*

39th Annual Conference of the Cognitive Science Society, 2217–2222. Austin, TX: Cognitive Science Society.

Hodgkin, A. L., and A. F. Huxley. 1952. A Quantitative Description of Membrane Current and Its Application to Conduction and Excitation in Nerve. *The Journal of Physiology* 117 (4): 500–544.

Hodos, W. 1961. Progressive Ratio as a Measure of Reward Strength. *Science* 134 (3483): 943–944.

Hoffman, R. E., and T. H. McGlashan. 2001. Book Review: Neural Network Models of Schizophrenia. *The Neuroscientist* 7 (5): 441–454.

Hoffman, R. E., and T. H. McGlashan. 2006. Using a Speech Perception Neural Network Computer Simulation to Contrast Neuroanatomic versus Neuromodulatory Models of Auditory Hallucinations. *Pharmacopsychiatry* 39 (February): 54–64.

Hoffman, R. E., U. Grasemann, R. Gueorguieva, D. Quinlan, D. Lane, and R. Miikkulainen. 2011. Using Computational Patients to Evaluate Illness Mechanisms in Schizophrenia. *Biological Psychiatry* 69 (10): 997–1005.

Hofstadter, D. 2007. *I Am a Strange Loop*. New York, NY: Basic Books.

Hofstadter, D. 2008. *Metamagical Themas: Questing for the Essence of Mind and Pattern*. New York, NY: Basic books.

Hollon, N. G., M. M. Arnold, J. O. Gan, M. E. Walton, and P. E. M. Phillips. 2014. Dopamine-Associated Cached Values Are Not Sufficient as the Basis for Action Selection. *Proceedings of the National Academy of Sciences* 111 (51): 18357–18362.

Holroyd, C. B., and M. G. H. Coles. 2002. The Neural Basis of Human Error Processing: Reinforcement Learning, Dopamine, and the Error-Related Negativity. *Psychological Review* 109 (4): 679–709.

Holroyd, C. B., and S. M. McClure. 2015. Hierarchical Control over Effortful Behavior by Rodent Medial Frontal Cortex: A Computational Model. *Psychological Review* 122 (1): 54–83.

Holroyd, C. B., S. Nieuwenhuis, N. Yeung, L. Nystrom, R. B. Mars, M. G. H. Coles, and J. D. Cohen. 2004. Dorsal Anterior Cingulate Cortex Shows fMRI Response to Internal and External Error Signals. *Nature Neuroscience* 7 (5): 497–498.

Holroyd, C. B., and N. Yeung. 2011. An Integrative Theory of Anterior Cingulate Cortex Function: Option Selection in Hierarchical Reinforcement Learning. In *Neural Basis of Motivational and Cognitive Control*, edited by R. B. Mars, 332–349. Cambridge, MA: The MIT Press.

Holroyd, C. B., N. Yeung, M. G. H. Coles, and J. D. Cohen. 2005. A Mechanism for Error Detection in Speeded Response Time Tasks. *Journal of Experimental Psychology: General* 134 (2): 163–191.

Homan, P., I. Levy, E. Feltham, C. Gordon, J. Hu, J. Li, R. H. Pietrzak, et al. 2019. Neural Computations of Threat in the Aftermath of Combat Trauma. *Nature Neuroscience* 22 (3): 470–476.

Homayoun, H., and B. Moghaddam. 2007. NMDA Receptor Hypofunction Produces Opposite Effects on Prefrontal Cortex Interneurons and Pyramidal Neurons. *Journal of Neuroscience* 27 (43): 11496–114500.

Hopfield, J. J. 1982. Neural Networks and Physical Systems with Emergent Collective Computational Abilities. *Proceedings of the National Academy of Sciences* 79 (8): 2554–2558.

Horga, G., T. V. Maia, R. Marsh, X. Hao, D. Xu, Y. Duan, G. Z. Tau, et al. 2015. Changes in Corticostriatal Connectivity during Reinforcement Learning in Humans. *Human Brain Mapping* 36 (2): 793–803.

Houthakker, H. S. 1950. Revealed Preference and the Utility Function. *Economica* 17 (66): 159.

Howe, M. W., and D. A. Dombeck. 2016. Rapid Signalling in Distinct Dopaminergic Axons during Locomotion and Reward. *Nature* 535 (7613): 505–510.

Howes, O. D., and S. Kapur. 2009. The Dopamine Hypothesis of Schizophrenia: Version III—The Final Common Pathway. *Schizophrenia Bulletin* 35 (3): 549–562.

Hsu, C.-W., L.-J. Wang, and P.-Y. Lin. 2018. Efficacy of Repetitive Transcranial Magnetic Stimulation for Tourette Syndrome: A Systematic Review and Meta-Analysis. *Brain Stimulation* 11 (5): 1110–1118.

Huk, A. C., and M. N. Shadlen. 2005. Neural Activity in Macaque Parietal Cortex Reflects Temporal Integration of Visual Motion Signals during Perceptual Decision Making. *Journal of Neuroscience* 25 (45): 10420–10436.

Hula, A., P. R. Montague, and P. Dayan. 2015. Monte Carlo Planning Method Estimates Planning Horizons during Interactive Social Exchange. *PLOS Computational Biology* 11 (6): e1004254.

Hursh, S. R. 2005. The Economics of Drug Abuse: A Quantitative Assessment of Drug Demand. *Molecular Interventions* 5 (1): 20–28.

Husain, M., and J. P. Roiser. 2018. Neuroscience of Apathy and Anhedonia: A Transdiagnostic Approach. *Nature Reviews Neuroscience* 19 (8): 470–484.

Huys, Q. J. M. 2018. Bayesian Approaches to Learning and Decision-Making. *Computational Psychiatry*, 247–271.

Huys, Q. J. M., N. D. Daw, and P. Dayan. 2015a. Depression: A Decision-Theoretic Analysis. *Annual Review of Neuroscience* 38 (1): 1–23.

Huys, Q. J. M., and P. Dayan. 2009. A Bayesian Formulation of Behavioral Control. *Cognition* 113 (3): 314–328.

Huys, Q. J. M., N. Eshel, E. O'Nions, L. Sheridan, P. Dayan, and J. P. Roiser. 2012. Bonsai Trees in Your Head: How the Pavlovian System Sculpts Goal-Directed Choices by Pruning Decision Trees. *PLoS Computational Biology* 8 (3): e1002410.

Huys, Q. J. M., M. Gölzer, E. Friedel, A. Heinz, R. Cools, P. Dayan, and R. J. Dolan. 2016a. The Specificity of Pavlovian Regulation Is Associated with Recovery from Depression. *Psychological Medicine* 46 (5): 1027–1035.

Huys, Q. J. M., M. Guitart-Masip, R. J. Dolan, and P. Dayan. 2015b. Decision-Theoretic Psychiatry. *Clinical Psychological Science* 3 (3): 400–421.

Huys, Q. J. M., T. V. Maia, and M. J. Frank. 2016b. Computational Psychiatry as a Bridge from Neuroscience to Clinical Applications. *Nature Neuroscience* 19 (3): 404–413.

Huys, Q. J. M., D. A. Pizzagalli, R. Bogdan, and P. Dayan. 2013. Mapping Anhedonia onto Reinforcement Learning: A Behavioural Meta-Analysis. *Biology of Mood & Anxiety Disorders* 3 (1): 12.

Huys, Q. J., J. Vogelstein, and P. Dayan. 2009. Psychiatry: Insights into Depression through Normative Decision-Making Models. In *Advances in Neural Information Processing Systems 17*, edited by L. K. Saul, Y. Weiss, and L. Bottou, 729–736. Defense Technical Information Center.

Hyman, S. E. 2010. The Diagnosis of Mental Disorders: The Problem of Reification. *Annual Review of Clinical Psychology* 6 (1): 155–179.

Hyman, S. E. 2012. Revolution Stalled. *Science Translational Medicine* 4 (155): 155cm11–155cm11.

Iglesias, S., S. Tomiello, M. Schneebeli, and K. E. Stephan. 2017. Models of Neuromodulation for Computational Psychiatry. *Wiley Interdisciplinary Reviews: Cognitive Science* 8 (3): e1420.

Iigaya, K., G. W. Story, Z. Kurth-Nelson, R. J. Dolan, and P. Dayan. 2016. The Modulation of Savouring by Prediction Error and Its Effects on Choice. *ELife* 5 (April).

Indovina, I., T. W. Robbins, A. O. Núñez-Elizalde, B. D. Dunn, and S. J. Bishop. 2011. Fear-Conditioning Mechanisms Associated with Trait Vulnerability to Anxiety in Humans. *Neuron* 69 (3): 563–571.

Insel, T., B. Cuthbert, M. Garvey, R. Heinssen, D. S. Pine, K. Quinn, C. Sanislow, and P. Wang. 2010. Research Domain Criteria (RDoC): Toward a New Classification Framework for Research on Mental Disorders. *American Journal of Psychiatry* 167 (7): 748–751.

Insel, T. R. 2012. Next-Generation Treatments for Mental Disorders. *Science Translational Medicine* 4 (155): 155ps19–155ps19.

Insel, T. R. 2015. The NIMH Experimental Medicine Initiative. *World Psychiatry* 14 (2): 151–153.

Insel, T. R., and B. N. Cuthbert. 2009. Endophenotypes: Bridging Genomic Complexity and Disorder Heterogeneity. *Biological Psychiatry* 66 (11): 988–989.

———. 2015. Brain Disorders? Precisely. *Science* 348 (6234): 499–500.

Itoi, K., and N. Sugimoto. 2010. The Brainstem Noradrenergic Systems in Stress, Anxiety and Depression. *Journal of Neuroendocrinology* 22 (5): 355–361.

Jackson, S. R., A. Parkinson, J. Jung, S. E. Ryan, P. S. Morgan, C. Hollis, and G. M. Jackson. 2011a. Compensatory Neural Reorganization in Tourette Syndrome. *Current Biology* 21 (7): 580–585.

Jackson, S. R., A. Parkinson, S. Y. Kim, M. Schüermann, and S. B. Eickhoff. 2011b. On the Functional Anatomy of the Urge-for-Action. *Cognitive Neuroscience* 2 (3–4): 227–243.

Jaffe, A., J. A. Z. Pham, I. Tarash, S. S. Getty, M. S. Fanselow, and J. D. Jentsch. 2014. The Absence of Blocking in Nicotine High-Responders as a Possible Factor in the Development of Nicotine Dependence? *The Open Addiction Journal* 7 (1): 8–16.

Jankovic, J. 2001. Tourette's Syndrome. *New England Journal of Medicine* 345 (16): 1184–1192.

Jardri, R., and S. Denève. 2013. Circular Inferences in Schizophrenia. *Brain: A Journal of Neurology* 136 (11): 3227–3241.

Jardri, R., S. Duverne, A. S. Litvinova, and S. Denève. 2017. Experimental Evidence for Circular Inference in Schizophrenia. *Nature Communications* 8 (1).

Jenkins, H. M., and B. R. Moore. 1973. The Form of the Auto-Shaped Response with Food or Water Reinforcers. *Journal of the Experimental Analysis of Behavior* 20 (2): 163–181.

Jepma, M., P. R. Murphy, M. R. Nassar, M. Rangel-Gomez, M. Meeter, and S. Nieuwenhuis. 2016. Catecholaminergic Regulation of Learning Rate in a Dynamic Environment. *PLOS Computational Biology* 12 (10): e1005171.

Jo, H. J., K. W. McCairn, W. S. Gibson, P. Testini, C. Z. Zhao, K. R. Gorny, J. P. Felmlee, et al. 2018. Global Network Modulation during Thalamic Stimulation for Tourette Syndrome. *NeuroImage: Clinical* 18: 502–509.

Joel, D., and I. Weiner. 2000. The Connections of the Dopaminergic System with the Striatum in Rats and Primates: An Analysis with Respect to the Functional and Compartmental Organization of the Striatum. *Neuroscience* 96 (3): 451–474.

Johansen, J. P., C. K. Cain, L. E. Ostroff, and J. E. LeDoux. 2011. Molecular Mechanisms of Fear Learning and Memory. *Cell* 147 (3): 509–524.

Johnson, J. D., W. Li, J. Li, and A. H. Klopf. 2001. A Computational Model of Learned Avoidance Behavior in a One-Way Avoidance Experiment. *Adaptive Behavior* 9 (2): 91–104.

Joshi, S., Y. Li, R. M. Kalwani, and J. I. Gold. 2016. Relationships between Pupil Diameter and Neuronal Activity in the Locus Coeruleus, Colliculi, and Cingulate Cortex. *Neuron* 89 (1): 221–234.

Juckel, G., F. Schlagenhauf, M. Koslowski, T. Wüstenberg, A. Villringer, B. Knutson, J. Wrase, and A. Heinz. 2006. Dysfunction of Ventral Striatal Reward Prediction in Schizophrenia. *NeuroImage* 29 (2): 409–416.

Jung, J., S. R. Jackson, A. Parkinson, and G. M. Jackson. 2013. Cognitive Control over Motor Output in Tourette Syndrome. *Neuroscience & Biobehavioral Reviews* 37 (6): 1016–1025.

Kable, J. W., and P. W. Glimcher. 2010. An "As Soon As Possible" Effect in Human Intertemporal Decision Making: Behavioral Evidence and Neural Mechanisms. *Journal of Neurophysiology* 103 (5): 2513–2531.

Kacelnik, A. 1997. Normative and Descriptive Models of Decision Making: Time Discounting and Risk Sensitivity. In *Ciba Foundation Symposium 208—Characterizing Human Psychological Adaptations*, edited by G. R. Bock and G. Cardew, 51–70. Chichester, England: Wiley.

Kahneman, D. 2011. *Thinking, Fast and Slow*. New York, NY: Farrar, Strauss, Giroux.

Kahneman, D., and A. Tversky. 1979. Prospect Theory: An Analysis of Decision under Risk. *Econometrica* 47 (2): 263–291.

Kalaska, J. F., and G. Rizzolatti. 2013. Voluntary Movement: The Primary Motor Cortex. In *Principles of Neural Science*, edited by E. R. Kandel, T. Schwartz, T. Jessell, S. Siegelbaum, and A. J. Hudspeth, 5th ed. Vol. 835–864. New York, NY: McGraw-Hill Professional.

Kamin, L. J. 1969. Predictability, Surprise, Attention, and Conditioning. In *Punishment and Aversive Behavior*, edited by B. A. Campbell and R. M. Church, 279–296. New York, NY: Appleton-Century-Crofts.

Kaplan, B. J., D. M. Dewey, S. G. Crawford, and B. N. Wilson. 2001. The Term Comorbidity Is of Questionable Value in Reference to Developmental Disorders. *Journal of Learning Disabilities* 34 (6): 555–565.

Kapur, S. 2003. Psychosis as a State of Aberrant Salience: A Framework Linking Biology, Phenomenology, and Pharmacology in Schizophrenia. *American Journal of Psychiatry* 160 (1): 13–23.

Karvelis, P., A. R. Seitz, S. M. Lawrie, and P. Seriès. 2018. Autistic Traits, but Not Schizotypy, Predict Increased Weighting of Sensory Information in Bayesian Visual Integration. ELife. May 14, 2018.

Kataoka, Y., P. S. A. Kalanithi, H. Grantz, M. L. Schwartz, C. Saper, J. F. Leckman, and F. M. Vaccarino. 2010. Decreased Number of Parvalbumin and Cholinergic Interneurons in the Striatum of Individuals with Tourette Syndrome. *The Journal of Comparative Neurology* 518 (3): 277–291.

Katthagen, T., C. Mathys, L. Deserno, H. Walter, N. Kathmann, A. Heinz, and F. Schlagenhauf. 2018. Modeling Subjective Relevance in Schizophrenia and Its Relation to Aberrant Salience. *PLOS Computational Biology* 14 (8): e1006319.

Keay, K. A., and R. Bandler. 2001. Parallel Circuits Mediating Distinct Emotional Coping Reactions to Different Types of Stress. *Neuroscience & Biobehavioral Reviews* 25 (7–8): 669–678.

Kelley, A. E., B. A. Baldo, and W. E. Pratt. 2005. A Proposed Hypothalamic-Thalamic-Striatal Axis for the Integration of Energy Balance, Arousal, and Food Reward. *The Journal of Comparative Neurology* 493 (1): 72–85.

Kendler, K. S., and A. Jablensky. 2011. Kraepelin's Concept of Psychiatric Illness. *Psychological Medicine* 41 (6): 1119–1126.

Keramati, M., A. Dezfouli, and P. Piray. 2011. Speed/Accuracy Trade-Off between the Habitual and the Goal-Directed Processes. *PLoS Computational Biology* 7 (5): e1002055.

Keramati, M., A. Durand, P. Girardeau, B. Gutkin, and S. H. Ahmed. 2017. Cocaine Addiction as a Homeostatic Reinforcement Learning Disorder. *Psychological Review* 124 (2): 130–153.

Keramati, M., and B. Gutkin. 2014. Homeostatic Reinforcement Learning for Integrating Reward Collection and Physiological Stability. *ELife* 3 (December).

Keramati, M., P. Smittenaar, R. J. Dolan, and P. Dayan. 2016. Adaptive Integration of Habits into Depth-Limited Planning Defines a Habitual-Goal–Directed Spectrum. *Proceedings of the National Academy of Sciences* 113 (45): 12868–12873.

Kéri, S., C. Szlobodnyik, G. Benedek, Z. Janka, and J. Gádoros. 2002. Probabilistic Classification Learning in Tourette Syndrome. *Neuropsychologia* 40 (8): 1356–1362.

Kerns, J. G. 2004. Anterior Cingulate Conflict Monitoring and Adjustments in Control. *Science* 303 (5660): 1023–1026.

Kessler, R. C., P. Berglund, O. Demler, R. Jin, D. Koretz, K. R. Merikangas, A. J. Rush, E. E. Walters, and P. S. Wang. 2003. The Epidemiology of Major Depressive Disorder: Results from the National Comorbidity Survey Replication. *JAMA* 289 (23): 3095–3105.

Khin, N. A., Y.-F. Chen, Y. Yang, P. Yang, and T. P. Laughren. 2011. Exploratory Analyses of Efficacy Data from Major Depressive Disorder Trials Submitted to the U.S. Food and Drug Administration in Support of New Drug Applications. *The Journal of Clinical Psychiatry* 72 (04): 464–472.

Khlestova, E., J. W. Johnson, J. H. Krystal, and J. Lisman. 2016. The Role of GluN2C-Containing NMDA Receptors in Ketamine's Psychotogenic Action and in Schizophrenia Models. *The Journal of Neuroscience* 36 (44): 11151–11157.

Kieras, D. E., and D. E. Meyer. 1997. An Overview of the E. P. I.C Architecture for Cognition and Performance With Application to Human-Computer Interaction. *Human–Computer Interaction* 12 (4): 391–438.

Killcross, S., and E. Coutureau. 2003. Coordination of Actions and Habits in the Medial Prefrontal Cortex of Rats. *Cerebral Cortex* 13 (4): 400–408.

Kious, B. M., J. Jimenez-Shahed, and D. R. Shprecher. 2016. Treatment-Refractory Tourette Syndrome. *Progress in Neuro-Psychopharmacology and Biological Psychiatry* 70 (October): 227–236.

Kishida, K. T., I. Saez, T. Lohrenz, M. R. Witcher, A. W. Laxton, S. B. Tatter, J. P. White, T. L. Ellis, P. E. M. Phillips, and P. R. Montague. 2016. Subsecond Dopamine Fluctuations in Human Striatum Encode Superposed Error Signals about Actual and Counterfactual Reward. *Proceedings of the National Academy of Sciences* 113 (1): 200–205.

Knowlton, B. J., L. R. Squire, and M. A. Gluck. 1994. Probabilistic Classification Learning in Amnesia. *Learning & Memory* 1 (2): 106–120.

Kocsis, L., and C. Szepesvári. 2006. Bandit Based Monte-Carlo Planning. In *Machine Learning: ECML 2006*, edited by J. Fürnkranz, T. Scheffer, and M. Spiliopoulou, 17: 282–293. Berlin, Germany: Springer.

Koechlin, E., C. Ody, and F. Kouneiher. 2003. The Architecture of Cognitive Control in the Human Prefrontal Cortex. *Science* 302 (5648): 1181–1185.

Koechlin, E., and C. Summerfield. 2007. An Information Theoretical Approach to Prefrontal Executive Function. *Trends in Cognitive Sciences* 11 (6): 229–235.

Koldewyn, K., D. Whitney, and S. M. Rivera. 2010. The Psychophysics of Visual Motion and Global Form Processing in Autism. *Brain* 133 (2): 599–610.

Koob, G. F. 2013. Addiction Is a Reward Deficit and Stress Surfeit Disorder. *Frontiers in Psychiatry* 4: 72.

Koob, G. F., and M. L. Moal. 2006. *Neurobiology of Addiction*. Cambridge, MA: Academic Press.

Kool, W., and M. Botvinick. 2014. A Labor/Leisure Tradeoff in Cognitive Control. *Journal of Experimental Psychology: General* 143 (1): 131–141.

Kotermanski, S. E., and J. W. Johnson. 2009. Mg2+ Imparts NMDA Receptor Subtype Selectivity to the Alzheimers Drug Memantine. *Journal of Neuroscience* 29 (9): 2774–2779.

Kourrich, S., P. E. Rothwell, J. R. Klug, and M. J. Thomas. 2007. Cocaine Experience Controls Bidirectional Synaptic Plasticity in the Nucleus Accumbens. *Journal of Neuroscience* 27 (30): 7921–7928.

Kozak, M. J., and B. N. Cuthbert. 2016. The NIMH Research Domain Criteria Initiative: Background, Issues, and Pragmatics. *Psychophysiology* 53 (3): 286–297.

Kreps, D. M., and E. L. Porteus. 1978. Temporal Resolution of Uncertainty and Dynamic Choice Theory. *Econometrica* 46 (1): 185.

Kristan, W. B., and P. Katz. 2006. Form and Function in Systems Neuroscience. *Current Biology* 16 (19): R828–31.

Krystal, J. H., D. C. D'Souza, D. Mathalon, E. Perry, A. Belger, and R. Hoffman. 2003. NMDA Receptor Antagonist Effects, Cortical Glutamatergic Function, and Schizophrenia: Toward a Paradigm Shift in Medication Development. *Psychopharmacology* 169 (3–4): 215–233.

Kumar, P., G. Waiter, T. Ahearn, M. Milders, I. Reid, and J. D. Steele. 2008. Abnormal Temporal Difference Reward-Learning Signals in Major Depression. *Brain* 131 (8): 2084–2093.

Kurth-Nelson, Z., W. Bickel, and A. D. Redish. 2012. A Theoretical Account of Cognitive Effects in Delay Discounting. *European Journal of Neuroscience* 35 (7): 1052–1064.

Kurth-Nelson, Z., and A. D. Redish. 2009. Temporal-Difference Reinforcement Learning with Distributed Representations. *PLoS ONE* 4 (10): e7362.

———. 2010. A Reinforcement Learning Model of Precommitment in Decision Making. *Frontiers in Behavioral Neuroscience* 4: 184.

———. 2012. Modeling Decision-Making Systems in Addiction. In *Computational Neuroscience of Drug Addiction*, edited by B. Gutkin and S. H. Ahmed, 163–187. New York, NY: Springer.

Kurzban, R. 2010. *Why Everyone (Else) Is a Hypocrite*. Princeton, NJ: Princeton University Press.

Laakso, A., H. Vilkman, J. Bergman, M. Haaparanta, O. Solin, E. Syvälahti, R. K. R. Salokangas, and J. Hietala. 2002. Sex Differences in Striatal Presynaptic Dopamine Synthesis Capacity in Healthy Subjects. *Biological Psychiatry* 52 (7): 759–763.

Lam, N. H., T. Borduqui, J. Hallak, A. C. Roque, A. Anticevic, J. H. Krystal, X.-J. Wang, and J. D. Murray. 2017. Effects of Altered Excitation–Inhibition Balance on Decision Making in a Cortical Circuit Model. *BioRxiv*, January, 100347.

Lammel, S., B. K. Lim, and R. C. Malenka. 2014. Reward and Aversion in a Heterogeneous Midbrain Dopamine System. *Neuropharmacology* 76 (Pt B): 351–359.

Lammel, S., B. K. Lim, C. Ran, K. W. Huang, M. J. Betley, K. M. Tye, K. Deisseroth, and R. C. Malenka. 2012. Input-Specific Control of Reward and Aversion in the Ventral Tegmental Area. *Nature* 491 (7423): 212–217.

Langdon, R., P. B. Ward, and M. Coltheart. 2008. Reasoning Anomalies Associated with Delusions in Schizophrenia. *Schizophrenia Bulletin* 36 (2): 321–330.

Langer, E. J. 1975. The Illusion of Control. *Journal of Personality and Social Psychology* 32 (2): 311–328.

Lapicque, L. É. 1907. Recherches Quantitatives Sur l'Excitation Des Nerfs Traitée Comme Une Polarisation. *Journal De Physiologie-Paris* 9: 620–635.

———. 1926. *L'Excitabilité en Fonction du Temps: La Chronaxie, Sa Signification et Sa Mesure*. Les Presses Universitaires de France.

Lawson, R. P., C. Mathys, and G. Rees. 2017. Adults with Autism Overestimate the Volatility of the Sensory Environment. *Nature Neuroscience* 20 (9): 1293–1299.

Lawson, R. P., G. Rees, and K. J. Friston. 2014. An Aberrant Precision Account of Autism. *Frontiers in Human Neuroscience* 8: 302.

Leckman, J. F., D. E. Walkter, and D. J. Cohen. 1993. Premonitory Urges in Tourette's Syndrome. *American Journal of Psychiatry* 150 (1): 98–102.

LeDoux, J. E., and D. S. Pine. 2016. Using Neuroscience to Help Understand Fear and Anxiety: A Two-System Framework. *American Journal of Psychiatry* 173 (11): 1083–1093.

Lee, D. 2013. Decision Making: From Neuroscience to Psychiatry. *Neuron* 78 (2): 233–248.

Lee, J., and S. Park. 2005. Working Memory Impairments in Schizophrenia: A Meta-Analysis. *Journal of Abnormal Psychology* 114 (4): 599–611.

Lee, R. 2017. Mistrustful and Misunderstood: A Review of Paranoid Personality Disorder. *Current Behavioral Neuroscience Reports* 4 (2): 151–165.

Lee, S. W., S. Shimojo, and J. P. O'Doherty. 2014. Neural Computations Underlying Arbitration between Model-Based and Model-Free Learning. *Neuron* 81 (3): 687–699.

Leptourgos, P., S. Denève, and R. Jardri. 2017. Can circular inference relate the neuropathological and behavioral aspects of schizophrenia? *Current Opinion in Neurobiology* 46, 154–161

Lener, M. S., M. J. Niciu, E. D. Ballard, M. Park, L. T. Park, A. C. Nugent, and C. A. Zarate. 2017. Glutamate and Gamma-Aminobutyric Acid Systems in the Pathophysiology of Major Depression and Antidepressant Response to Ketamine. *Biological Psychiatry* 81 (10): 886–897.

Lennington, J. B., G. Coppola, Y. Kataoka-Sasaki, T. V. Fernandez, D. Palejev, Y. Li, A. Huttner, et al. 2016. Transcriptome Analysis of the Human Striatum in Tourette Syndrome. *Biological Psychiatry* 79 (5): 372–382.

Lenoir, M., F. Serre, L. Cantin, and S. H. Ahmed. 2007. Intense Sweetness Surpasses Cocaine Reward. *PLoS ONE* 2 (8): e698.

Lerner, T. N., and A. C. Kreitzer. 2011. Neuromodulatory Control of Striatal Plasticity and Behavior. *Current Opinion in Neurobiology* 21 (2): 322–327.

Lesh, T. A., T. A. Niendam, M. J. Minzenberg, and C. S. Carter. 2011. Cognitive Control Deficits in Schizophrenia: Mechanisms and Meaning. *Neuropsychopharmacology* 36 (1): 316–338.

Parks, D. S. Levine, R. W., and D. L. Long. 1998. *Fundamentals of Neural Network Modeling: Neuropsychology and Cognitive Neuroscience*. Cambridge, MA: MIT Press.

Li, J., and N. D. Daw. 2011. Signals in Human Striatum Are Appropriate for Policy Update Rather than Value Prediction. *Journal of Neuroscience* 31 (14): 5504–5511.

Li, Jian, D. Schiller, G. Schoenbaum, E. A. Phelps, and N. D. Daw. 2011. Differential Roles of Human Striatum and Amygdala in Associative Learning. *Nature Neuroscience* 14 (10): 1250–1252.

Li, Y., J.-S. Zhang, F. Wen, X.-Y. Lu, C.-M. Yan, F. Wang, and Y.-H. Cui. 2019. Premonitory Urges Located in the Tongue for Tic Disorder: Two Case Reports and Review of Literature. *World Journal of Clinical Cases* 7 (12): 1508–1514.

Liao, W., Y. Yu, H.-H. Miao, Y.-X. Feng, G.-J. Ji, and J.-H. Feng. 2017. Inter-Hemispheric Intrinsic Connectivity as a Neuromarker for the Diagnosis of Boys with Tourette Syndrome. *Molecular Neurobiology* 54 (4): 2781–2789.

Lieder, I., V. Adam, O. Frenkel, S. Jaffe-Dax, M. Sahani, and M. Ahissar. 2019. Perceptual Bias Reveals Slow-Updating in Autism and Fast-Forgetting in Dyslexia. *Nature Neuroscience* 22 (2): 256–64.

Lilienfeld, S. O., I. D. Waldman, and A. C. Israel. 1994. A Critical Examination of the Use of the Term and Concept of Comorbidity in Psychopathology Research. *Clinical Psychology: Science and Practice* 1 (1): 71–83.

Lindquist, K. A., and L. F. Barrett. 2012. A Functional Architecture of the Human Brain: Emerging Insights from the Science of Emotion. *Trends in Cognitive Sciences* 16 (11): 533–540.

Linscott, R. J., and J. van Os. 2010. Systematic Reviews of Categorical Versus Continuum Models in Psychosis: Evidence for Discontinuous Subpopulations Underlying a Psychometric

Continuum. Implications for DSM-V, DSM-VI, and DSM-VII. *Annual Review of Clinical Psychology* 6 (1): 391–419.

Lissek, S., D. S. Pine, and C. Grillon. 2006. The Strong Situation: A Potential Impediment to Studying the Psychobiology and Pharmacology of Anxiety Disorders. *Biological Psychology* 72 (3): 265–270.

Lissek, S., A. S. Powers, E. B. McClure, E. A. Phelps, G. Woldehawariat, C. Grillon, and D. S. Pine. 2005. Classical Fear Conditioning in the Anxiety Disorders: A Meta-Analysis. *Behaviour Research and Therapy* 43 (11): 1391–1424.

Lissek, S., S. Rabin, R. E. Heller, D. Lukenbaugh, M. Geraci, D. S. Pine, and C. Grillon. 2010. Overgeneralization of Conditioned Fear as a Pathogenic Marker of Panic Disorder. *American Journal of Psychiatry* 167 (1): 47–55.

Liu, J.-L., J.-T. Liu, J. K. Hammitt, and S.-Y. Chou. 1999. The Price Elasticity of Opium in Taiwan, 1914–1942. *Journal of Health Economics* 18 (6): 795–810.

Ljungberg, T., P. Apicella, and W. Schultz. 1992. Responses of Monkey Dopamine Neurons during Learning of Behavioral Reactions. *Journal of Neurophysiology* 67 (1): 145–163.

Llinás, R., F. J. Urbano, E. Leznik, R. R. Ramírez, and H. J. F. van Marle. 2005. Rhythmic and Dysrhythmic Thalamocortical Dynamics: GABA Systems and the Edge Effect. *Trends in Neurosciences* 28 (6): 325–333.

Lloyd, K., and P. Dayan. 2016. Safety out of Control: Dopamine and Defence. *Behavioral and Brain Functions* 12 (May): 15.

Lodge, D. J., and A. A. Grace. 2011. Hippocampal Dysregulation of Dopamine System Function and the Pathophysiology of Schizophrenia. *Trends in Pharmacological Sciences* 32 (9): 507–513.

Loewenstein, G. 1987. Anticipation and the Valuation of Delayed Consumption. *The Economic Journal* 97 (387): 666–684.

———. 2000. Emotions in Economic Theory and Economic Behavior. *American Economic Review* 90 (2): 426–432.

Lohrenz, T., K. McCabe, C. F. Camerer, and P. R. Montague. 2007. Neural Signature of Fictive Learning Signals in a Sequential Investment Task. *Proceedings of the National Academy of Sciences* 104 (22): 9493–9498.

Loomes, G., and R. Sugden. 1982. Regret Theory: An Alternative Theory of Rational Choice Under Uncertainty. *The Economic Journal* 92 (368): 805–824.

Maatz, A., P. Hoff, and J. Angst. 2015. Eugen Bleulers Schizophrenia—a Modern Perspective. *Dialogues in Clinical Neuroscience* 17 (1): 43.

MacCorquodale, K., and P. E. Meehl. 1948. On a Distinction between Hypothetical Constructs and Intervening Variables. *Psychological Review* 55 (2): 95–107.

Mackintosh, NJ. 1983. *Conditioning and Associative Learning.* Oxford, England: Clarendon Press.

MacLeod, C., E. Rutherford, L. Campbell, G. Ebsworthy, and L. Holker. 2002. Selective Attention and Emotional Vulnerability: Assessing the Causal Basis of Their Association through the Experimental Manipulation of Attentional Bias. *Journal of Abnormal Psychology* 111 (1): 107–123.

Madden, G. J., and W. K. Bickel. 2010. *Impulsivity: The Behavioral and Neurological Science of Discounting.* Washington, D.C.: APA Books.

Mahadevan, S. 1996. Average Reward Reinforcement Learning: Foundations, Algorithms, and Empirical Results. *Machine Learning* 22 (1–3): 159–195.

Maia, T. V. 2009. Reinforcement Learning, Conditioning, and the Brain: Successes and Challenges. *Cognitive, Affective, & Behavioral Neuroscience* 9 (4): 343–364.

Maia, T. V. 2010. Two-Factor Theory, the Actor–Critic Model, and Conditioned Avoidance. *Learning & Behavior* 38 (1): 50–67.

———. 2015. Introduction to the Series on Computational Psychiatry. *Clinical Psychological Science* 3 (3): 374–377.

Maia, T. V., and V. A. Conceição. 2017. The Roles of Phasic and Tonic Dopamine in Tic Learning and Expression. *Biological Psychiatry* 82 (6): 401–412.

———. 2018. Dopaminergic Disturbances in Tourette Syndrome: An Integrative Account. *Biological Psychiatry* 84 (5): 332–344.

Maia, T. V., R. E. Cooney, and B. S. Peterson. 2008. The Neural Bases of Obsessive-Compulsive Disorder in Children and Adults. *Development and Psychopathology* 20 (4): 1251–1283.

Maia, T. V., and M. J. Frank. 2011. From Reinforcement Learning Models to Psychiatric and Neurological Disorders. *Nature Neuroscience* 14 (2): 154–162.

———. 2017. An Integrative Perspective on the Role of Dopamine in Schizophrenia. *Biological Psychiatry* 81 (1): 52–66.

Maier, S. F., and M. E. Seligman. 1976. Learned Helplessness: Theory and Evidence. *Journal of Experimental Psychology: General* 105 (1): 3–46.

Mailman, R., and V. Murthy. 2010. Third Generation Antipsychotic Drugs: Partial Agonism or Receptor Functional Selectivity? *Current Pharmaceutical Design* 16 (5): 488–501.

Maj, M. 2005. "Psychiatric Comorbidity": An Artefact of Current Diagnostic Systems? *British Journal of Psychiatry* 186 (3): 182–184.

Makris, N., J. Biederman, M. C. Monuteaux, and L. J. Seidman. 2009. Towards Conceptualizing a Neural Systems-Based Anatomy of Attention-Deficit/Hyperactivity Disorder. *Developmental Neuroscience* 31 (1–2): 36–49.

Marks, K. R., D. N. Kearns, C. J. Christensen, A. Silberberg, and S. J. Weiss. 2010. Learning That a Cocaine Reward Is Smaller than Expected: A Test of Redish's Computational Model of Addiction. *Behavioural Brain Research* 212 (2): 204–207.

Marr, D. 1982. *Vision: A Computational Investigation into the Human Representation and Processing of Visual Information.* Cambridge, MA: The MIT Press.

Marsh, R., G. M. Alexander, M. G. Packard, H. Zhu, J. C. Wingard, G. Quackenbush, and B. S. Peterson. 2004. Habit Learning in Tourette Syndrome: A Translational Neuroscience Approach to a Developmental Psychopathology. *Archives of General Psychiatry* 61 (12): 1259.

Martino, D., C. Ganos, and Y. Worbe. 2018. Neuroimaging Applications in Tourettes Syndrome. In *International Review of Neurobiology*, 143:65–108. Elsevier.

Mason, L., E. Eldar, and R. B. Rutledge. 2017. Mood Instability and Reward Dysregulation-A Neurocomputational Model of Bipolar Disorder. *JAMA Psychiatry* 74 (12): 1275–1276.

Mathews, A., and C. MacLeod. 2005. Cognitive Vulnerability to Emotional Disorders. *Annual Review of Clinical Psychology* 1 (1): 167–195.

Mathys, C., J. Daunizeau, K. Friston, and K. Stephan. 2011. A Bayesian Foundation for Individual Learning under Uncertainty. *Frontiers in Human Neuroscience* 5: 39.

Mathys, C. D., E. I. Lomakina, J. Daunizeau, S. Iglesias, K. H. Brodersen, K. J. Friston, and K. E. Stephan. 2014. Uncertainty in Perception and the Hierarchical Gaussian Filter. *Frontiers in Human Neuroscience* 8: 825.

Matsumoto, M., and O. Hikosaka. 2007. Lateral Habenula as a Source of Negative Reward Signals in Dopamine Neurons. *Nature* 447 (7148): 1111–1115.

———. 2009. Two Types of Dopamine Neuron Distinctly Convey Positive and Negative Motivational Signals. *Nature* 459 (7248): 837–841.

Mattar, M. G., and N. D. Daw. 2018. Prioritized memory access explains planning and hippocampal replay. *Nature Neuroscience* 21(11): 1609.

Mayberg, H. S. 2014. Neuroimaging and Psychiatry: The Long Road from Bench to Bedside. *Hastings Center Report* 44 (s2): S31–36.

Mayer, J. S., and S. Park. 2012. Working Memory Encoding and False Memory in Schizophrenia and Bipolar Disorder in a Spatial Delayed Response Task. *Journal of Abnormal Psychology* 121 (3): 784–794.

Mazzoni, P., A. Hristova, and J. W. Krakauer. 2007. Why Don't We Move Faster? Parkinson's Disease, Movement Vigor, and Implicit Motivation. *Journal of Neuroscience* 27 (27): 7105–7116.

McClure, S. M., and W. K. Bickel. 2014. A Dual-Systems Perspective on Addiction: Contributions from Neuroimaging and Cognitive Training. *Annals of the New York Academy of Sciences* 1327 (1): 62–78.

McCulloch, W. S., and W. Pitts. 1943. A Logical Calculus of the Ideas Immanent in Nervous Activity. *The Bulletin of Mathematical Biophysics* 5 (4): 115–133.

McCutcheon, James E., S. R. Ebner, A. L. Loriaux, and M. F. Roitman. 2012. Encoding of Aversion by Dopamine and the Nucleus Accumbens. *Frontiers in Neuroscience* 6.

McCutcheon, James Edgar. 2015. The Role of Dopamine in the Pursuit of Nutritional Value. *Physiology & Behavior* 152 (December): 408–415.

McGuire, J. F., J. Piacentini, E. A. Brennan, A. B. Lewin, T. K. Murphy, B. J. Small, and E. A. Storch. 2014. A Meta-Analysis of Behavior Therapy for Tourette Syndrome. *Journal of Psychiatric Research* 50 (March): 106–112.

McNaughton, N., and P. J. Corr. 2004. A Two-Dimensional Neuropsychology of Defense: Fear/ Anxiety and Defensive Distance. *Neuroscience & Biobehavioral Reviews* 28 (3): 285–305.

Meier, M. H., A. Caspi, A. Reichenberg, R. S. E. Keefe, H. L. Fisher, H. Harrington, R. Houts, R. Poulton, and T. E. Moffitt. 2014. Neuropsychological Decline in Schizophrenia From the Premorbid to the Postonset Period: Evidence From a Population-Representative Longitudinal Study. *American Journal of Psychiatry* 171 (1): 91–101.

Mejias, J. F., J. D. Murray, H. Kennedy, and X.-J. Wang. 2016. Feedforward and Feedback Frequency-Dependent Interactions in a Large-Scale Laminar Network of the Primate Cortex. *Science Advances* 2 (11): e1601335.

Meltzer, H. Y., and S. M. Stahl. 1976. The Dopamine Hypothesis of Schizophrenia: A Review. *Schizophrenia Bulletin* 2 (1): 19–76.

Meyer, R. E., and S. M. Mirin. 1979. *The Heroin Stimulus.* New York, NY: Plenum Publishing.

Milne, E., J. Swettenham, P. Hansen, R. Campbell, H. Jeffries, and K. Plaisted. 2002. High Motion Coherence Thresholds in Children with Autism. *Journal of Child Psychology and Psychiatry* 43 (2): 255–263.

Minsky, M., and S. A. Papert. 1969. *Perceptrons: An Introduction to Computational Geometry.* Cambridge, MA: The MIT Press.

Mirenowicz, J., and W. Schultz. 1996. Preferential Activation of Midbrain Dopamine Neurons by Appetitive Rather than Aversive Stimuli. *Nature* 379 (6564): 449–451.

Mkrtchian, A., J. Aylward, P. Dayan, J. P. Roiser, and O. J. Robinson. 2017. Modeling Avoidance in Mood and Anxiety Disorders Using Reinforcement Learning. *Biological Psychiatry* 82 (7): 532–539.

Mobbs, D., P. Petrovic, J. L. Marchant, D. Hassabis, N. Weiskopf, B. Seymour, R. J. Dolan, and C. D. Frith. 2007. When Fear Is Near: Threat Imminence Elicits Prefrontal-Periaqueductal Gray Shifts in Humans. *Science* 317 (5841): 1079–1083.

Mogwitz, S., J. Buse, N. Wolff, and V. Roessner. 2018. Update on the Pharmacological Treatment of Tics with Dopamine-Modulating Agents. *ACS Chemical Neuroscience* 9 (4): 651–672.

Montague, P. R. 2007. Neuroeconomics: A View from Neuroscience. *Functional Neurology* 22 (4): 219.

Montague, P., P. Dayan, and T. Sejnowski. 1996. A Framework for Mesencephalic Dopamine Systems Based on Predictive Hebbian Learning. *The Journal of Neuroscience* 16 (5): 1936–1947.

Montague, P. R., R. J. Dolan, K. J. Friston, and P. Dayan. 2012. Computational Psychiatry. *Trends in Cognitive Sciences* 16 (1): 72–80.

Moran, R., M. Keramati, P. Dayan and R. J. Dolan. 2019. Retrospective model-based inference guides model-free credit assignment, *Nature Communications*, 10(1): 750.

Morand-Beaulieu, S., S. Grot, J. Lavoie, J. B. Leclerc, D. Luck, and M. E. Lavoie. 2017. The Puzzling Question of Inhibitory Control in Tourette Syndrome: A Meta-Analysis. *Neuroscience & Biobehavioral Reviews* 80 (September): 240–262.

Morris, L. S., K. Baek, P. Kundu, N. A. Harrison, M. J. Frank, and V. Voon. 2016. Biases in the Explore-Exploit Tradeoff in Addictions: The Role of Avoidance of Uncertainty. *Neuropsychopharmacology: Official Publication of the American College of Neuropsychopharmacology* 41 (4): 940–948.

Morris, S. E., and B. N. Cuthbert. 2012. Research Domain Criteria: Cognitive Systems, Neural Circuits, and Dimensions of Behavior. *Dialogues in Clinical Neuroscience* 14 (1): 29–37.

Moutoussis, M., R. P. Bentall, W. El-Deredy, and P. Dayan. 2011. Bayesian Modelling of Jumping-to-Conclusions Bias in Delusional Patients. *Cognitive Neuropsychiatry* 16 (5): 422–447.

Moutoussis, M., R. P. Bentall, J. Williams, and P. Dayan. 2008. A Temporal Difference Account of Avoidance Learning. *Network: Computation in Neural Systems* 19 (2): 137–160.

Moutoussis, M., N. Shahar, T. U. Hauser, and R. J. Dolan. 2018. Computation in Psychotherapy, or How Computational Psychiatry Can Aid Learning-Based Psychological Therapies. *Computational Psychiatry* 2 (February): 50–73.

Mowrer, O. 1947. On the Dual Nature of Learning—a Re-interpretation of "Conditioning" and "Problem-Solving." *Harvard Educational Review* 17 (2): 102–150.

Mrazek, D. A., J. C. Hornberger, C. A. Altar, and I. Degtiar. 2014. A Review of the Clinical, Economic, and Societal Burden of Treatment-Resistant Depression: 1996–2013. *Psychiatric Services* 65 (8): 977–987.

Murray, J. D., A. Anticevic, M. Gancsos, M. Ichinose, P. R. Corlett, J. H. Krystal, and X.-J. Wang. 2014. Linking Microcircuit Dysfunction to Cognitive Impairment: Effects of Disinhibition Associated with Schizophrenia in a Cortical Working Memory Model. *Cerebral Cortex* 24 (4): 859–872.

Murray, John D., J. Jaramillo, and X.-J. Wang. 2017. Working Memory and Decision-Making in a Frontoparietal Circuit Model. *The Journal of Neuroscience* 37 (50): 12167–12186.

Murschall, A., and W. Hauber. 2006. Inactivation of the Ventral Tegmental Area Abolished the General Excitatory Influence of Pavlovian Cues on Instrumental Performance. *Learning & Memory* 13 (2): 123–126.

Myerson, J., and L. Green. 1995. Discounting of Delayed Rewards: Models of Individual Choice. *Journal of the Experimental Analysis of Behavior* 64 (3): 263–276.

Nagel, R. 1995. Unraveling in Guessing Games: An Experimental Study. *The American Economic Review* 85 (5): 1313–1326.

Nakamura, K., and T. Ono. 1986. Lateral Hypothalamus Neuron Involvement in Integration of Natural and Artificial Rewards and Cue Signals. *Journal of Neurophysiology* 55 (1): 163–181.

Naqvi, N. H., and A. Bechara. 2010. The Insula and Drug Addiction: An Interoceptive View of Pleasure, Urges, and Decision-Making. *Brain Structure and Function* 214 (5–6): 435–450.

Nassar, M. R., K. M. Rumsey, R. C. Wilson, K. Parikh, B. Heasly, and J. I. Gold. 2012. Rational Regulation of Learning Dynamics by Pupil-Linked Arousal Systems. *Nature Neuroscience* 15 (7): 1040–1046.

Navratilova, E., and F. Porreca. 2014. Reward and Motivation in Pain and Pain Relief. *Nature Neuroscience* 17 (10): 1304–1312.

Nee, D. E., and J. W. Brown. 2013. Dissociable Frontal–Striatal and Frontal–Parietal Networks Involved in Updating Hierarchical Contexts in Working Memory. *Cerebral Cortex* 23 (9): 2146–2158.

Nee, D. E., and M. D'Esposito. 2016. The Hierarchical Organization of the Lateral Prefrontal Cortex. *ELife* 5 (March).

Nespoli, E., F. Rizzo, T. Boeckers, U. Schulze, and B. Hengerer. 2018. Altered Dopaminergic Regulation of the Dorsal Striatum Is Able to Induce Tic-like Movements in Juvenile Rats. Edited by Joohyung Lee. *PLOS ONE* 13 (4): e0196515.

Neumann, W., A. Horn, S. Ewert, J. Huebl, C. Brücke, C. Slentz, G. Schneider, and A. A. Kühn. 2017. A Localized Pallidal Physiomarker in Cervical Dystonia. *Annals of Neurology* 82 (6): 912–924.

Neumann, W.-J., J. Huebl, C. Brücke, R. Lofredi, A. Horn, A. Saryyeva, K. Müller-Vahl, J. K. Krauss, and A. A. Kühn. 2018. Pallidal and Thalamic Neural Oscillatory Patterns in Tourettes Syndrome: Pallido-Thalamic Activity in Tourettes Syndrome. *Annals of Neurology* 84 (4): 505–514.

Neuner, I., F. Schneider, and N. J. Shah. 2013. Functional Neuroanatomy of Tics. In *International Review of Neurobiology*, 112:35–71. Elsevier.

Newell, A., and H. A. Simon. 1961. Computer Simulation of Human Thinking: A Theory of Problem Solving Expressed as a Computer Program Permits Simulation of Thinking Processes. *Science* 134 (3495): 2011–2017.

Newell, Allen, and H. A. Simon. 1972. *Human Problem Solving*. Englewood Cliffs, NJ: Prentice-Hall.

Ng, A. Y., D. Harada, and S. Russell. 1999. Policy Invariance under Reward Transformations: Theory and Application to Reward Shaping. In *Proceedings of the Sixteenth International Conference on Machine Learning*, edited by I. Bratko and S. Dzeroski, 99:278–287. San Francisco, CA: Morgan Kaufmann.

Nitschke, J. B., I. Sarinopoulos, K. L. Mackiewicz, H. S. Schaefer, and R. J. Davidson. 2006. Functional Neuroanatomy of Aversion and Its Anticipation. *NeuroImage* 29 (1): 106–116.

Niv, Y., N. D. Daw, D. Joel, and P. Dayan. 2007. Tonic Dopamine: Opportunity Costs and the Control of Response Vigor. *Psychopharmacology* 191 (3): 507–520.

Niv, Y., M. O. Duff, and P. Dayan. 2005. Dopamine, Uncertainty and T. D. Learning. *Behavioral and Brain Functions* 1 (1): 6.

Niv, Y., D. Joel, and P. Dayan. 2006. A Normative Perspective on Motivation. *Trends in Cognitive Sciences* 10 (8): 375–381.

Niyogi, R. K., Y.-A. Breton, R. B. Solomon, K. Conover, P. Shizgal, and P. Dayan. 2014. Optimal Indolence: A Normative Microscopic Approach to Work and Leisure. *Journal of The Royal Society, Interface* 11 (91): 20130969.

Niyogi, R. K., P. Shizgal, and P. Dayan. 2014. Some Work and Some Play: Microscopic and Macroscopic Approaches to Labor and Leisure. *PLoS Computational Biology* 10 (12): e1003894.

Norman, D. A., and T. Shallice. 1986. Attention to Action: Willed and Automatic Control of Behavior. In *Consciousness and Self-Regulation: Advances in Research and Theory*, edited by R. J. Davidson, G. E. Schwartz, and D. Shapiro, 1–18. New York, NY: Plenum Publishing.

Norman, L. J., C. Carlisi, S. Lukito, H. Hart, D. Mataix-Cols, J. Radua, and K. Rubia. 2016. Structural and Functional Brain Abnormalities in Attention-Deficit/Hyperactivity Disorder and Obsessive-Compulsive Disorder: A Comparative Meta-Analysis. *JAMA Psychiatry* 73 (8): 815.

Nour, M. M., T. Dahoun, P. Schwartenbeck, R. A. Adams, T. H. B. FitzGerald, C. Coello, M. B. Wall, R. J. Dolan, and O. D. Howes. 2018. Dopaminergic Basis for Signaling Belief Updates, but Not Surprise, and the Link to Paranoia. *Proceedings of the National Academy of Sciences* 115 (43): E10167–E10176.

O'Connell, R. G., M. N. Shadlen, K. Wong-Lin, and S. P. Kelly. 2018. Bridging Neural and Computational Viewpoints on Perceptual Decision-Making. *Trends in Neurosciences* 41 (11): 838–852.

O'Doherty, J., P. Dayan, J. Schultz, R. Deichman, K. J. Friston, and R. J. Dolan. 2004. Dissociable Roles of Ventral and Dorsal Striatum in Instrumental Conditioning. *Science* 304 (5669): 452–454.

O'Donnell, P. 2012. Cortical Disinhibition in the Neonatal Ventral Hippocampal Lesion Model of Schizophrenia: New Vistas on Possible Therapeutic Approaches. *Pharmacology & Therapeutics* 133 (1): 19–25.

O'Keefe, J., and L. Nadel. 1978. *The Hippocampus as a Cognitive Map*. Oxford, England: Clarendon Press.

Olds, J., and P. Milner. 1954. Positive Reinforcement Produced by Electrical Stimulation of Septal Area and Other Regions of Rat Brain. *Journal of Comparative and Physiological Psychology* 47 (6): 419–427.

Olshausen, B. A., and D. J. Field. 1997. Sparse Coding with an Overcomplete Basis Set: A Strategy Employed by V1? *Vision Research* 37 (23): 3311–3325.

O'Neill, E. 1956. *Long Day's Journey into Night*. London, England: Jonathan Cape.

O'Reilly, R. C. 2006. Biologically Based Computational Models of High-Level Cognition. *Science* 314 (5796): 91–94.

O'Reilly, R. C., T. S. Braver, and J. D. Cohen. 1999. A Biologically Based Computational Model of Working Memory. In *Models of Working Memory: Mechanisms of Active Maintenance and Executive Control*, edited by A. Miyake and P. Shah, 375–411. Cambridge, England: Cambridge University Press.

O'Reilly, R. C., and M. J. Frank. 2006. Making Working Memory Work: A Computational Model of Learning in the Prefrontal Cortex and Basal Ganglia. *Neural Computation* 18 (2): 283–328.

O'Reilly, R. C., M. J. Frank, T. E. Hazy, and B. Watz. 2007. PVLV: The Primary Value and Learned Value Pavlovian Learning Algorithm. *Behavioral Neuroscience* 121 (1): 31–49.

O'Reilly, R. C., S. A. Herd, and W. M. Pauli. 2010. Computational Models of Cognitive Control. *Current Opinion in Neurobiology* 20 (2): 257–261.

O'Reilly, R. C., and Y. Munakata. 2000. *Computational Explorations in Cognitive Neuroscience*. Cambridge, MA: The MIT Press.

Oudeyer, P.-Y., F. Kaplan, and V. V. Hafner. 2007. Intrinsic Motivation Systems for Autonomous Mental Development. *IEEE Transactions on Evolutionary Computation* 11 (2): 265–286.

Palmer, C. J., R. P. Lawson, and J. Hohwy. 2017. Bayesian Approaches to Autism: Towards Volatility, Action, and Behavior. *Psychological Bulletin* 143 (5): 521–542.

Palminteri, S., and M. Pessiglione. 2017. Opponent Brain Systems for Reward and Punishment Learning. In *Decision Neuroscience*, 291–303. Elsevier.

Palminteri, S., D. Justo, C. Jauffret, B. Pavlicek, A. Dauta, C. Delmaire, V. Czernecki, et al. 2012. Critical Roles for Anterior Insula and Dorsal Striatum in Punishment-Based Avoidance Learning. *Neuron* 76 (5): 998–1009.

Palminteri, S., M. Lebreton, Y. Worbe, D. Grabli, A. Hartmann, and M. Pessiglione. 2009. Pharmacological Modulation of Subliminal Learning in Parkinson's and Tourette's Syndromes. *Proceedings of the National Academy of Sciences* 106 (45): 19179–19184.

Palminteri, S., M. Lebreton, Y. Worbe, A. Hartmann, S. Lehéricy, M. Vidailhet, D. Grabli, and M. Pessiglione. 2011. Dopamine-Dependent Reinforcement of Motor Skill Learning: Evidence from Gilles de La Tourette Syndrome. *Brain* 134 (8): 2287–2301.

Panlilio, L. V., E. B. Thorndike, and C. W. Schindler. 2007. Blocking of Conditioning to a Cocaine-Paired Stimulus: Testing the Hypothesis That Cocaine Perpetually Produces a Signal of Larger-than-Expected Reward. *Pharmacology, Biochemistry, and Behavior* 86 (4): 774–777.

Parke, J., and M. Griffiths. 2004. Gambling Addiction and the Evolution of the "Near Miss." *Addiction Research and Theory* 12 (5): 407–411.

Patzelt, E. H., C. A. Hartley, and S. J. Gershman. 2018. Computational Phenotyping: Using Models to Understand Individual Differences in Personality, Development, and Mental Illness. *Personality Neuroscience* 1.

Paulus, M. P., Q. J. M. Huys, and T. V. Maia. 2016. A Roadmap for the Development of Applied Computational Psychiatry. *Biological Psychiatry: Cognitive Neuroscience and Neuroimaging* 1 (5): 386–392.

Pe, M. L., J. Vandekerckhove, and P. Kuppens. 2013. A Diffusion Model Account of the Relationship between the Emotional Flanker Task and Rumination and Depression. *Emotion* 13 (4): 739–747.

Pearce, J. M., and G. Hall. 1980. A Model for Pavlovian Learning: Variations in the Effectiveness of Conditioned but Not of Unconditioned Stimuli. *Psychological Review* 87 (6): 532–552.

Pechtel, P., S. J. Dutra, E. L. Goetz, and D. A. Pizzagalli. 2013. Blunted Reward Responsiveness in Remitted Depression. *Journal of Psychiatric Research* 47 (12): 1864–1869.

Pedersen, M. L., M. J. Frank, and G. Biele. 2017. The Drift Diffusion Model as the Choice Rule in Reinforcement Learning. *Psychonomic Bulletin & Review* 24 (4): 1234–1251.

Pellicano, E., and D. Burr. 2012. When the World Becomes Too Real: A Bayesian Explanation of Autistic Perception. *Trends in Cognitive Sciences* 16 (10): 504–510.

Perepletchikova, F., T. A. Treat, and A. E. Kazdin. 2007. Treatment Integrity in Psychotherapy Research: Analysis of the Studies and Examination of the Associated Factors. *Journal of Consulting and Clinical Psychology* 75 (6): 829–841.

Perry, A. N., C. Westenbroek, and J. B. Becker. 2013. The Development of a Preference for Cocaine over Food Identifies Individual Rats with Addiction-Like Behaviors. *PLoS ONE* 8 (11): e79465.

Peters, E., and P. Garety. 2006. Cognitive Functioning in Delusions: A Longitudinal Analysis. *Behaviour Research and Therapy* 44 (4): 481–514.

Peters, J., and C. Büchel. 2010. Episodic Future Thinking Reduces Reward Delay Discounting through an Enhancement of Prefrontal-Mediotemporal Interactions. *Neuron* 66 (1): 138–148.

Petrides, M. 2005. Lateral Prefrontal Cortex: Architectonic and Functional Organization. *Philosophical Transactions of the Royal Society B: Biological Sciences* 360 (1456): 781–795.

Petry, N. M. 2012. *Contingency Management for Substance Abuse Treatment*. New York, NY: Routledge.

Pezzulo, G., F. Rigoli, and F. Chersi. 2013. The Mixed Instrumental Controller: Using Value of Information to Combine Habitual Choice and Mental Simulation. *Frontiers in Psychology* 4: 92.

Piray, P., M. M. Keramati, A. Dezfouli, C. Lucas, and A. Mokri. 2010. Individual Differences in Nucleus Accumbens Dopamine Receptors Predict Development of Addiction-Like Behavior: A Computational Approach. *Neural Computation* 22 (9): 2334–2368.

Pizzagalli, D. A. 2014. Depression, Stress, and Anhedonia: Toward a Synthesis and Integrated Model. *Annual Review of Clinical Psychology* 10 (1): 393–423.

Pizzagalli, D. A., A. E. Evins, E. C. Schetter, M. J. Frank, P. E. Pajtas, D. L. Santesso, and M. Culhane. 2008a. Single Dose of a Dopamine Agonist Impairs Reinforcement Learning in Humans: Behavioral Evidence from a Laboratory-Based Measure of Reward Responsiveness. *Psychopharmacology* 196 (2): 221–232.

Pizzagalli, D. A., E. Goetz, M. Ostacher, D. V. Iosifescu, and R. H. Perlis. 2008b. Euthymic Patients with Bipolar Disorder Show Decreased Reward Learning in a Probabilistic Reward Task. *Biological Psychiatry* 64 (2): 162–168.

Pizzagalli, D. A., D. Iosifescu, L. A. Hallett, K. G. Ratner, and M. Fava. 2008c. Reduced Hedonic Capacity in Major Depressive Disorder: Evidence from a Probabilistic Reward Task. *Journal of Psychiatric Research* 43 (1): 76–87.

Pizzagalli, D. A., A. L. Jahn, and J. P. O'Shea. 2005. Toward an Objective Characterization of an Anhedonic Phenotype: A Signal-Detection Approach. *Biological Psychiatry* 57 (4): 319–327.

Pogorelov, V., M. Xu, H. R. Smith, G. F. Buchanan, and C. Pittenger. 2015. Corticostriatal Interactions in the Generation of Tic-like Behaviors after Local Striatal Disinhibition. *Experimental Neurology* 265 (March): 122–128.

Poldrack, R. A. 2007. Region of Interest Analysis for FMRI. *Social Cognitive and Affective Neuroscience* 2 (1): 67–70.

Polyn, S. M., K. A. Norman, and M. J. Kahana. 2009. A Context Maintenance and Retrieval Model of Organizational Processes in Free Recall. *Psychological Review* 116 (1): 129–156.

Posner, M. I., and C. R. Snyder. 1975. Attention and Cognitive Control. In *Information Processing and Cognition: The Loyola Symposium*, edited by R. L. Solso, 55–85. Hillsdale, NJ: Lawrence Erlbaum Associates Inc.

Postuma, R. B., and A. Dagher. 2006. Basal Ganglia Functional Connectivity Based on a Meta-Analysis of 126 Positron Emission Tomography and Functional Magnetic Resonance Imaging Publications. *Cerebral Cortex* 16 (10): 1508–1521.

Powers, A. R., C. Mathys, and P. R. Corlett. 2017. Pavlovian Conditioning–Induced Hallucinations Result from Overweighting of Perceptual Priors. *Science* 357 (6351): 596–600.

Powers, M. B., J. M. Halpern, M. P. Ferenschak, S. J. Gillihan, and E. B. Foa. 2010. A Meta-Analytic Review of Prolonged Exposure for Posttraumatic Stress Disorder. *Clinical Psychology Review* 30 (6): 635–641.

Preskorn, S. H. 2010a. CNS Drug Development: Part II: Advances from the 1960s to the 1990s. *Journal of Psychiatric Practice®* 16 (6): 413–415.

———. 2010b. CNS Drug Development: Part I: The Early Period of CNS Drugs. *Journal of Psychiatric Practice* 16 (5): 334–339.

Price, A. L. 2009. Distinguishing the Contributions of Implicit and Explicit Processes to Performance of the Weather Prediction Task. *Memory & Cognition* 37 (2): 210–222.

Pulcu, E., and M. Browning. 2017. Correction: Affective Bias as a Rational Response to the Statistics of Rewards and Punishments. *ELife* 6 (October): e27879.

———. 2019. The Misestimation of Uncertainty in Affective Disorders. *Trends in Cognitive Sciences* 23 (10): 865–875.

Puterman, M. L. 2005. *Markov Decision Processes: Discrete Stochastic Dynamic Programming*. Hoboken, NJ: John Wiley & Sons, Inc.

Qi, Z., G. Miller, and E. Voit. 2010. Computational Modeling of Synaptic Neurotransmission as a Tool for Assessing Dopamine Hypotheses of Schizophrenia. *Pharmacopsychiatry* 43 (S 01): S50–60.

Quadt, L., H. D. Critchley, and S. N. Garfinkel. 2018. The Neurobiology of Interoception in Health and Disease: Neuroscience of Interoception. *Annals of the New York Academy of Sciences* 1428 (1): 112–128.

Rabin, M., and R. H. Thaler. 2001. Anomalies: Risk Aversion. *Journal of Economic Perspectives* 15 (1): 219–232.

Raby, C. R., D. M. Alexis, A. Dickinson, and N. S. Clayton. 2007. Planning for the Future by Western Scrub-Jays. *Nature* 445 (7130): 919–921.

Radua, J., A. Schmidt, S. Borgwardt, A. Heinz, F. Schlagenhauf, P. McGuire, and P. Fusar-Poli. 2015. Ventral Striatal Activation During Reward Processing in Psychosis. *JAMA Psychiatry* 72 (12): 1243.

Rae, C. L., D. E. O. Larsson, S. N. Garfinkel, and H. D. Critchley. 2019. Dimensions of Interoception Predict Premonitory Urges and Tic Severity in Tourette Syndrome. *PsyArXiv*, June.

Rae, C. L., L. Polyanska, C. D. Gould van Praag, J. Parkinson, S. Bouyagoub, Y. Nagai, A. K. Seth, N. A. Harrison, S. N. Garfinkel, and H. D. Critchley. 2018. Face Perception Enhances Insula and Motor Network Reactivity in Tourette Syndrome. *Brain* 141 (11): 3249–3261.

Raines, J. M., K. R. Edwards, M. F. Sherman, C. I. Higginson, J. B. Winnick, K. Navin, J. M. Gettings, F. Conteh, S. M. Bennett, and M. W. Specht. 2018. Premonitory Urge for Tics Scale (PUTS): Replication and Extension of Psychometric Properties in Youth with Chronic Tic Disorders (CTDs). *Journal of Neural Transmission* 125 (4): 727–734.

Rall, W., J. M. Brookhart, V. B. Mountcastle, E. R. Kandel, S. R. Geiger, and American Physiological Society. 1977. Core Conductor Theory and Cable Properties of Neurons. In *The Nervous System, Vol. 1, Cellular Biology of Neurons*, 39–97. Bethesda, MD: American Physiological Society.

Rangel, A., C. Camerer, and P. R. Montague. 2008. A Framework for Studying the Neurobiology of Value-Based Decision Making. *Nature Reviews Neuroscience* 9 (7): 545–556.

Rao, R. P. N., and D. H. Ballard. 1999. Predictive Coding in the Visual Cortex: A Functional Interpretation of Some Extra-Classical Receptive-Field Effects. *Nature Neuroscience* 2 (1): 79–87.

Rao, S. G., G. V. Williams, and P. S. Goldman-Rakic. 2000. Destruction and Creation of Spatial Tuning by Disinhibition: GABA(A) Blockade of Prefrontal Cortical Neurons Engaged by Working Memory. *The Journal of Neuroscience* 20 (1): 485–494.

Ratcliff, R. 1978. A Theory of Memory Retrieval. *Psychological Review* 85 (2): 59–108.

Ratcliff, R., P. L. Smith, S. D. Brown, and G. McKoon. 2016. Diffusion Decision Model: Current Issues and History. *Trends in Cognitive Sciences* 20 (4): 260–281.

Ratcliff, R., and F. Tuerlinckx. 2002. Estimating Parameters of the Diffusion Model: Approaches to Dealing with Contaminant Reaction Times and Parameter Variability. *Psychonomic Bulletin & Review* 9 (3): 438–481.

Rawson, P. 2005. *A Handbook of Short-Term Psychodynamic Psychotherapy*. London, England: Karnac Books.

Raymond, J. G., J. D. Steele, and P. Seriès. 2017. Modeling Trait Anxiety: From Computational Processes to Personality. *Frontiers in Psychiatry* 8 (1).

Redish, A. D. 2004. Addiction as a Computational Process Gone Awry. *Science* 306 (5703): 1944–1947.

Redish, A. D. 2013. *The Mind within the Brain: How We Make Decisions and How Those Decisions Go Wrong*. Oxford, England: Oxford University Press.

———. 2016. Vicarious Trial and Error. *Nature Reviews Neuroscience* 17 (3): 147–159.

Redish, A. D., and J. A. Gordon. 2016. *Computational Psychiatry: New Perspectives on Mental Illness*. Cambridge, MA: The MIT Press.

Redish, A. D., S. Jensen, and A. Johnson. 2008. A Unified Framework for Addiction: Vulnerabilities in the Decision Process: And Discussion. *Behavioral and Brain Sciences* 31 (4): 415–487.

Redish, A. D., S. Jensen, A. Johnson, and Z. Kurth-Nelson. 2007. Reconciling Reinforcement Learning Models with Behavioral Extinction and Renewal: Implications for Addiction, Relapse, and Problem Gambling. *Psychological Review* 114 (3): 784–805.

Redish, A. D., and A. Johnson. 2007. A Computational Model of Craving and Obsession. *Annals of the New York Academy of Sciences* 1104 (1): 324–339.

Regier, P. S., and A. D. Redish. 2015. Contingency Management and Deliberative Decision-Making Processes. *Frontiers in Psychiatry* 6 (June): 0076.

Rescorla, R. A., and R. L. Solomon. 1967. Two-Process Learning Theory: Relationships between Pavlovian Conditioning and Instrumental Learning. *Psychological Review* 74 (3): 151–182.

Rescorla, R. A., and A. R. Wagner. 1972. A Theory of Pavlovian Conditioning: Variations in the Effectiveness of Reinforcement and Nonreinforcement. In *Classical Conditioning II:*

Current Research and Theory, edited by A. H. Black and W. F. Prokasy, 2:64–99. New York, NY: Appleton-Century-Crofts.

Reynolds, J. R., and R. C. O'Reilly. 2009. Developing PFC Representations Using Reinforcement Learning. *Cognition* 113 (3): 281–292.

Reynolds, J. R., R. C. O'Reilly, J. D. Cohen, and T. S. Braver. 2012. The Function and Organization of Lateral Prefrontal Cortex: A Test of Competing Hypotheses. *PLoS ONE* 7 (2): e30284.

Reynolds, S. M., and K. C. Berridge. 2001. Fear and Feeding in the Nucleus Accumbens Shell: Rostrocaudal Segregation of GABA-Elicited Defensive Behavior versus Eating Behavior. *The Journal of Neuroscience* 21 (9): 3261–3270.

———. 2002. Positive and Negative Motivation in Nucleus Accumbens Shell: Bivalent Rostrocaudal Gradients for GABA-Elicited Eating, Taste "Liking"/"Disliking" Reactions, Place Preference/Avoidance, and Fear. *The Journal of Neuroscience* 22 (16): 7308–7320.

———. 2008. Emotional Environments Retune the Valence of Appetitive versus Fearful Functions in Nucleus Accumbens. *Nature Neuroscience* 11 (4): 423–425.

Rick, S., and G. Loewenstein. 2008. Intangibility in Intertemporal Choice. *Philosophical Transactions of the Royal Society B: Biological Sciences* 363 (1511): 3813–3824.

Ridderinkhof, K. R., M. Ullsperger, E. A. Crone, and S. Nieuwenhuis. 2004. The Role of the Medial Frontal Cortex in Cognitive Control. *Science* 306 (5695): 443–447.

Rizzo, R., A. Pellico, P. R. Silvestri, F. Chiarotti, and F. Cardona. 2018. A Randomized Controlled Trial Comparing Behavioral, Educational, and Pharmacological Treatments in Youths With Chronic Tic Disorder or Tourette Syndrome. *Frontiers in Psychiatry* 9 (March): 100.

Rizzolatti, G., and J. F. Kalaska. 2013. Voluntary Movement: The Parietal and Premotor Cortex. In *Principles of Neural Science*, edited by E. R. Kandel, T. Schwartz, T. Jessell, S. Siegelbaum, and A. J. Hudspeth, 5th ed. Vol. 865–893. New York, NY: McGraw-Hill Professional.

Rizzolatti, G., and P. L. Strick. 2013. Cognitive Functions of the Premotor Systems. In *Principles of Neural Science*, edited by E. R. Kandel, T. Schwartz, T. Jessell, S. Siegelbaum, and A. J. Hudspeth, 5th ed. Vol. 412–425. New York, NY: McGraw-Hill Professional.

Robertson, M. M., V. Eapen, H. S. Singer, D. Martino, J. M. Scharf, P. Paschou, V. Roessner, et al. 2017. Gilles de La Tourette Syndrome. *Nature Reviews Disease Primers* 3 (1): 16097.

Robins, E., and S. B. Guze. 1970. Establishment of Diagnostic Validity in Psychiatric Illness: Its Application to Schizophrenia. *American Journal of Psychiatry* 126 (7): 983–987.

Robinson, M. J. F., and K. C. Berridge. 2013. Instant Transformation of Learned Repulsion into Motivational "Wanting." *Current Biology* 23 (4): 282–289.

Robinson, T. E., and K. C. Berridge. 2003. Addiction. *Annual Review of Psychology* 54 (1): 25–53.

Robinson, T. E., and S. B. Flagel. 2009. Dissociating the Predictive and Incentive Motivational Properties of Reward-Related Cues through the Study of Individual Differences. *Biological Psychiatry* 65 (10): 869–873.

Rock, P. L., J. P. Roiser, W. J. Riedel, and A. D. Blackwell. 2014. Cognitive Impairment in Depression: A Systematic Review and Meta-Analysis. *Psychological Medicine* 44 (10): 2029–2040.

Roe, R. M., J. R. Busemeyer, and J. T. Townsend. 2001. Multialternative Decision Field Theory: A Dynamic Connectionist Model of Decision Making. *Psychological Review* 108 (2): 370–392.

Roesch, M. R., D. J. Calu, and G. Schoenbaum. 2007. Dopamine Neurons Encode the Better Option in Rats Deciding between Differently Delayed or Sized Rewards. *Nature Neuroscience* 10 (12): 1615–1624.

Rogers, T. T., and J. L. McClelland. 2004. *Semantic Cognition: A Parallel Distributed Processing Approach*. Cambridge, MA: The MIT Press.

Roiser, J. P, R. Elliott, and B. J. Sahakian. 2012. Cognitive Mechanisms of Treatment in Depression. *Neuropsychopharmacology* 37 (1): 117–136.

Roiser, J. P., O. D. Howes, C. A. Chaddock, E. M. Joyce, and P. McGuire. 2013. Neural and Behavioral Correlates of Aberrant Salience in Individuals at Risk for Psychosis. *Schizophrenia Bulletin* 39 (6): 1328–1336.

Roiser, J. P., K. E. Stephan, H. E. M. den Ouden, T. R. E. Barnes, K. J. Friston, and E. M. Joyce. 2009. Do Patients with Schizophrenia Exhibit Aberrant Salience? *Psychological Medicine* 39 (2): 199–209.

Roitman, J. D., and M. N. Shadlen. 2002. Response of Neurons in the Lateral Intraparietal Area during a Combined Visual Discrimination Reaction Time Task. *The Journal of Neuroscience* 22 (21): 9475–9489.

Roitman, M. F., R. A. Wheeler, R. M. Wightman, and R. M. Carelli. 2008. Real-Time Chemical Responses in the Nucleus Accumbens Differentiate Rewarding and Aversive Stimuli. *Nature Neuroscience* 11 (12): 1376–1377.

Rolls, E. T., and G. Deco. 2011. A Computational Neuroscience Approach to Schizophrenia and Its Onset. *Neuroscience & Biobehavioral Reviews* 35 (8): 1644–1653.

Rolls, E. T., and F. Grabenhorst. 2008. The Orbitofrontal Cortex and Beyond: From Affect to Decision-Making. *Progress in Neurobiology* 86 (3): 216–244.

Rolls, E. T., M. Loh, G. Deco, and G. Winterer. 2008. Computational Models of Schizophrenia and Dopamine Modulation in the Prefrontal Cortex. *Nature Reviews Neuroscience* 9 (9): 696–709.

Rosenberg, A., J. S. Patterson, and D. E. Angelaki. 2015. A Computational Perspective on Autism. *Proceedings of the National Academy of Sciences of the United States of America* 112 (30): 9158–9165.

Rosenblatt, F. 1958. The Perceptron: A Probabilistic Model for Information Storage and Organization in the Brain. *Psychological Review* 65 (6): 386–408.

Rotaru, D. C., H. Yoshino, D. A. Lewis, G. B. Ermentrout, and G. Gonzalez-Burgos. 2011. Glutamate Receptor Subtypes Mediating Synaptic Activation of Prefrontal Cortex Neurons: Relevance for Schizophrenia. *Journal of Neuroscience* 31 (1): 142–156.

Roth, A. E. 2002. The Economist as Engineer: Game Theory, Experimentation, and Computation as Tools for Design Economics. *Econometrica* 70 (4): 1341–1378.

Rothenhoefer, K. M., V. D. Costa, R. Bartolo, R. Vicario-Feliciano, E. A. Murray, and B. B. Averbeck. 2017. Effects of Ventral Striatum Lesions on Stimulus-Based versus Action-Based Reinforcement Learning. *The Journal of Neuroscience* 37 (29): 6902–6914.

Rothwell, P. E., J. C. Gewirtz, and M. J. Thomas. 2010. Episodic Withdrawal Promotes Psychomotor Sensitization to Morphine. *Neuropsychopharmacology* 35 (13): 2579–2589.

Rubinov, M., and E. Bullmore. 2013. Fledgling Pathoconnectomics of Psychiatric Disorders. *Trends in Cognitive Sciences* 17 (12): 641–647.

Rumelhart, D. E., G. E. Hinton, and R. J. Williams. 1986. Learning Representations by Back-Propagating Errors. *Nature* 323 (6088): 533–536.

Rumelhart, D. E., J. L. McClelland, and PDP Group. 1987. *Parallel Distributed Processing: Explorations in the Microstructure of Cognition, Volume 1, Foundations.* Cambridge, MA: The MIT Press.

Rumelhart, D. E., P. Smolensky, J. L. McClelland, and G. E. Hinton. 1986. Schemata and Sequential Thought Processes in PDP Models. In *Parallel Distributed Processing: Explorations in the Microstructure, Vol. 2: Psychological and Biological Models,* edited by D. E. Rumelhart and J. L. McClelland. Cambridge, MA: The MIT Press.

Rupprechter, S., A. Stankevicius, Q. J. M. Huys, J. D. Steele, and P. Seriès. 2018. Major Depression Impairs the Use of Reward Values for Decision-Making. *Scientific Reports* 8 (1): 1–8.

Russell, J. A., and L. F. Barrett. 1999. Core Affect, Prototypical Emotional Episodes, and Other Things Called Emotion: Dissecting the Elephant. *Journal of Personality and Social Psychology* 76 (5): 805–819.

Rutledge, R. B., A. M. Chekroud, and Q. J. Huys. 2019. Machine Learning and Big Data in Psychiatry: Toward Clinical Applications. *Current Opinion in Neurobiology* 55 (April): 152–159.

Sackett, D. A., M. P. Saddoris, and R. M. Carelli. 2017. Nucleus Accumbens Shell Dopamine Preferentially Tracks Information Related to Outcome Value of Reward. *Eneuro* 4 (3): eNEURO.0058-17.2017.

Salamone, J. D., M. Pardo, S. E. Yohn, L. López-Cruz, N. San Miguel, and M. Correa. 2016. Mesolimbic Dopamine and the Regulation of Motivated Behavior. In *Behavioral Neuroscience of Motivation,* edited by E. H. Simpson and P. D. Balsam, 231–257. Current Topics in Behavioral Neurosciences 27. Berlin, Germany: Springer.

Salvador, A., Y. Worbe, C. Delorme, G. Coricelli, R. Gaillard, T. W. Robbins, A. Hartmann, and S. Palminteri. 2017. Specific Effect of a Dopamine Partial Agonist on Counterfactual Learning: Evidence from Gilles de La Tourette Syndrome. *Scientific Reports* 7 (1): 6292.

Sambrani, T., E. Jakubovski, and K. R. Müller-Vahl. 2016. New Insights into Clinical Characteristics of Gilles de La Tourette Syndrome: Findings in 1032 Patients from a Single German Center. *Frontiers in Neuroscience* 10 (September).

Samejima, K. 2005. Representation of Action-Specific Reward Values in the Striatum. *Science* 310 (5752): 1337–1340.

Samuel, A. L. 1959. Some Studies in Machine Learning Using the Game of Checkers. *IBM Journal of Research and Development* 3 (3): 210–229.

Samuelson, P. A. 1938. A Note on the Pure Theory of Consumers Behaviour. *Economica* 5 (17): 61–71.

Samuelson, Paul A. 1937. Some Aspects of the Pure Theory of Capital. *The Quarterly Journal of Economics* 51 (3): 469–496.

———. 1948. Consumption Theory in Terms of Revealed Preference. *Economica* 15 (60): 243–253.

Sanislow, C. A., M. Ferrante, J. Pacheco, M. V. Rudorfer, and S. E. Morris. 2019. Advancing Translational Research Using NIMH Research Domain Criteria and Computational Methods. *Neuron* 101 (5): 779–782.

Sanislow, C. A., D. S. Pine, K. J. Quinn, M. J. Kozak, M. A. Garvey, R. K. Heinssen, P. S.-E. Wang, and B. N. Cuthbert. 2010. Developing Constructs for Psychopathology Research: Research Domain Criteria. *Journal of Abnormal Psychology* 119 (4): 631–639.

Schacter, D. L., D. R. Addis, D. Hassabis, V. C. Martin, R. N. Spreng, and K. K. Szpunar. 2012. The Future of Memory: Remembering, Imagining, and the Brain. *Neuron* 76 (4): 677–694.

Schall, J. D. 2004. On Building a Bridge between Brain and Behavior. *Annual Review of Psychology* 55 (1): 23–50.

Schlagenhauf, F., Q. J. M. Huys, L. Deserno, M. A. Rapp, A. Beck, H.-J. Heinze, R. Dolan, and A. Heinz. 2014. Striatal Dysfunction during Reversal Learning in Unmedicated Schizophrenia Patients. *NeuroImage* 89 (April): 171–180.

Schmaal, L., D. P. Hibar, P. G. Sämann, G. B. Hall, B. T. Baune, N. Jahanshad, J. W. Cheung, et al. 2017. Cortical Abnormalities in Adults and Adolescents with Major Depression Based on Brain Scans from 20 Cohorts Worldwide in the ENIGMA Major Depressive Disorder Working Group. *Molecular Psychiatry* 22 (6): 900–909.

Schmack, K., A. Gomez-Carrillo de Castro, M. Rothkirch, M. Sekutowicz, H. Rossler, J.-D. Haynes, A. Heinz, P. Petrovic, and P. Sterzer. 2013. Delusions and the Role of Beliefs in Perceptual Inference. *Journal of Neuroscience* 33 (34): 13701–13712.

Schmidhuber, J. 2010. Formal Theory of Creativity, Fun, and Intrinsic Motivation (1990–2010). *IEEE Transactions on Autonomous Mental Development* 2 (3): 230–247.

Schneider, W., and J. M. Chein. 2003. Controlled and Automatic Processing: Behavior, Theory, and Biological Mechanisms. *Cognitive Science* 27 (3): 525–559.

Schoenbaum, G., M. R. Roesch, and T. A. Stalnaker. 2006. Orbitofrontal Cortex, Decision-Making and Drug Addiction. *Trends in Neurosciences* 29 (2): 116–124.

Schultz, W., P. Dayan, and P. R. Montague. 1997. A Neural Substrate of Prediction and Reward. *Science* 275 (5306): 1593–1599.

Schultz, Wolfram. 1998. Predictive Reward Signal of Dopamine Neurons. *Journal of Neurophysiology* 80 (1): 1–27.

———. 2002. Getting Formal with Dopamine and Reward. *Neuron* 36 (2): 241–263.

———. 2016. Dopamine Reward Prediction Error Coding. *Dialogues in Clinical Neuroscience* 18 (1): 23.

Schwartenbeck, P., T. H. B. FitzGerald, and R. Dolan. 2016. Neural Signals Encoding Shifts in Beliefs. *NeuroImage* 125 (January): 578–586.

Seeman, P. 1987. Dopamine Receptors and the Dopamine Hypothesis of Schizophrenia. *Synapse* 1 (2): 133–152.

Seligman, M. E. P. 1972. Learned Helplessness. *Annual Review of Medicine* 23 (1): 407–412.

Seriès, P. 2019. Post-Traumatic Stress Disorder as a Disorder of Prediction. *Nature Neuroscience* 22 (3): 334–336.

Seriès, P., and A. R. Seitz. 2013. Learning What to Expect (in Visual Perception). *Frontiers in Human Neuroscience* 7: 668.

Seriès, P., and M. Sprevak. 2014. Intelligent Machines and the Human Brain. In *Philosophy and the Sciences for Everyone*, edited by M. Massimi, 86–102. New York, NY: Routledge.

Seymour, B., J. P. O'Doherty, P. Dayan, M. Koltzenburg, A. K. Jones, R. J. Dolan, K. J. Friston, and R. S. Frackowiak. 2004. Temporal Difference Models Describe Higher-Order Learning in Humans. *Nature* 429 (6992): 664–667.

Seymour, B., J. P. O'Doherty, M. Koltzenburg, K. Wiech, R. Frackowiak, K. Friston, and R. Dolan. 2005. Opponent Appetitive-Aversive Neural Processes Underlie Predictive Learning of Pain Relief. *Nature Neuroscience* 8 (9): 1234–1240.

Shadlen, M. N., and W. T. Newsome. 2001. Neural Basis of a Perceptual Decision in the Parietal Cortex (Area LIP) of the Rhesus Monkey. *Journal of Neurophysiology* 86 (4): 1916–1936.

Shadmehr, R., J. J. Orban de Xivry, M. Xu-Wilson, and T.-Y. Shih. 2010. Temporal Discounting of Reward and the Cost of Time in Motor Control. *Journal of Neuroscience* 30 (31): 10507–10516.

Shannon, C. E. 1948. A Mathematical Theory of Communication. *Bell System Technical Journal* 27 (3): 379–423.

Sharp, P. B., and E. Eldar. 2019. Computational Models of Anxiety: Nascent Efforts and Future Directions. *Current Directions in Psychological Science* 28 (2): 170–176. https://doi.org/10.1177/0963721418818441.

Sharpe, M. J., C. Y. Chang, M. A. Liu, H. M. Batchelor, L. E. Mueller, J. L. Jones, Y. Niv, and G. Schoenbaum. 2017. Dopamine Transients Are Sufficient and Necessary for Acquisition of Model-Based Associations. *Nature Neuroscience* 20 (5): 735–742.

Shay, C. F., M. Ferrante, G. W. Chapman, and M. E. Hasselmo. 2016. Rebound Spiking in Layer II Medial Entorhinal Cortex Stellate Cells: Possible Mechanism of Grid Cell Function. *Neurobiology of Learning and Memory* 129 (March): 83–98.

Shedler, J. 2010. The Efficacy of Psychodynamic Psychotherapy. *American Psychologist* 65 (2): 98–109.

Sheffer, C. E., D. R. Christensen, R. Landes, L. P. Carter, L. Jackson, and W. K. Bickel. 2014. Delay Discounting Rates: A Strong Prognostic Indicator of Smoking Relapse. *Addictive Behaviors* 39 (11): 1682–1689.

Shen, W., M. Flajolet, P. Greengard, and D. J. Surmeier. 2008. Dichotomous Dopaminergic Control of Striatal Synaptic Plasticity. *Science* 321 (5890): 848–851.

Shenhav, A., M. M. Botvinick, and J. D. Cohen. 2013. The Expected Value of Control: An Integrative Theory of Anterior Cingulate Cortex Function. *Neuron* 79 (2): 217–240.

Shenhav, A., S. Musslick, F. Lieder, W. Kool, T. L. Griffiths, J. D. Cohen, and M. M. Botvinick. 2017. Toward a Rational and Mechanistic Account of Mental Effort. *Annual Review of Neuroscience* 40 (1): 99–124.

Shephard, E., M. J. Groom, and G. M. Jackson. 2019. Implicit Sequence Learning in Young People with Tourette Syndrome with and without Co-occurring Attention-Deficit/Hyperactivity Disorder. *Journal of Neuropsychology* 13 (3): 529–549.

Shephard, E., G. M. Jackson, and M. J. Groom. 2016. Electrophysiological Correlates of Reinforcement Learning in Young People with Tourette Syndrome with and without Co-Occurring ADHD Symptoms. *International Journal of Developmental Neuroscience* 51 (June): 17–27.

Shiffrin, R. M., and W. Schneider. 1977. Controlled and Automatic Human Information Processing: II. Perceptual Learning, Automatic Attending and a General Theory. *Psychological Review* 84 (2): 127–190.

Shima, K., M. Isoda, H. Mushiake, and J. Tanji. 2007. Categorization of Behavioural Sequences in the Prefrontal Cortex. *Nature* 445 (7125): 315–318.

Siegle, G. J., and M. E. Hasselmo. 2002. Using Connectionist Models to Guide Assessment of Psychological Disorder. *Psychological Assessment* 14 (3): 263–278.

Siegle, G. J., S. R. Steinhauer, and M. E. Thase. 2004. Pupillary Assessment and Computational Modeling of the Stroop Task in Depression. *International Journal of Psychophysiology* 52 (1): 63–76.

Sigurdsson, H. P., S. E. Pépés, G. M. Jackson, A. Draper, P. S. Morgan, and S. R. Jackson. 2018. Alterations in the Microstructure of White Matter in Children and Adolescents with Tourette Syndrome Measured Using Tract-Based Spatial Statistics and Probabilistic Tractography. *Cortex* 104 (July): 75–89.

Simmons, J. M., and K. J. Quinn. 2014. The NIMH Research Domain Criteria (RDoC) Project: Implications for Genetics Research. *Mammalian Genome* 25 (1–2): 23–31.

Simon, H. 1962. The Architecture of Complexity. *Proceedings of the American Philosophical Society* 106 (6): 467.

Simonyan, K., H. Cho, A. Hamzehei Sichani, E. Rubien-Thomas, and M. Hallett. 2017. The Direct Basal Ganglia Pathway Is Hyperfunctional in Focal Dystonia. *Brain* 140 (12): 3179–3190.

Singh, S., A. G. Barto, and N. Chentanez. 2005. Intrinsically Motivated Reinforcement Learning. In *Advances in Neural Information Processing Systems 17*, edited by L. K. Saul, Y. Weiss, and L. Bottou, 1281–1288. Defense Technical Information Center.

Sinha, P., M. M. Kjelgaard, T. K. Gandhi, K. Tsourides, A. L. Cardinaux, D. Pantazis, S. P. Diamond, and R. M. Held. 2014. Autism as a Disorder of Prediction. *Proceedings of the National Academy of Sciences of the United States of America* 111 (42): 15220–15225.

Skinner, B. F. 1938. *The Behavior of Organisms*. New York, NY: Appleton-Century-Crofts.

Slifstein, M., E. van de Giessen, J. Van Snellenberg, J. L. Thompson, R. Narendran, R. Gil, E. Hackett, et al. 2015. Deficits in Prefrontal Cortical and Extrastriatal Dopamine Release in Schizophrenia. *JAMA Psychiatry* 72 (4): 316–324.

Smieskova, R., J. P. Roiser, C. A. Chaddock, A. Schmidt, F. Harrisberger, K. Bendfeldt, A. Simon, et al. 2015. Modulation of Motivational Salience Processing during the Early Stages of Psychosis. *Schizophrenia Research* 166 (1–3): 17–23.

Smith, P. L., and R. Ratcliff. 2004. Psychology and Neurobiology of Simple Decisions. *Trends in Neurosciences* 27 (3): 161–168.

Snider, S. E., H. U. Deshpande, J. M. Lisinski, M. N. Koffarnus, S. M. LaConte, and W. K. Bickel. 2018. Working Memory Training Improves Alcohol Users Episodic Future Thinking: A Rate-Dependent Analysis. *Biological Psychiatry: Cognitive Neuroscience and Neuroimaging* 3 (2): 160–167.

Snitz, B. E., A. MacDonald, and C. S. Carter. 2006. Cognitive Deficits in Unaffected First-Degree Relatives of Schizophrenia Patients: A Meta-Analytic Review of Putative Endophenotypes. *Schizophrenia Bulletin* 32 (1): 179–194.

Snyder, H. R. 2013. Major Depressive Disorder Is Associated with Broad Impairments on Neuropsychological Measures of Executive Function: A Meta-Analysis and Review. *Psychological Bulletin* 139 (1): 81–132.

Snyder, H. R., A. Miyake, and B. L. Hankin. 2015. Advancing Understanding of Executive Function Impairments and Psychopathology: Bridging the Gap between Clinical and Cognitive Approaches. *Frontiers in Psychology* 6 (March).

Snyder, S. H. 1976. The Dopamine Hypothesis of Schizophrenia: Focus on the Dopamine Receptor. *The American Journal of Psychiatry* 133 (2): 197–202.

Soares-Cunha, C., B. Coimbra, N. Sousa, and A. J. Rodrigues. 2016. Reappraising Striatal D_1-and D_2-Neurons in Reward and Aversion. *Neuroscience & Biobehavioral Reviews* 68 (September): 370–386.

Solomon, R. L., and J. D. Corbit. 1974. An Opponent-Process Theory of Motivation: I. Temporal Dynamics of Affect. *Psychological Review* 81 (2): 119–145.

Soltani, A., and X.-J. Wang. 2009. Synaptic Computation Underlying Probabilistic Inference. *Nature Neuroscience* 13 (1): 112–119.

Solway, A., and M. M. Botvinick. 2012. Goal-Directed Decision Making as Probabilistic Inference: A Computational Framework and Potential Neural Correlates. *Psychological Review* 119 (1): 120–154.

Solway, A., C. Diuk, N. Córdova, D. Yee, A. G. Barto, Y. Niv, and M. M. Botvinick. 2014. Optimal Behavioral Hierarchy. *PLoS Computational Biology* 10 (8): e1003779.

Sowell, E. R., E. Kan, J. Yoshii, P. M. Thompson, R. Bansal, D. Xu, A. W. Toga, and B. S. Peterson. 2008. Thinning of Sensorimotor Cortices in Children with Tourette Syndrome. *Nature Neuroscience* 11 (6): 637–639.

Spencer, K. 2009. The Functional Consequences of Cortical Circuit Abnormalities on Gamma Oscillations in Schizophrenia: Insights from Computational Modeling. *Frontiers in Human Neuroscience* 3.

Spitzer, R. L., J. B. Williams, and A. E. Skodol. 1980. DSM-III: The Major Achievements and an Overview. *The American Journal of Psychiatry* 137 (2): 151–164.

Stankevicius, A., Q. J. M. Huys, A. Kalra, and P. Seriès. 2014. Optimism as a Prior Belief about the Probability of Future Reward. *PLoS Computational Biology* 10 (5): e1003605.

Starc, M., J. D. Murray, N. Santamauro, A. Savic, C. Diehl, Y. T. Cho, V. Srihari, et al. 2017. Schizophrenia Is Associated with a Pattern of Spatial Working Memory Deficits Consistent with Cortical Disinhibition. *Schizophrenia Research* 181 (March): 107–116.

Steele, J. D., and M. P. Paulus. 2019. Pragmatic Neuroscience for Clinical Psychiatry. *The British Journal of Psychiatry* 215 (1): 404–408.

Stein, J. S., A. N. Tegge, J. K. Turner, and W. K. Bickel. 2018. Episodic Future Thinking Reduces Delay Discounting and Cigarette Demand: An Investigation of the Good-Subject Effect. *Journal of Behavioral Medicine* 41 (2): 269–276.

Steinacher, A., and K. A. Wright. 2013. Relating the Bipolar Spectrum to Dysregulation of Behavioural Activation: A Perspective from Dynamical Modelling. *PLoS ONE* 8 (5): e63345.

Steinberg, T., S. Shmuel Baruch, A. Harush, R. Dar, D. Woods, J. Piacentini, and A. Apter. 2010. Tic Disorders and the Premonitory Urge. *Journal of Neural Transmission* 117 (2): 277–284.

Stephan, K. E., T. Baldeweg, and K. J. Friston. 2006. Synaptic Plasticity and Dysconnection in Schizophrenia. *Biological Psychiatry* 59 (10): 929–939.

Stephan, K. E., K. J. Friston, and C. D. Frith. 2009. Dysconnection in Schizophrenia: From Abnormal Synaptic Plasticity to Failures of Self-Monitoring. *Schizophrenia Bulletin* 35 (3): 509–527.

Stephan, K. E., and C. Mathys. 2014. Computational Approaches to Psychiatry. *Current Opinion in Neurobiology* 25 (April): 85–92.

Stephan, K. E., W. D. Penny, J. Daunizeau, R. J. Moran, and K. J. Friston. 2009. Bayesian Model Selection for Group Studies. *NeuroImage* 46 (4): 1004–1017.

Stephens, D. W., and J. R. Krebs. 1986. *Foraging Theory*. Princeton, NJ: Princeton University Press.

Sterzer, P., R. A. Adams, P. Fletcher, C. Frith, S. M. Lawrie, L. Muckli, P. Petrovic, P. Uhlhaas, M. Voss, and P. R. Corlett. 2018. The Predictive Coding Account of Psychosis. *Biological Psychiatry* 84 (9): 634–643.

Stocker, A. A., and E. P. Simoncelli. 2006. Noise Characteristics and Prior Expectations in Human Visual Speed Perception. *Nature Neuroscience* 9 (4): 578–585.

Strauss, G. P., and J. M. Gold. 2012. A New Perspective on Anhedonia in Schizophrenia. *American Journal of Psychiatry* 169 (4): 364–373.

Strauss, G. P., B. M. Robinson, J. A. Waltz, M. J. Frank, Z. Kasanova, E. S. Herbener, and J. M. Gold. 2010. Patients with Schizophrenia Demonstrate Inconsistent Preference Judgments for Affective and Nonaffective Stimuli. *Schizophrenia Bulletin* 37 (6): 1295–1304.

Strauss, G. P., J. A. Waltz, and J. M. Gold. 2014. A Review of Reward Processing and Motivational Impairment in Schizophrenia. *Schizophrenia Bulletin* 40 (Suppl. 2): S107–16.

Stuke, H., H. Stuke, V. A. Weilnhammer, and K. Schmack. 2017. Psychotic Experiences and Overhasty Inferences Are Related to Maladaptive Learning. *PLOS Computational Biology* 13 (1): e1005328.

Sulzer, D., S. J. Cragg, and M. E. Rice. 2016. Striatal Dopamine Neurotransmission: Regulation of Release and Uptake. *Basal Ganglia* 6 (3): 123–148.

Sun, R. 2008. *The Cambridge Handbook of Computational Psychology*. Cambridge, England: Cambridge University Press.

Sutton, R. S. 1988. Learning to Predict by the Methods of Temporal Differences. *Machine Learning* 3 (1): 9–44.

———. 1990. Integrated Architectures for Learning, Planning, and Reacting Based on Approximating Dynamic Programming. In *Proceedings of the Seventh International Conference on Machine Learning*, edited by M. B. Morgan, 216–224. San Francisco, CA: Morgan Kaufmann.

Sutton, R. S., and A. G. Barto. 1998. *Reinforcement Learning: An Introduction*. Cambridge, MA: The MIT Press.

Syed, E. C. J., L. L. Grima, P. J. Magill, R. Bogacz, P. Brown, and M. E. Walton. 2016. Action Initiation Shapes Mesolimbic Dopamine Encoding of Future Rewards. *Nature Neuroscience* 19 (1): 34–36.

Szechtman, H., W. Sulis, and D. Eilam. 1998. Quinpirole Induces Compulsive Checking Behavior in Rats: A Potential Animal Model of Obsessive-Compulsive Disorder (OCD). *Behavioral Neuroscience* 112 (6): 1475–1485.

Szita, I., and A. Lőrincz. 2008. The Many Faces of Optimism. In *Proceedings of the 25th International Conference on Machine Learning*, edited by W. Cohen, A. McCallum, and S. Roweis, 1048–1055. New York, NY: ACM Press.

Teller, D. Y. 1984. Linking Propositions. *Vision Research* 24 (10): 1233–1246.

Tenenbaum, J. B., T. L. Griffiths, and C. Kemp. 2006. Theory-Based Bayesian Models of Inductive Learning and Reasoning. *Trends in Cognitive Sciences* 10 (7): 309–318.

Teufel, C., and P. C. Fletcher. 2016. The Promises and Pitfalls of Applying Computational Models to Neurological and Psychiatric Disorders. *Brain* 139 (10): 2600–2608.

Teufel, C., N. Subramaniam, V. Dobler, J. Perez, J. Finnemann, P. R. Mehta, I. M. Goodyer, and P. C. Fletcher. 2015. Shift toward Prior Knowledge Confers a Perceptual Advantage in Early Psychosis and Psychosis-Prone Healthy Individuals. *Proceedings of the National Academy of Sciences* 112 (43): 13401–13406.

The ESSTS Guidelines Group, V. Roessner, K. J. Plessen, A. Rothenberger, A. G. Ludolph, R. Rizzo, L. Skov, et al. 2011a. European Clinical Guidelines for Tourette Syndrome and Other Tic Disorders. Part II: Pharmacological Treatment. *European Child & Adolescent Psychiatry* 20 (4): 173–196.

The ESSTS Guidelines Group, C. Verdellen, J. van de Griendt, A. Hartmann, and T. Murphy. 2011b. European Clinical Guidelines for Tourette Syndrome and Other Tic Disorders. Part III: Behavioural and Psychosocial Interventions. *European Child & Adolescent Psychiatry* 20 (4): 197–207.

Thenganatt, M. A., and J. Jankovic. 2016. Recent Advances in Understanding and Managing Tourette Syndrome. *F1000Research* 5 (February): 152.

Tian, J., R. Huang, J. Y. Cohen, F. Osakada, D. Kobak, C. K. Machens, E. M. Callaway, N. Uchida, and M. Watabe-Uchida. 2016. Distributed and Mixed Information in Monosynaptic Inputs to Dopamine Neurons. *Neuron* 91 (6): 1374–1389.

Tiffany, S. T. 1999. Cognitive Concepts of Craving. *Alcohol Research and Health* 23 (3): 215–224.

Toda, M., and A. Abi-Dargham. 2007. Dopamine Hypothesis of Schizophrenia: Making Sense of It All. *Current Psychiatry Reports* 9 (4): 329–336.

Tolman, E. C. 1948. Cognitive Maps in Rats and Men. *Psychological Review* 55 (4): 189–208.

Treadway, M. T., N. A. Bossaller, R. C. Shelton, and D. H. Zald. 2012. Effort-Based Decision-Making in Major Depressive Disorder: A Translational Model of Motivational Anhedonia. *Journal of Abnormal Psychology* 121 (3): 553–558.

Treadway, M. T., and D. H. Zald. 2013. Parsing Anhedonia: Translational Models of Reward-Processing Deficits in Psychopathology. *Current Directions in Psychological Science* 22 (3): 244–249.

Tremblay, L., Y. Worbe, S. Thobois, V. Sgambato-Faure, and J. Féger. 2015. Selective Dysfunction of Basal Ganglia Subterritories: From Movement to Behavioral Disorders. *Movement Disorders* 30 (9): 1155–1170.

Trimmer, P. C., A. D. Higginson, T. W. Fawcett, J. M. McNamara, and A. I. Houston. 2015. Adaptive Learning Can Result in a Failure to Profit from Good Conditions: Implications for Understanding Depression. *Evolution, Medicine, and Public Health* 2015 (1): 123–135.

Trope, Y., and N. Liberman. 2010. Construal-Level Theory of Psychological Distance. *Psychological Review* 117 (2): 440–463.

Tsibulsky, V. L., and A. B. Norman. 1999. Satiety Threshold: A Quantitative Model of Maintained Cocaine Self-Administration. *Brain Research* 839 (1): 85–93.

Turchin, P. 2003. *Historical Dynamics: Why States Rise and Fall.* Princeton, N. J.: Princeton University Press.

Turner, B. M., B. U. Forstmann, E.-J. Wagenmakers, S. D. Brown, P. B. Sederberg, and M. Steyvers. 2013. A Bayesian Framework for Simultaneously Modeling Neural and Behavioral Data. *NeuroImage* 72 (May): 193–206.

Tversky, A., and D. Kahneman. 1992. Advances in Prospect Theory: Cumulative Representation of Uncertainty. *Journal of Risk and Uncertainty* 5 (4): 297–323.

Uhlhaas, P. J. 2013. Dysconnectivity, Large-Scale Networks and Neuronal Dynamics in Schizophrenia. *Current Opinion in Neurobiology* 23 (2): 283–290.

Uhlhaas, P. J., and W. Singer. 2010. Abnormal Neural Oscillations and Synchrony in Schizophrenia. *Nature Reviews Neuroscience* 11 (2): 100–113.

Üstün, T. B., J. L. Ayuso-Mateos, S. Chatterji, C. Mathers, and C. J. L. Murray. 2004. Global Burden of Depressive Disorders in the Year 2000. *British Journal of Psychiatry* 184 (5): 386–392.

Vaghi, M. M., F. Luyckx, A. Sule, N. A. Fineberg, T. W. Robbins, and B. De Martino. 2017. Compulsivity Reveals a Novel Dissociation between Action and Confidence. *Neuron* 96 (2): 348–354.e4.

Vaidya, C. J., S. A. Bunge, N. M. Dudukovic, C. A. Zalecki, G. R. Elliott, and J. D. E. Gabrieli. 2005. Altered Neural Substrates of Cognitive Control in Childhood ADHD: Evidence From Functional Magnetic Resonance Imaging. *American Journal of Psychiatry* 162 (9): 1605–1613.

Vallesi, A., F. Canalaz, M. Balestrieri, and P. Brambilla. 2015. Modulating Speed-Accuracy Strategies in Major Depression. *Journal of Psychiatric Research* 60 (January): 103–108.

Valton, V., P. Karvelis, K. L. Richards, A. R. Seitz, S. M. Lawrie, and P. Seriès. 2019. Acquisition of Visual Priors and Induced Hallucinations in Chronic Schizophrenia. *Brain* 142 (8): 2523–2537.

Van de Cruys, S., K. Evers, R. Van der Hallen, L. Van Eylen, B. Boets, L. de-Wit, and J. Wagemans. 2014. Precise Minds in Uncertain Worlds: Predictive Coding in Autism. *Psychological Review* 121 (4): 649–675.

Van de Griendt, J. M. T. M., C. W. J. Verdellen, M. K. van Dijk, and M. J. P. M. Verbraak. 2013. Behavioural Treatment of Tics: Habit Reversal and Exposure with Response Prevention. *Neuroscience & Biobehavioral Reviews* 37 (6): 1172–1177.

Van der Meer, M., Z. Kurth-Nelson, and A. D. Redish. 2012. Information Processing in Decision-Making Systems. *The Neuroscientist* 18 (4): 342–359.

Van Meel, C. S. D. J. Heslenfeld, J. Oosterlaan, and J. A. Sergeant. 2007. Adaptive Control Deficits in Attention-Deficit/Hyperactivity Disorder (ADHD): The Role of Error Processing. *Psychiatry Research* 151 (3): 211–220.

Vassena, E., C. B. Holroyd, and W. H. Alexander. 2017. Computational Models of Anterior Cingulate Cortex: At the Crossroads between Prediction and Effort. *Frontiers in Neuroscience* 11 (June).

Velanova, K., L. L. Jacoby, M. E. Wheeler, M. P. McAvoy, S. E. Petersen, and R. L. Buckner. 2003. Functional-Anatomic Correlates of Sustained and Transient Processing Components Engaged during Controlled Retrieval. *The Journal of Neuroscience* 23 (24): 8460–8470.

Venton, B. J., H. Zhang, P. A. Garris, P. E. M. Phillips, D. Sulzer, and R. M. Wightman. 2003. Real-Time Decoding of Dopamine Concentration Changes in the Caudate-Putamen during Tonic and Phasic Firing: Decoding Dopamine Neurotransmission. *Journal of Neurochemistry* 87 (5): 1284–1295.

Verharen, J. P. H., U. N. Danner, S. Schröder, E. Aarts, A. A. van Elburg, and R. A. H. Adan. 2019. Insensitivity to Losses: A Core Feature in Patients with Anorexia Nervosa? *Biological Psychiatry: Cognitive Neuroscience and Neuroimaging* 0 (0).

Vierling-Claassen, D., P. Siekmeier, S. Stufflebeam, and N. Kopell. 2008. Modeling GABA Alterations in Schizophrenia: A Link between Impaired Inhibition and Altered Gamma and Beta Range Auditory Entrainment. *Journal of Neurophysiology* 99 (5): 2656–2671.

Vigo, D., G. Thornicroft, and R. Atun. 2016. Estimating the True Global Burden of Mental Illness. *The Lancet Psychiatry* 3 (2): 171–178.

Vinckier, F., R. Gaillard, S. Palminteri, L. Rigoux, A. Salvador, A. Fornito, R. Adapa, M. O. Krebs, M. Pessiglione, and P. C. Fletcher. 2016. Confidence and Psychosis: A Neuro-Computational Account of Contingency Learning Disruption by NMDA Blockade. *Molecular Psychiatry* 21 (7): 946–955.

Volman, S. F., S. Lammel, E. B. Margolis, Y. Kim, J. M. Richard, M. F. Roitman, and M. K. Lobo. 2013. New Insights into the Specificity and Plasticity of Reward and Aversion Encoding in the Mesolimbic System. *Journal of Neuroscience* 33 (45): 17569–17576.

Volman, V., M. M. Behrens, and T. J. Sejnowski. 2011. Downregulation of Parvalbumin at Cortical GABA Synapses Reduces Network Gamma Oscillatory Activity. *Journal of Neuroscience* 31 (49): 18137–18148.

Voon, V., K. Derbyshire, C. Rück, M. A. Irvine, Y. Worbe, J. Enander, L. R. N. Schreiber, et al. 2015. Disorders of Compulsivity: A Common Bias towards Learning Habits. *Molecular Psychiatry* 20 (3): 345–352.

Vos, T., A. D. Flaxman, M. Naghavi, R. Lozano, C. Michaud, M. Ezzati, K. Shibuya, J. A. Salomon, S. Abdalla, and V. Aboyans. 2012. Years Lived with Disability (YLDs) for 1160 Sequelae of 289

Diseases and Injuries 1990–2010: A Systematic Analysis for the Global Burden of Disease Study 2010. *The Lancet* 380 (9859): 2163–2196.

Wagenaar, W. A. 1988. *Paradoxes of Gambling Behaviour*. Hillsdale, N. J.: Lawrence Erlbaum Associates Inc.

Wakefield, J. C. 1992. The Concept of Mental Disorder: On the Boundary between Biological Facts and Social Values. *American Psychologist* 47 (3): 373–388.

Walker, E. R., R. E. McGee, and B. G. Druss. 2015. Mortality in Mental Disorders and Global Disease Burden Implications. *JAMA Psychiatry* 72 (4): 334–341.

Wallace, R. 2017. *Computational Psychiatry: A Systems Biology Approach to the Epigenetics of Mental Disorders*. New York, NY: Springer.

Wanat, M. J., C. M. Kuhnen, and P. E. M. Phillips. 2010. Delays Conferred by Escalating Costs Modulate Dopamine Release to Rewards But Not Their Predictors. *Journal of Neuroscience* 30 (36): 12020–12027.

Wang, H., G. G. Stradtman, X.-J. Wang, and W.-J. Gao. 2008. A Specialized NMDA Receptor Function in Layer 5 Recurrent Microcircuitry of the Adult Rat Prefrontal Cortex. *Proceedings of the National Academy of Sciences* 105 (43): 16791–16796.

Wang, M., Y. Yang, C.-J. Wang, N. J. Gamo, L. E. Jin, J. A. Mazer, J. H. Morrison, X.-J. Wang, and A. F. T. Arnsten. 2013. NMDA Receptors Subserve Persistent Neuronal Firing during Working Memory in Dorsolateral Prefrontal Cortex. *Neuron* 77 (4): 736–749.

Wang, X.-J. 1999. Synaptic Basis of Cortical Persistent Activity: The Importance of NMDA Receptors to Working Memory. *The Journal of Neuroscience* 19 (21): 9587–9603.

———. 2001. Synaptic Reverberation Underlying Mnemonic Persistent Activity. *Trends in Neurosciences* 24 (8): 455–463.

———. 2002. Probabilistic Decision Making by Slow Reverberation in Cortical Circuits. *Neuron* 36 (5): 955–968.

———. 2008. Decision Making in Recurrent Neuronal Circuits. *Neuron* 60 (2): 215–234.

———. 2010. Neurophysiological and Computational Principles of Cortical Rhythms in Cognition. *Physiological Reviews* 90 (3): 1195–1268.

———. 2013. The Prefrontal Cortex as a Quintessential "Cognitive-Type" Neural Circuit. In *Principles of Frontal Lobe Function*, edited by D. T. Stuss and R. T. Knight, 226–248. New York, NY: Oxford University Press.

Wang, X.-J., and H. Kennedy. 2016. Brain Structure and Dynamics across Scales: In Search of Rules. *Current Opinion in Neurobiology* 37 (April): 92–98.

Wang, X.-J., and J. H. Krystal. 2014. Computational Psychiatry. *Neuron* 84 (3): 638–654.

Wang, X.-J., J. Tegner, C. Constantinidis, and P. S. Goldman-Rakic. 2004. Division of Labor among Distinct Subtypes of Inhibitory Neurons in a Cortical Microcircuit of Working Memory. *Proceedings of the National Academy of Sciences* 101 (5): 1368–1373.

Warwick, Z. S., and H. P. Weingarten. 1994. Dissociation of Palatability and Calorie Effects in Learned Flavor Preferences. *Physiology & Behavior* 55 (3): 501–504.

Watkins, C. J. C. H. 1989. Learning from Delayed Rewards. PhD thesis, Cambridge, England: Cambridge University.

Watson, J. B. 1913. Psychology as the Behaviorist Views It. *Psychological Review* 20 (2): 158–177.

Wen, H., Y. Liu, I. Rekik, S. Wang, Z. Chen, J. Zhang, Y. Zhang, Y. Peng, and H. He. 2017a. Multi-Modal Multiple Kernel Learning for Accurate Identification of Tourette Syndrome Children. *Pattern Recognition* 63 (March): 601–611.

———. 2018. Combining Disrupted and Discriminative Topological Properties of Functional Connectivity Networks as Neuroimaging Biomarkers for Accurate Diagnosis of Early Tourette Syndrome Children. *Molecular Neurobiology* 55 (4): 3251–3269.

Wen, H., Y. Liu, I. Rekik, S. Wang, J. Zhang, Y. Zhang, Y. Peng, and H. He. 2017b. Disrupted Topological Organization of Structural Networks Revealed by Probabilistic Diffusion Tractography in Tourette Syndrome Children: Disrupted Structural Networks of T. S. Children. *Human Brain Mapping* 38 (8): 3988–4008.

Wenzel, J. M., N. A. Rauscher, J. F. Cheer, and E. B. Oleson. 2015. A Role for Phasic Dopamine Release within the Nucleus Accumbens in Encoding Aversion: A Review of the Neurochemical Literature. *ACS Chemical Neuroscience* 6 (1): 16–26.

Westbrook, A., and T. S. Braver. 2015. Cognitive Effort: A Neuroeconomic Approach. *Cognitive, Affective, & Behavioral Neuroscience* 15 (2): 395–415.

———. 2016. Dopamine Does Double Duty in Motivating Cognitive Effort. *Neuron* 89 (4): 695–710.

White, C. N., R. A. Curl, and J. F. Sloane. 2016. Using Decision Models to Enhance Investigations of Individual Differences in Cognitive Neuroscience. *Frontiers in Psychology* 7 (February): 81.

White, C. N., R. Ratcliff, M. W. Vasey, and G. McKoon. 2010a. Anxiety Enhances Threat Processing without Competition among Multiple Inputs: A Diffusion Model Analysis. *Emotion* 10 (5): 662–677.

———. 2010b. Using Diffusion Models to Understand Clinical Disorders. *Journal of Mathematical Psychology* 54 (1): 39–52.

White, C. N., K. Skokin, B. Carlos, and A. Weaver. 2016. Using Decision Models to Decompose Anxiety-Related Bias in Threat Classification. *Emotion* 16 (2): 196–207.

Whiteford, H. A., A. J. Ferrari, L. Degenhardt, V. Feigin, and T. Vos. 2015. The Global Burden of Mental, Neurological and Substance Use Disorders: An Analysis from the Global Burden of Disease Study 2010. *PLOS ONE* 10 (2): e0116820.

Wightman, R. M., and D. L. Robinson. 2002. Transient Changes in Mesolimbic Dopamine and Their Association with "Reward." *Journal of Neurochemistry* 82 (4): 721–735.

Wilder, B., and C. Brackett. 1945. *The Lost Weekend*. Film. Paramount Pictures, Los Angeles, CA.

Willcutt, E. G., A. E. Doyle, J. T. Nigg, S. V. Faraone, and B. F. Pennington. 2005. Validity of the Executive Function Theory of Attention-Deficit/Hyperactivity Disorder: A Meta-Analytic Review. *Biological Psychiatry* 57 (11): 1336–1346.

Williams, D. R., and H. Williams. 1969. Auto-Maintenance in the Pigeon: Sustained Pecking despite Contingent Non-Reinforcement. *Journal of the Experimental Analysis of Behavior* 12 (4): 511–520.

Williams, J., and P. Dayan. 2005. Dopamine, Learning, and Impulsivity: A Biological Account of Attention-Deficit/Hyperactivity Disorder. *Journal of Child and Adolescent Psychopharmacology* 15 (2): 160–179.

Willner, P. 2017. The Chronic Mild Stress (CMS) Model of Depression: History, Evaluation and Usage. *Neurobiology of Stress* 6 (February): 78–93.

Wilson, M. 1993. DSM-III and the Transformation of American Psychiatry: A History. *American Journal of Psychiatry* 150 (3): 399–410.

Wilson, R. C., and A. G. E Collins. 2019. Ten Simple Rules for the Computational Modeling of Behavioral Data. *eLife* 8:e49547.

Wong, K.-F., A. C. Huk, M. N. Shadlen, and X.-J. Wang. 2007. Neural Circuit Dynamics Underlying Accumulation of Time-Varying Evidence during Perceptual Decision Making. *Frontiers in Computational Neuroscience* 1:6.

Wong, K.-F., and X.-J. Wang. 2006. A Recurrent Network Mechanism of Time Integration in Perceptual Decisions. *Journal of Neuroscience* 26 (4): 1314–1328.

Wong, K. K., M. L. T. M. Müller, H. Kuwabara, S. A. Studenski, and N. I. Bohnen. 2012. Gender Differences in Nigrostriatal Dopaminergic Innervation Are Present at Young-to-Middle but Not at Older Age in Normal Adults. *Journal of Clinical Neuroscience* 19 (1): 183–184.Woods, D. W., J. Piacentini, M. B. Himle, and S. Chang. 2005. Premonitory Urge for Tics Scale (PUTS): Initial Psychometric Results and Examination of the Premonitory Urge Phenomenon in Youths with Tic Disorders. *Journal of Developmental & Behavioral Pediatrics* 26 (6): 397–403.

Worbe, Y., S. Palminteri, A. Hartmann, M. Vidailhet, S. Lehéricy, and M. Pessiglione. 2011. Reinforcement Learning and Gilles de La Tourette Syndrome: Dissociation of Clinical Phenotypes and Pharmacological Treatments. *Archives of General Psychiatry* 68 (12): 1257.

Worbe, Y., N. Baup, D. Grabli, M. Chaigneau, S. Mounayar, K. McCairn, J. Féger, and L. Tremblay. 2009. Behavioral and Movement Disorders Induced by Local Inhibitory Dysfunction in Primate Striatum. *Cerebral Cortex* 19 (8): 1844–1856.

Worbe, Y., E. Gerardin, A. Hartmann, R. Valabrégue, M. Chupin, L. Tremblay, M. Vidailhet, O. Colliot, and S. Lehéricy. 2010. Distinct Structural Changes Underpin Clinical Phenotypes in Patients with Gilles de La Tourette Syndrome. *Brain* 133 (12): 3649–3660.

Worbe, Y., S. Lehericy, and A. Hartmann. 2015a. Neuroimaging of Tic Genesis: Present Status and Future Perspectives. *Movement Disorders* 30 (9): 1179–1183.

Worbe, Y., C. Malherbe, A. Hartmann, M. Pélégrini-Issac, A. Messé, M. Vidailhet, S. Lehéricy, and H. Benali. 2012. Functional Immaturity of Cortico-Basal Ganglia Networks in Gilles de La Tourette Syndrome. *Brain* 135 (6): 1937–1946.

Worbe, Y., L. Marrakchi-Kacem, S. Lecomte, R. Valabregue, F. Poupon, P. Guevara, A. Tucholka, et al. 2015b. Altered Structural Connectivity of Cortico-Striato-Pallido-Thalamic Networks in Gilles de La Tourette Syndrome. *Brain* 138 (2): 472–482.

Worbe, Y., S. Palminteri, G. Savulich, N. D. Daw, E. Fernandez-Egea, T. W. Robbins, and V. Voon. 2015c. Valence-Dependent Influence of Serotonin Depletion on Model-Based Choice Strategy. *Molecular Psychiatry* 21 (5): 624–629.

World Health Organization. 1992. *The ICD-10 Classification of Mental and Behavioural Disorders: Clinical Descriptions and Diagnostic Guidelines.* Geneva: World Health Organization.

Wylie, S. A., K. R. Ridderinkhof, T. R. Bashore, and W. P. M. van den Wildenberg. 2010. The Effect of Parkinson's Disease on the Dynamics of On-Line and Proactive Cognitive Control during Action Selection. *Journal of Cognitive Neuroscience* 22 (9): 2058–2073.

Yang, G. J., J. D. Murray, G. Repovs, M. W. Cole, A. Savic, M. F. Glasser, C. Pittenger, et al. 2014. Altered Global Brain Signal in Schizophrenia. *Proceedings of the National Academy of Sciences* 111 (20): 7438–7443.

Yang, G. J., J. D. Murray, X.-J. Wang, D. C. Glahn, G. D. Pearlson, G. Repovs, J. H. Krystal, and A. Anticevic. 2015. Functional Hierarchy Underlies Preferential Connectivity Disturbances in Schizophrenia. *Proceedings of the National Academy of Sciences* 113 (2): E219–28.

Yang, G. R., J. D. Murray, and X.-J. Wang. 2016. A Dendritic Disinhibitory Circuit Mechanism for Pathway-Specific Gating. *Nature Communications* 7 (1): E219–28.

Yin, H. H., and B. J. Knowlton. 2006. The Role of the Basal Ganglia in Habit Formation. *Nature Reviews Neuroscience* 7(6): 464–476.

Young, H. F., and R. P. Bentall. 1997. Probabilistic Reasoning in Deluded, Depressed and Normal Subjects: Effects of Task Difficulty and Meaningful versus Non-Meaningful Material. *Psychological Medicine* 27 (2): 455–465.

Yu, A. J., and P. Dayan. 2005. Uncertainty, Neuromodulation, and Attention. *Neuron* 46 (4): 681–692.

Zanos, P., Moaddel, R, Morris, P., Georgiou, P., Fischel, J, and Elmer, G. I., Alkondon M, et al 2016. NMDAR Inhibition-Independent Antidepressant Actions of Ketamine Metabolites. *Nature* 533 (7604):481–486.

Ziegler, S., M. L. Pedersen, A. M. Mowinckel, and G. Biele. 2016. Modelling ADHD: A Review of ADHD Theories through Their Predictions for Computational Models of Decision-Making and Reinforcement Learning. *Neuroscience and Biobehavioral Reviews* 71 (December): 633–656.

Zipser, D., B. Kehoe, G. Littlewort, and J. Fuster. 1993. A Spiking Network Model of Short-Term Active Memory. *The Journal of Neuroscience* 13 (8): 3406–3420.

Zorowitz, S., I. Momennejad, and N. D. Daw. 2019. Anxiety, Avoidance, and Sequential Evaluation. *BioRxiv*, August, 724492.

Zorumski, C. F., Y. Izumi, and S. Mennerick. 2016. Ketamine: NMDA Receptors and Beyond. *The Journal of Neuroscience* 36 (44): 11158–11164.

Zylberberg, J., and B. W. Strowbridge. 2017. Mechanisms of Persistent Activity in Cortical Circuits: Possible Neural Substrates for Working Memory. *Annual Review of Neuroscience* 40 (1): 603–627.

Index